PHILIP L. HILLSMAN, M. D.

Cocaine, Marijuana, Designer Drugs: Chemistry, Pharmacology, and Behavior

Editors

Kinfe K. Redda
Associate Professor
College of Pharmacy and
Pharmaceutical Sciences
Florida A & M University
Tallahassee, Florida

Charles A. Walker
Chancellor and Professor of Pharmacology
University of Arkansas
Pine Bluff, Arkansas

Gene Barnett
Division of Cardio-Renal Drug Products
Food and Drug Administration
Rockville, Maryland

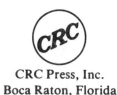

CRC Press, Inc.
Boca Raton, Florida

Library of Congress Cataloging-in-Publication Data

Cocaine, marijuana, designer drugs : chemistry, pharmacology and
    behavior / editors, Kinfe K. Redda, Charles A. Walker, Gene Barnett.
        p. cm.
        Based on the Eleventh Annual Clinical Pharmacy Symposium organized
and conducted by the College of Pharmacy and Pharmaceutical
Sciences, Florida Agricultural and Mechanical University in
Tallahassee, Florida, held during March 6-10, 1986.
        Includes bibliographies and index.
        ISBN 0-8493-6853-7
        1. Substance abuse--Congresses. 2. Cocaine--Physiological effect-
-Congresses. 3. Marijuana--Physiological effect--Comgresses.
4. Designer drugs--Physiological effect--Congresses.
5. Psychopharmacology--Congresses. I. Redda, Kinfe K. II Walker,
Charles A. III Barnett, Gene. IV. Clinical Pharmacy Syposium
(11th : 1986 : Tallahassee, Fla.)
RM316.C63 1989
616.86'3--dc19

88-10529
CIP

Direct all inquiries to CRC Press, Inc., 2000 Corporate Blvd., N.W., Boca Raton, Florida, 33431.

© 1989 by CRC Press, Inc.
Second Printing, 1990

International Standard Book Number 0-8493-6853-7

Library of Congress Card Number 88-10529
Printed in the United States

THE EDITORS

Kinfe "Ken" Redda, Ph.D., is at present an Associate Professor of Medicinal Chemistry at the College of Pharmacy and Pharmaceutical Sciences, Florida A & M University (FAMU), Tallahassee. He obtained his Ph.D. degree from the Faculty of Pharmacy and Pharmaceutical Sciences, University of Alberta, Edmonton, in 1978. After completing 2 years of postdoctoral research fellowships in Canada in the area of synthetic medicinal chemistry, Dr. Redda was appointed Assistant Professor of Medicinal Chemistry at the College of Pharmacy, Medical Sciences Campus, University of Puerto Rico (UPR) in San Juan. Dr. Redda was involved in teaching, research, and service at UPR for 5 years.

Beginning in January 1985, he was appointed to his present position at FAMU. Since then, Dr. Redda has also been serving as a member of the Biomedical Research Review Committee, the initial review group responsible for reviewing research and training grants submitted to the National Institute on Drug Abse (NIDA). At FAMU, he is now serving as the Principal Investigator and Program Director of the NASA-sponsored and FAMU-administered Space Life Sciences Training Program (SLSTP). Moreover, he is the Program Director of the Minority Biomedical Research Support (MBRS) Program at FAMU.

Dr. Redda has been a recipient of several honors and awards for his scholarly activities including the "Investor's Medal" awarded by the Canadian Patents and Development, Ltd., in recognition of having made an invention on which a patent was issued in 1978. He has also received the Chancellors Certificate for being the most outstanding faculty member in the College of Pharmacy, UPR, in 1982.

To date, Dr. Redda has received national research and training grants totaling over $1.2 million. He is a registered pharmacist and a member of several national scientific, professional, and civic organizations and has published 3 book chapters and nearly 20 articles in prestigious scientific journals.

Charles A. Walker, Ph.D., is presently Chancellor of the University of Arkansas at Pine Bluff. He obtained a B.S. in General Science from Arkansas AM & N College in 1957, an M.S. in Nutrition and Biochemistry from Washington State University in 1959, and a Ph.D. in Neuropharmacology from Loyola University of Chicago, Stritch School of Medicine, in 1969. He completed postdoctorate training (summers) at the University of California, Harvard, and Woods Hole-NASA, Ames, CA.

Dr. Walker is a member of numerous organizations including Sigma Xi, American Association for the Advancement of Science, New York Academy of Sciences, International Society for Chronobiology, American Institute of Chemistry (Fellow), Phi Zeta, American Society for Pharmacology and Experimental Therapeutics, Aerospace Medical Association, Professional Directory of American Men and Women in Science, Society for Research on Civilization Diseases and Environment, APhA, FPA, FSHP, Academy of Pharmaceutical Sciences, Tallahassee Jaycees Kappa Psi Pharmaceutical Fraternity, NAACP, AACP, and Urban League.

Of his special accomplishments, Dr. Walker developed the first Ph.D. program in the history of Florida A & M University in the area of Pharmaceutical Sciences. He developed two endowments for the university: one for pharmacy practitioners to result in $4 million, and one for the Eminent Scholars Program of $1 million. Total committed for the next 4 years — $6 million.

An accomplished scientist, Dr. Walker has published 40 scientific publications in refereed journals, 4 books (symposia proceedings) and 14 book chapters, and 54 abstracts of presentations at scientific meetings.

Gene Barnett, Ph.D., is presently serving as an associate of the Director of the Food and Drug Administration's (FDA) Division of Cardio-Renal Drug Products in the area of drug pharmacokinetics. He obtained his M.S. degree from Stanford University and his Ph.D. from Indiana University in the area of physical chemistry. Between 1966 and 1976, Dr. Barnett was actively involved in teaching and research in several institutions in the U.S. — Cornell University, Denver University, and the University of California at San Francisco — and in Latin American universities in Mexico, Brazil, and Chile.

Between 1976 and 1986, Dr. Barnett served in the Research Division of the National Institute on Drug Abuse (NIDA) in the capacity of an administrator and technical director dealing with aspects of pharmacodynamics, biopharmaceutics, and pharmacokinetics as applied to chemical structure-activity relationships. In addition to his other active duties, Dr. Barnett has also been involved as a research scientist in the Laboratory of Mathematical Biology, National Cancer Institute at Bethesda, MD, since 1983. Besides, he serves as an expert consultant to several prestigious North American pharmaceutical institutions of teaching and research.

Dr. Barnett is an accomplished scientist with national and international reputation. He has published 5 monographs, 7 chapters in scientific books, and he is the author of more than 35 research papers. He has presented his research work in numerous national and international conferences.

ACKNOWLEDGMENT

The editors acknowledge their gratitude to the College of Pharmacy and Pharmaceutical Sciences, Florida A & M University (FAMU) in Tallahassee for providing a forum in which numerous health professionals, social workers, and scientists were assembled to exchange ideas during the 11th Annual Clinical Symposium held at FAMU in March 1986. The proceedings of the symposium encouraged and stimulated the development and final completion of this publication. Special thanks goes to Mr. Leonard L. Inge and Dr. Larry D. Fannin who served as members of the Symposium Organizing Committee. The editors would also like to express their gratitude to Ms. Jamesina M. Watson and Ms. Marie L. Delinois for helping type several of the manuscripts.

Kinfe K. Redda, Ph.D.
Charles A. Walker, Ph.D.
Gene Barnett, Ph.D.

CONTRIBUTORS

Sayed M. H. Al-Habet, Ph.D.
Center for Anti-Inflammatory Research
College of Pharmacy and Pharmaceutical
 Science
Florida A & M University
Tallahassee, Florida

John J. Ambre, M.D., Ph.D.
Associate Professor
Department of Medicine
Northwestern University Medical School
Chicago, Illinois

Gene Barnett, Ph.D.
Division of Cardio-Renal Drug Products
Food and Drug Administration
Rockville, Maryland
 and
Advanced Scientific Computer
 Laboratory, PRI
National Cancer Institute, FCRF
Frederick, Maryland

Carol Bohach, B.S.
Department of Family Medicine
University of Miami School of Medicine
Miami, Florida

Roger M. Brown, Ph.D.
Chief
Neuroscience Research Branch
Division of Preclinical Research
National Institute on Drug Abuse
Rockville, Maryland

Jordi Cami, M.D., Ph.D.
Director
Department of Pharmacology and
 Toxicology
Municipal Institute of Medical Research
Barcelona, Spain

Nicola G. Cascella, M.D.
Addiction Research Center
National Institute on Drug Abuse
Rockville, Maryland

Neal Castagnoli, Jr., Ph.D.
Division of Toxicology
Schools of Pharmacy and Medicine
University of California
San Francisco, California

C. Nora Chiang, Ph.D.
Division of Preclinical Research
National Institute on Drug Abuse
Rockville, Maryland

James Cleary, Ph.D.
Geriatric Research, Education, and
 Clinical Center
Veterans Administration Medical Center
Minneapolis, Minnesota
 and
Research Associate
Department of Psychology
University of Minnesota
Minneapolis, Minnesota

Randall L. Commissaris, Ph.D.
Associate Professor
Department of Pharmaceutical Sciences
Wayne State University College of
 Pharmacy
Detroit, Michigan

Hala N. ElSohly, Ph.D.
Research Associate Professor
Research Institute of Pharmaceutical
 Sciences
School of Pharmacy
University of Mississippi
University, Mississippi

Mahmoud A. ElSohly, Ph.D.
Research Professor
Research Institute of Pharmaceutical
 Sciences
School of Pharmacy
University of Mississippi
University, Mississippi

Syed Husain, Ph.D.
Associate Professor
Department of Pharmacology
University of North Dakota
Grand Forks, North Dakota

Elaine M. Johnson, Ph.D.
Department of Health and Human
  Services
Former Deputy Director
National Institute on Drug Abuse
Rockville, Maryland

Karen M. Kumor, M.D.
Addiction Research Center
National Institute on Drug Abuse
Rockville, Maryland

Henry J. Lee, Ph.D.
Center for Anti-Inflammatory Research
College of Pharmacy and Pharmaceutical
  Science
Florida A & M University
Tallahassee, Florida

Kenneth D. McIntire, Ph.D.
Associate Professor and Chairman
Department of Psychology
University of Wisconsin
Eau Claire, Wisconsin

David E. Nichols, Ph.D.
Professor
Department of Medicinal Chemistry and
  Pharmacognosy
School of Pharmacy and Pharmacal
  Sciences
Purdue University
West Lafayette, Indiana

Rao S. Rapaka, Ph.D.
Research Technology Branch
National Institute on Drug Abuse
Rockville, Maryland

Kinfe K. Redda, Ph.D.
Associate Professor
College of Pharmacy and Pharmaceutical
  Sciences
Florida A & M University
Tallahassee, Florida

Maria-Elena Rodriguez, M.D.
UCLA Drug Abuse Research Group
Neuropsychiatric Institute
University of California
Los Angeles, California

Michael A. Sherer, M.D.
American Neurosciences
Rockville, Maryland

Thomas P. Singer, Ph.D.
Molecular Biology Division
Veterans Administration Medical Center
San Francisco, California

Anthony Trevor, Ph.D.
Departments of Pharmacology and
  Pharmacy
University of California
San Francisco, California

Charles A. Walker, Ph.D.
Chancellor and Professor of
  Pharmacology
University of Arkansas
Pine Bluff, Arkansas

TABLE OF CONTENTS

Chapter 1

INTRODUCTION

Kinfe K. Redda and Charles A. Walker

The publication of this book was triggered by the 11th Annual Clinical Pharmacy Symposium organized and conducted by the College of Pharmacy and Pharmaceutical Sciences, Florida Agricultural and Mechanical University in Tallahassee, Florida, held during March 6 to 10, 1986. The symposium provided a forum in which several nationally known health professionals, social workers, and scientists gathered together and discussed and analyzed the scientific and social issues of "drug abuse". Ms. Elaine M. Johnson, Acting Deputy Director, National Institute on Drug Abuse, of the Alcohol, Drug Abuse, and Mental Health Administration, Rockville, Maryland, was the keynote speaker of the opening session and addressed the national perspective of drug abuse. The theme of the symposium focused primarily on the subject of cocaine and marijuana.

After the symposium was successfully completed, the editors organized, compiled, and edited manuscripts of the symposium proceedings and decided to expand the scope of the discussion to include relevant and timely topics such as "designer drugs" (controlled substances analogues) and uses, misuses, and abuses of anabolic steroids by athletes. Contributed research monographs dealing with these particular subjects were requested from colleagues who did not attend the symposium and, thus, the effort led to the ultimate development and publication of this work.

The topic "drug abuse" is certainly of extraordinary timeliness. "Drug abuse" can be viewed from several points of view: sociological, psychological, medical, legal, and moral. The definition of drug abuse varies, depending on one's orientation. A generally accepted definition of drug abuse is the excessive and persistent self-administration of a chemical substance without regard for medically or culturally accepted patterns.[1]

Drug abuse, also referred to as chemical abuse or substance abuse, is viewed as the use of those agents to the extent that they interfere with the health and the "normal" social functioning of an individual. Often times, drug misuse is confused with drug abuse and is placed within the broad definition of "drug abuse". However, some distinction has to be made in that drug misuse refers to the administration of appropriately prescribed drugs, but in improper dosage or for inappropriate purposes.[1,2]

Chemicals of abuse are so insidious and pervasive that an alarming number of people, professional athletes, entertainers, members of the health profession, and many others, are engaged in their use with the illusion of being euphoric: self-confident, energetic, invulnerable, and masterful. For example, cocaine use, for a brief ecstatic moment, can make you feel brilliant and that you will live forever. What may not be apparent is the fact that it can also kill you. Cocaine intoxication has recently been referred to as "pharmacological Russian roulette", because an amount that can bring an ecstatic moment to one individual can cause fatal massive heart failure in another.[3] Moreover, cocaine use invariably leads to intoxicant-related problems such as disruption of family life, accidents, fires, homicides, suicides, drownings, loss of productivity, loss of jobs, or legal difficulties.[4]

Drug abusers tend to "drop out" of general society. They tend to congregate and "hang out" together, possibly in very unsanitary conditions. Burglary, pandering, and prostitution may become a way of life to secure money for a "fix". The drug habit can be very expensive since they are illegally obtained.[1] Such "colonies" provide fertile breeding grounds for the rapid spread of acquired immune deficiency syndrome (AIDS) which has reached epidemic proportions in the U.S. at the present time.

By the latest government estimate, the U.S. drug habit has risen to $110 billion a year! It is known that one of every six American teenage youngsters will have sampled cocaine before senior prom night in high school. It is also known that there are more than five million regular cocaine users in the U.S. About 20 to 25 million have tried cocaine at least once, and there are nearly 600 cocaine-related deaths yearly. Of all college students, 30% have tried cocaine by their 4th year and 42% have tried marijuana. Of the U.S. population, 25% has tried marijuana at least once, and about 9% smoke it regularly. There are about one half million estimated hard core heroine users.[5]

Cocaine, an alkaloid derived from the waxy leaves of the tropical shrub *Ethryroxylum coca* is available in salt form as cocaine hydrochloride (powder, "snow") and cocaine free base (rock cocaine, "crack"). It has basically two major pharmacological effects: the blockade of sodium channels and the blockade of catecholamine reuptake in the brain. There has been compelling clinical evidence that cocaine use can worsen preexisting weaknesses of the heart as well as trigger powerful attacks. Habitual cocaine users usually face anxiousness, depression, hallucinations, and psychosis after an initial euphoric high. These effects could eventually slide into full-blown paranoid schizophrenia and possibly permanent brain damage.[3]

The marijuana plant *(Cannabis sativa)* contains a variety of cannabinoid derivatives, which, together with alcohol, constitute the most widely abused drugs of the world. Use of *Cannabis* has increased sharply in the U.S. during the past 20 years, particularly among adolescents and preadolescents. Many such young users are experimenting with drugs as they experiment with other things. Although most youthful experimenters do not become habitual users, many continue to use drugs. The reasons are varied and probably not identical for any two users. The younger children who become drug abusers rebel against society before they have completed the developmental tasks of adolescents. Not having completed these, the individuals may exhibit even greater psychiatric difficulties than those who became drug abusers at a later age.[1] As marijuana use has become part of the experience of growing up and, in many parts of the world, a part of adult social life, scientists are finding out that *Cannabis* may share with nicotine and alcohol a potential for carcinogenicity, among other hazardous health consequences.[6] The marijuana cigarette, known to contain a complex mixture of toxic chemical compounds, mainly delivers the tetrahydrocannabinoid (THC) products into the blood stream rapidly during inhalation. Recent studies indicate that development of true tolerance in man to the behavioral and pharmacological effects of THC has been observed after prolonged administration of high doses of THC.[7-10]

Recently, clandestinely synthesized new chemical compounds referred to as "designer drugs" have attracted intense public attention. These compounds are prepared by innovative chemists by utilizing the structure-activity relationships of known psychoactive drugs. Some derivatives are known to be 10 to 1000 times more active than the known so-called recreational drugs. However, their use, abuse, purity, pharmacokinetics, and toxicity behavior are not yet well documented in the literature. Fentanyl, for example, which is a synthetic derivative of heroine, is 100 times as strong as morphine, and 20 to 40 times as strong as heroine; its medicinal analogues, sufentanyl and lofentanyl, are, respectively, 2000 and 6000 times as strong as morphine. The danger of designer drugs lies in the fact that every abusable drug can have several synthetic analogues that can be stronger, cheaper, and more deadly and varied in effect than the original.

When they first hit the street, most designer drugs are as legal as common salt. The skilled designer chemist "fiddles" with the chemical structure of a drug of abuse slightly in such a way as to avoid the regulations that ban its use, but maintains or increases its potency. According to the Federal Controlled Substances Act of 1970, a compound is legal until declared otherwise. Designer drugs are just the latest bad news about the drug culture developing in many countries. Law enforcement agencies keep making record numbers of arrests and confiscations of various substances of abuse, but they are hardly making a dent in controlling the staggering amount of designer drugs.

The use of anabolic steroids by athletes has recently raised many controversies in the world of sports. The concerns deal primarily with the uses, misuses, and abuses of the male hormone testosterone and its synthetic derivatives. Testesterone stimulates the build-up of muscles that men experience at puberty, in addition to mediating the development of adult male sexual characteristics. Athletes who want to increase muscle mass usually find physicians who are willing to prescribe anabolic steroids. Athletes involved in body building, weightlifting, and football are particularly attracted to effects of the muscle-building (anabolic) effects of testosterone. Despite their popularity among athletes, there is a sharp disagreement among scientists as to whether anabolic steroids actually improve physical performance. Many investigators believe that there are so many interfering factors like nutrition, environment, psychological outlook, and that anabolic steroids work in some people, but not in others. The side effects of these hormones range from annoying skin diseases (e.g., acne) to deadly liver tumors, sterility, and coronary heart failure. Other undesirable effects documented in the literature are related to the sex hormone properties of the derivatives: baldness and changes in sexual desire. Some men experience enlargement of the breasts.[12]

The publication is entitled *Cocaine, Marijuana, Designer Drugs: Chemistry, Pharmacology, and Behavior* to reflect the emphasis placed on these particular topics. It is hoped to increase the understanding of chemical abuse and is primarily addressed to the scientific community, health care practitioners, social workers, and psychologists.

REFERENCES

1. **Sheridan, E., Patterson, H. R., and Gustafson, E. A., Eds.,** The problem of drug abuse, *Falconer's the Drug, the Nurse, the Patient, 7th ed.,* W. B. Saunders, Philadelphia, 1985, chap. 7.
2. **Rogers, P. G.,** Drug abuse in our society, *J. Am. Pharm. Assoc.,* NS 8, 3, 1968.
3. **Maranto, G.,** Coke, the random killer, *Discover,* 6, 16, 1985.
4. **Senay, E. C.,** *Substance Abuse Disorders in Clinical Practice,* John Wright-PSG Littleton, Mass., 1985, 127.
5. 1985 Data, President's Commission on Organized Crime, National Institute on Drug Abuse, Institute for Social Research, Rockville, Md., 1985.
6. **Senay, E. C.,** *Substance Abuse Disorders in Clinical Practice,* John Wright-PSG Littleton, Mass., 1985, 117.
7. Marijuana and Health, Annu. Rep. to the U.S. Congress, National Institute on Drug Abuse, Rockville, Maryland, 1984.
8. **Ohlsson, A., Agurell, S., Londgren, J. E., Gillespie, H. K., and Hollister, L. E.,** Pharmacokinetic studies of *delta*-1-tetrahydrocannabinol in man, *Pharmacokinetics and Pharmacodynamics of Psychoactive Drugs,* Biomedical Publications, Foster City, Calif., 1985, 75.
9. **Hunt, C. A. and Jones, R. T.,** Tolerance and disposition of tetrahydrocannabinol in man, *J. Pharm. Exp. Ther.,* 215, 35, 1980.
10. **Londgren, J. E., Ohlsson, A., Agurell, S., Hollister, L. E., and Gillespie, H. K.,** Clinical effects and plasma levels of *delta*-9-tetrahydrocannabinol in heavy and light users of Cannabis, *Psychopharmacology,* 74, 208, 1981.
11. **Gallagher, W.,** The looming menace of designer drugs, *Discover,* August, 24, 1986.
12. **Zurer, P. S.,** Drugs in sports, *Chemical and Engineering News,* April 30, 1984.

Chapter 2

THE NATIONAL PERSPECTIVE OF DRUG ABUSE

Elaine M. Johnson

TABLE OF CONTENTS

I. THE DIMENSIONS OF THE NATIONAL PROBLEM

There can be no doubt that drug abuse is one of the gravest problems facing the U.S. today. Although the number of Americans using drugs has somewhat stabilized, the level of drug use remains very high and unacceptable. In fact, the use of some drugs is still increasing among certain groups within the population.

In order to better understand the nature and extent of the problem, the National Institute on Drug Abuse (NIDA) supports several national surveys. These studies include a national household survey, usually conducted every 3 years, and an annual nationwide survey of drug use among high school seniors. NIDA also maintains a nationwide drug abuse-monitoring system known as The Drug Abuse Warning Network (DAWN) in hospital emergency rooms in 27 large urban areas across the U.S. The emergency room data are supplemented in many cities with a medical examiner system which charts trends in deaths caused by or related to drug abuse.

The National Household Survey on Drug Abuse reflects the magnitude of the problem in the U.S. Our latest survey completed in 1985 reveals that 18 million Americans are currently using marijuana; 6 million Americans are currently using cocaine; 3 million Americans use other stimulants; and over 2 million Americans are using sedatives without a prescription.

Data from the National High School Senior Survey indicated that the number of young Americans using drugs increased dramatically in the 2 decades from 1960 to 1979. This upward trend peaked and then began to recede for many drugs between 1979 and 1987.

The use of some drugs showed little change in 1987. These include LSD, heroin, and opiates other than heroin; and there was some evidence of a continuing gradual increase in the use of inhalants. Because of the major problem with cocaine, it deserves special mention, and I would like to discuss in particular the serious consequences it poses for us.

It was found that *cocaine* use by high school seniors declined substantially for the first time in 1987 among virtually all of the subgroups examined. These included both males and females, the college- and the noncollege bound, and students from rural and urban areas in all regions of America.

Data from the DAWN show that between 1983 and 1987 there was a five- to sixfold increase in the number of emergency mentions of cocaine and of medical examiner reports of cocaine-related deaths. The number of cocaine-related deaths reported by medical examiners increased from 323 in 1983 to 1538 in 1987. We believe we are now seeing the tragic results of the cocaine use that began its sharp use in the late 1970s and in the 1980s.

Although the majority of people still snort or inhale cocaine, those entering emergency rooms are also injecting the drug. Injection of cocaine now reflects 26.1% of emergency room cocaine visits. In addition, smoking (freebasing) increased substantially from 1.3% of admissions in 1981 to 29.9% in 1987.

Until the etiology of cocaine dependence is completely understood, it will be impossible to determine in advance who is most vulnerable to cocaine addiction. Everyone who uses the drug must be considered at risk.

Now we are also disturbed by the evidence that youths have been experimenting with drugs at younger and younger ages since 1975. For marijuana, alcohol, and cigarettes — the "gateway drugs" — the average age at first use now is at the junior high school level. While drug abuse rates vary from community to community and there are some differences in the extent and pattern of use by sex, race-ethnicity, and social class, no group has been found to have an immunity.

Drug abuse does more than threaten the health and social well-being of the individual user. To take a very dramatic example, as a result of sharing needles, a high percentage of intravenous drug abusers are now carriers of the AIDS virus; these users can then transmit the virus to their sexual partners and, in the case of pregnant women, to their children. Drug use also has been found to be highly correlated with both violent and nonviolent crimes by juveniles and adults. It is estimated that in 1980, drug-using *adult offenders* alone accounted for costs to society of $16.9 billion. Finally, drug use by persons in key jobs affecting health and public safety is a growing concern, as is the role of drug use in decreasing productivity among workers in general.

II. THE FEDERAL STRATEGY

Because drug abuse is such a complex problem — one which involves scientific, economic, legal, and public policy issues — it demands a highly complex and comprehensive solution. The goal of the drug abuse policy of the Federal Government is to eliminate both drug abuse and its adverse consequences. The 1984 National Strategy for Prevention of Drug Abuse and Drug Trafficking, developed by the White House Office of Drug Abuse Policy and signed by the President, is still in force and divides the national effort into two components: a demand reduction program and a supply reduction program.

The demand reduction program is intended to (1) dissuade the nonuser from experimenting with drugs; (2) deter the occasional user or experimenter from progressing to the abuse of drugs; (3) make treatment available for abusers of drugs who seek it; and (4) help the former abuser regain a place as a productive member of society. The supply reduction program is intended to (1) make drugs difficult to obtain, expensive, risky to possess, sell, or consume, and (2) thereby reduce the number of experimenters and chronic users.

In all, 33 federal agencies participate in the National Strategy and its two-pronged approach to drug abuse. However, a key element of the 1984 National Strategy is the continuing partnership between government and the private sector. The strategy promotes the involvement of parents and volunteers in teaching young people, especially elementary school children, to develop healthy behavior and positive goals and to be aware of the risks involved in using drugs. In coordination with federal agencies, private business, labor organizations, the media, and the entertainment and sports industries are using their unique resources to deglamorize drug-taking behavior, promote positive images of a drug-free life for young people, and disseminate accurate, up-to-date information regarding the dangers of drug use.

With regard to treatment, the strategy promotes integration of drug abuse services into the general health care system. It also calls for each local community to support treatment facilities and approaches appropriate to its special needs.

III. THE NIDA ROLE

The efforts of the National Institute on Drug Abuse, a component of the Department of Health and Human Services, are a significant part of this multifaceted approach to reducing the personal and societal costs of drug abuse. It is the lead federal agency responsible for drug abuse health issues, focusing on the demand reduction side. Prior to 1981, the institute had a broad mandate that included providing direct financial assistance for drug abuse education, training, treatment, and rehabilitation, as well as conducting both an intramural and extramural research program.

With the passage of Title XX of Public Law 97-35 (The Alcohol and Drug Abuse and Mental Health Services Block Grant) in 1981, full responsibility for carrying out treatment and prevention service functions was transferred to the states. The current role of NIDA in the area of demand reduction, as set forth both in the National Strategy and the Alcohol and Drug Abuse Amendments of 1983 (Public Law 98-24), is to (1) develop and disseminate new knowledge about drug abuse, its prevention and treatment, and (2) exercise national leadership in encouraging and assisting the private sector, the states, and local governments to implement and support prevention, intervention, and treatment programs in their communities. In addition, NIDA research on the abuse liability and risks associated with specific drugs support the supply reduction program by providing the information necessary to control drugs under the Controlled Substances Act.

IV. THE NIDA RESEARCH PROGRAM

The NIDA research program has several important components. Through its *epidemiological research* program, the institute has developed a unique capability for reliably assessing the nature and extent of the drug abuse problem of the nation and its trends over time. As already mentioned, in order to track the incidence and prevalence of drug abuse, NIDA supports two ongoing epidemiological surveys, the National Household Survey on Drug Abuse and the High School Senior Survey. The NIDA Drug Abuse Warning Network (DAWN) monitors information on the negative health consequences of drug use through emergency rooms and medical examiner reports. In addition to these major efforts, NIDA also supports a number of special epidemiological studies.

About half of the NIDA research program consists of *basic research* which seeks to develop new knowledge about the mechanisms of action of drugs, their sites of action, especially in the brain and central nervous system, and their pharmacology. Recent advances in receptor research under sponsorship of NIDA grants have done much to advance our basic knowledge about how drugs act in the body and how their effects are produced. Other research conducted by NIDA focuses on the hazards of various drugs, ranging from the adverse biological effects of drugs on body systems to their psychobehavioral effects on learning, performance, and cognition and their social effects. From this type or research we have learned, for example, that acute intoxication with marijuana interferes with many aspects of mental functioning and poses a major impediment to classroom performance. The drug also has serious acute effects on perception and coordination performance, both of which are involved in driving and many of the tasks of daily living.

NIDA-funded scientists are also involved in the development of new compounds, the prediction of drug action, the determination of metabolic pathways of drugs, and the development of assay methods for detecting drugs in body fluids. This last area has had great practical use for law enforcement agencies and for businesses concerned about drug use by their job applicants and employees. NIDA sponsored a conference on Drug Abuse in the Workplace, which highlighted the most current information on various drug detection technologies and brought together a wide range of companies to discuss how these technologies could best be used both to safeguard the public and to help drug-abusing individuals.

Research in all of these areas is conducted both through extramural grants and contracts and at the NIDA intramural research facility, the Addiction Research Center (ARC). In 1985, the ARC, which began as the research division of the U.S. Narcotic Farm in Lexington, Kentucky, celebrated its 50th anniversary and the dedication of its new facilities in Baltimore. The ARC represents the largest single interdisciplinary team working on the problems of drug abuse. It employs neuroscientists, analytic chemists, biochemists, pharmacologists, behavioral pharmacologists, psychologists, and psychiatrists. They work on problems ranging from effects of drugs on the immune system to the psychological responses to cocaine withdrawal.

Prevention and treatment research are a major part of the NIDA research program. The current research program of the NIDA in support of prevention includes several broad areas: (1) research on causes of use and abuse; (2) research on trends in use; (3) research on the abuse potential of drugs; (4) research on the risks and consequences of using various drugs; and (5) research on methods of prevention and early intervention. The first area of research seeks to expand understanding of the factors that inhibit or contribute to the risk of drug abuse in later life. Better understanding of these factors, or the etiology of drug abuse, assists substantially in the development or refinement of preventive interventions. The second area, research on trends in use, helps identify prevention priorities and enables prevention programs to target high-risk groups. The third area, research on abuse potential of drugs, permits the development of appropriate guidelines for the use of drugs and permits the scheduling of certain drugs in order to restrict access to them. The fourth area, research on the risks and consequences associated with particular drugs, provides the information necessary in the development of accurate information on drug abuse, central to so many prevention efforts. The final area, preventive intervention research, looks at how effective different prevention programs are in deterring or delaying the onset of various drug abuse behavior patterns. This research focuses on youth, since adolescence is the time during which most drug use is initiated.

The treatment research program at NIDA is focused on those persons who are already heavily involved in drug abuse and who are suffering the consequences of that involvement. In recent years, there has been a substantial increase not only in the number of casual users and of dependent individuals, but in the variety of drugs they are using. Multiple drug use has become the rule rather than the exception. As patterns of drug abuse have become more diverse and complex, finding the most effective treatments has become a much more complex task. In addition, as with other biobehavioral problems, the population seeking treatment for drug abuse is heterogeneous. The individuals vary along demographic dimensions such as social class, age, employment, and other drug experiences. To further complicate the problem, psychopathology is often associated as an antecedent to or consequence of substance abuse. Thus, there is a need to match the therapy with the needs of the patient.

NIDA has concentrated its treatment research efforts on the development of innovative, effective, and cost-efficient therapeutic approaches. Recent areas of emphasis included interrelations between drug abuse and other biobehavioral disorders (e.g., eating disorders and stimulant abuse), special problems related to particular agents (e.g., cocaine) or forms of drug abuse, development and evaluation of new agents used as adjuncts in treatment (e. g., LAAM, naltrexone, nicotine gum), as well as the complex interactions between behavioral, pharmacological, and treatment variables in determining long-term outcome.

V. PRIORITY AREAS FOR RESEARCH

Within these ongoing areas of NIDA research, there are a number of special areas of research which may be of particular interest today and which we consider of top priority. *Cocaine,* which is not only an extremely dangerous and addictive drug, but one of the few which is increasing in use, has been a special focus of our research during the last several years. We regard cocaine as a significant public health problem, both in terms of the number of users and the serious adverse consequences for which these users are at risk. In addition to its continuing efforts to track trends in cocaine use and to refine our data sources to get an even more accurate picture of the dimensions of the problem, NIDA is devoting an increasing proportion of its resources to research aimed at understanding exactly how cocaine works, what its effects are, and what treatment and prevention approaches are most efficacious in dealing with this particular drug. In 1984, for example, the institute funded approximately 23 grants related to cocaine and other stimulants.

A number of important findings have emerged from our research on cocaine. We now know, for example, that cocaine is one of the most powerfully addictive drugs, exerting its effect by acting directly on the reward or pleasure centers of the brain. This action produces an intense desire to experience the effects of cocaine again. The positive reinforcing properties of cocaine have been demonstrated in every species of animal tested. In addition, if access to the drug is not limited, there is evidence that some animals will self-administer cocaine to the point of toxicity and death, selecting cocaine in preference to food and water. By contrast, animals will not self-administer opiates, even heroin, to the point of such toxicity.

To encourage additional research, in 1984 NIDA distributed a new research announcement to the field inviting applications for studies to broaden understanding of cocaine use and help identify effective strategies for treatment and prevention. This research is to focus on a number of areas, including etiology, biomedical aspects, neuroscience, behavioral pharmacology, treatment, and prevention. This represents a significant expansion in our research portfolio on cocaine.

Last year, NIDA published "Cocaine: Pharmacology, Effects, and Treatment of Abuse". The monograph discusses the scientific evidence that cocaine is powerfully addictive and describes how it activates reward circuits in the brain. It also discusses current and experimental treatment for cocaine abuse. In July of 1984, NIDA held a national symposium on cocaine for the purpose of developing a comprehensive description of patterns and consequences of cocaine use in this country. Prominent clinicians, researchers, and epidemiologists presented papers which were published in another monograph entitled "Cocaine Use in America: Epidemiologic and Clinical Perspectives", which was released in early Fall, 1985.

Research into the treatment of cocaine abuse is an important priority area for NIDA. The treatment of cocaine use presents special challenges, and NIDA intends to carry out more studies on the natural history of cocaine abuse and on methods that may be effective in its treatment. We have learned a good deal about several approaches which work for many individuals. These include psychotherapy, behavior modification, self-help strategies, and various pharmacotherapies.

The use of *controlled substance analogues,* which have the unfortunate street name of "designer drugs", is another area of research currently receiving emphasized focus at NIDA. In recognition of the danger that these drugs pose, NIDA is supporting a number of research projects that are designed to detect and monitor the use of these drugs and the extent to which the use spreads to other geographic areas; assess the basic mechanism of drug actions, toxicity, and clinical pathology; determine more precisely the health consequences of using these drugs; and disseminate information to the medical community, treatment and prevention programs, and to the public at large. For example, NIDA-funded researchers have demonstrated the neurotoxicity of one class of these drugs — the methamphetamines — which includes both MDA (known on the street as "Adam" and MDMA (or "Ecstasy"). They have also learned that the dose of these drugs that produces psychological effects is not far removed from the dose needed to induce neural damage, and thus we believe it very possible that the individuals abusing these methamphetamine derivatives are indeed inducing brain damage.

In spite of pending legislation that will automatically bring all so-called "designer drugs" under the Controlled Substances Act, it seems likely that clandestine laboratories will continue to produce new and toxic compounds. The institute plans to work closely with the DEA to contain the potentially disastrous consequences of designer drugs by expanding its research into the structure and behavioral pharmacology of these compounds, and by developing educational activities that will contribute to preventing their use and abuse.

NIDA has been gravely concerned about the *relationship between intravenous drug abuse and AIDS.* Based on national data, approximately 65% of the cases of AIDS are among nonintravenous drug-using, homosexual men, 8% are among homosexual intravenous drug users, and approximately 17% are among heterosexual intravenous drug users. Put another way, individuals with a history of intravenous drug use make up approximately 25% of the total number of reported AIDS cases. When we look at certain areas of the country, the relationship between intravenous drug use and AIDS is even more dramatic. For example, in the New York area, 38% of reported AIDS cases are among those with a history of intravenous drug use. Pediatric cases represent less than $1^1/_2\%$ of the total AIDS cases; however, 52% of these children are the offspring of intravenous drug users. Many people also fail to appreciate that there are significant numbers of women who are developing AIDS or are infected with the AIDS virus; many of these are women with a history of using intravenous drugs.

The activities of NIDA in the area of AIDS have focused on three principal populations: intravenous drug users currently infected with the AIDS virus; other drug users at high risk of and concerned about the disease; and drug abuse treatment and service providers. In the area of research, we are continuing support for and plan to fund additional studies on the role of drug use and the interaction of drugs of abuse on the immune system. We are also encouraging studies to develop and expand our understanding of the epidemiology of AIDS. This research will focus on the etiology, risk-factors, and natural history of AIDS among populations at risk for developing the disease due to drug abuse or contact with drug abusers. Because intravenous drug users are the second largest group of AIDS victims, NIDA will focus its research on treatment as the most effective way to decrease needle sharing among individuals who are at risk for transmitting the AIDS virus to others.

Treatment research is an area that we consider a priority. As more is known through research about those treatment methods that are both successful and cost effective, emphasis will be given to the compulsive drug abusers who engage in aggressive behavior and crime, and who are the least responsive to education and information on the dangers of drug use.

Finally, we are interested in the entire question of *biological vulnerability to drug abuse.* We now know from research over the past decade that heredity is a factor in vulnerability for developing alcoholism, and recent findings indicate that there are gender differences in this vulnerability — boys appear more at risk than girls. The NIDA future research program includes studies of possible connections between aggressive behavior in childhood, and later drug abuse and violence. Other emphasis will include the influence of the environment (social interaction, sensory stimulation, stress), the effect of nutrition that may influence the metabolism of important neurotransmitters, and the special problems of school dropouts, behavioral problem children, children of users, ethnic and minority populations that may place them more at risk for drug use and abuse.

VI. NATIONAL LEADERSHIP ACTIVITIES

As important as we consider our research activities to be, the national leadership role of NIDA in the area of drug abuse prevention and treatment goes beyond its lead role in funding and carrying out research in these areas. A major part of the mission of the institute is to provide guidance and assistance to drug abuse prevention and treatment efforts at the state and community levels. In carrying out this responsibility, NIDA pursues a number of different but related activities. They include technical assistance to groups in both the public and private sector, identification and replication of model prevention and treatment programs, dissemination of prevention and treatment research findings to schools, parent groups, primary health care providers, and law enforcement personnel through publications and workshops, and public education through the development of written information and national media campaigns. All of these activities build on the knowledge gained through our research activities.

In the area of AIDS, for instance, education and prevention programs targeted at specific audiences are a major element of our strategy. Clearly, drug users, particularly intravenous drug users, need to know about the risks to themselves, their sex partners, and families when they use intravenous drugs. Right now we have no way of predicting which individuals carrying the virus will develop AIDS. At present, it appears that over a 5-year period approximately 5 to 10% of those infected with the virus will go on to develop AIDS, and 20 to 25% will probably develop AIDS-related complex. We have reason to believe that the intravenous drug user who uses frequently is at greater risk than one who uses infrequently. Nevertheless, even the occasional user of intravenous drugs, whether heroin, cocaine, amphetamines, or some other substance, is at risk for contracting the virus and subsequently AIDS itself. This point must be stressed and is the cornerstone of our efforts in prevention and education regarding AIDS and intravenous drug use.

In the area of AIDS, we are developing and disseminating information to specific high-risk subgroups and the general public about the relationship between drug abuse, the spread of the AIDS virus, and the risks for subsequently developing AIDS. A "NIDA Capsule", or fact sheet, on the subject of AIDS and drug abuse has been developed and has been distributed both to the press and to state drug abuse agencies. It describes AIDS, the methods by which the disease is transmitted, and specific ways to reduce risk of infection with the virus. Other publications are being planned, including flyers, booklets, and posters to be printed in both English and Spanish.

We are undertaking a number of other activities aimed at better informing treatment and service providers about suitable procedures for serving drug abuse clients infected, or at risk for becoming infected, with the AIDS virus. We have developed a repository of findings and materials about AIDS and intravenous drug use and have initiated monthly mailings to state agency directors of recent findings and new materials that may be useful in planning service delivery and prevention activities.

Because it is important to address the fears of both the clients and the staffs of drug abuse treatment programs, we are developing training materials and programs for State drug abuse agencies, drug treatment programs, criminal justice detention systems, and other relevant health care agencies which serve intravenous drug users and/or their families. A series of workshops will discuss such topics as AIDS and the drug abuse treatment environment, counseling clients exposed to the AIDS virus, whether or not they are symptomatic, and treatment of these clients in residential programs. Though specific procedures and policies will, of course, have to vary from state to state, we hope to establish consensus around a number of issues. NIDA will also provide on-site technical assistance on AIDS and drug abuse to drug abuse treatment programs.

In other areas as well, we consider the dissemination of our research findings as important as the research itself, and we have been developing a number of mechanisms — in addition to monographs and other publications — for getting them out to the practitioners who can make use of them. For example, during 1985, NIDA held a series of workshops — in Portland, Boston, Atlanta, Los Angeles, New York, Dallas, and Chicago — designed to disseminate new research-based treatment models to practitioners. Each workshop had four emphases: treatment of cocaine dependence, treatment of adolescent substance abusers, providing aftercare/self-help services, and evaluating one's own service delivery. In April 1985, in Milwaukee, the Wisconsin Institute of Drug Abuse and the Tellurian Society, with NIDA as cosponsor, held a national symposium on cocaine. Surgeon General Dr. C. Everett Koop gave the keynote address, "Cocaine and Health", and former NIDA Director Dr. William Pollin spoke on the topic, "Cocaine — A Powerfully Addictive Drug". Other NIDA staff and a number of NIDA-supported researchers presented information on current activities and findings in cocaine research, prevention, and treatment. More than 400 health professionals, law enforcement personnel, alcohol and drug abuse professionals, researchers, and industrial representatives have attended our meetings.

NIDA has been developing how-to manuals for delivery of treatment services; these manuals include information on such topics as diagnosis, aftercare, and vocational rehabilitation. We are now publishing and disseminating to the field *NIDA Notes*, which give capsule accountings of recent findings significant to planners, service providers, and the public in a language and format useful to them. The institute will be holding five prevention evaluation workshops for service providers and the general public involved in prevention activities. There will be additional workshops on needs of assessment/monitoring in the community and financing treatment in this new economic era.

During the past 3 years, NIDA has been involved in two major national media campaigns designed to get the most accurate and current information about drug abuse — the information which our research provides — to carefully targeted audiences. The 1983—1985 NIDA Drug Abuse Prevention Media Campaign was developed to reach parents and young people with drug abuse prevention messages through a broad range of media materials. The campaign was designed to motivate parents to learn about drugs, talk to their children about the drug problem, and join with other parents to fight drug abuse in the community. Equally important, NIDA wanted to motivate young people to take their own action to resist peer pressure to use drugs, and, accordingly, a major theme of the campaign was "Just Say No". This message was integrated into radio and television public service announcements distributed to broadcasters nationally and into print materials distributed to organizations and agencies throughout the country.

In 1985, NIDA launched Phase II of this highly successful campaign by expanding its target audiences to include minority, inner-city young people, ages 10 to 14, and their families. Phase II used subway transit ads with antidrug messages and new radio and television public service announcements, featuring black and Hispanic narrators and appropriate urban settings. In addition, the drug information flyers used in the campaign were translated into Spanish. The Phase II strategy was supplemented with a unique project, a music video aimed at teenagers, which forcefully brings across the message that you can be drug free and still successful and accepted by your peers. This "Just Say No" video has been widely aired on television and made available on free-loan for use by community groups of parents and young people.

NIDA launched another major media campaign focused on cocaine. The primary audience of the campaign was young employed adults, 18 to 35 years old; future target audiences will include high school and college students. The media campaign encouraged young people and other potential users to resist the pressure to use cocaine and provided serious, authoritative information about the known health consequences of the drug. Families, friends, employers, and co-workers were secondary target audiences.

Needham, Harper Worldwide, the volunteer ad agency for the recent "Just Say No" prevention campaign, also worked with the National Ad Council on this project. In addition to television and radio spots, the campaign included print ads and articles in newspapers and magazines, transit ads, information bulletins and fact sheets, posters and other collateral materials, and exhibits at meetings and conferences. A number of major corporations worked with NIDA to help mobilize corporate America to participate in the campaign. Two magazines — *Fortune* and *Institutional Investor* — offered assistance in marketing the campaign. We believe the campaign was successful in changing societal attitudes toward cocaine by increasing awareness of the substance as a dangerous dependence-producing drug and in changing societal attitudes toward it.

Chapter 3

BEHAVIORAL PHARMACOLOGY OF DRUG ABUSE

James P. Cleary and Kenneth D. McIntire

TABLE OF CONTENTS

I. INTRODUCTION

The observation that chemical substances can affect the behavior of an organism surely predates recorded history. Additionally, pharmacologists and other scientists have used behavior as a convenient dependent variable to investigate drug action for the last several hundred years. However, the integration of pharmacology with a general, systematic analysis of behavior is relatively recent. Despite the fact that Pavlov and colleagues used drugs in the investigation of conditioned reflexes,[1] modern behavioral pharmacology can probably be traced to a seminal paper by Peter Dews.[2] The significance of this early paper was the demonstration that the effect of a drug was dependent upon environmental and/or behavioral factors present when the drug was administered. The finding that the behavioral effects of a drug can be influenced by the scheduling of environmental events had an immediate impact on interest in the experimental analysis of drug/behavior relations. Prior to 1955, there were a total of 30 reported research articles related to drug effects on "learned animal behavior". Between 1955 and 1963, there were 281 research articles.[3] By 1968, the now classic *Behavioral Pharmacology,* by Thompson and Schuster, was published as the first major text integrating behavioral principles and drug research. Subsequently, the number of research articles and books devoted to the experimental analysis of drug/behavior relations has proliferated to the point that behavioral pharmacology can stand as a separate discipline which can contribute to the understanding of behavioral principles as well as drug action.

The present chapter summarizes the contribution of behavioral pharmacology (BP) to the analysis of chemical abuse, with an emphasis on cocaine and majijuana. However, our discussion will be facilitated if it is preceded with a brief presentation of the background and conceptual framework used to describe behavior/environment relations in BP. This emphasis on the relationships between behavior, drugs, and environmental circumstances contrasts BP with other disciplines which may use behavior to analyze drug effects. For example, pharmacologists may use behavior as a dependent variable to clarify physiological or chemical mechanisms of drug action, e.g., presence of morphine-induced emesis as a response used to indicate opiate receptors. In such instances, the drug/behavior relation is used to infer events and phenomena at a different level of analysis, i.e., the subject's behavior tells us something about neurophysiology or neurochemistry. But behavior may also serve as a dependent variable whose *primary* explanation is in terms of the conditions producing and maintaining the behavior itself. Such an explanation of drug/behavior interaction is at the heart of BP and involves analysis of antecedent and consequent environmental events and the principals that govern their functional relationship to behavior. This approach deemphasizes effects produced by the intrinsic characteristics of the drug and substitutes environmental history and current context as major determinants of an effect of a drug. As orderly relations continue to emerge between the scheduling of environmental events and the occurrence of behavior, nonreductionistic, environmental explanations of behavior become increasingly useful.

A more detailed examination of Dews' 1955[2] study may clarify some of the points discussed above. In this study, pigeons were trained to peck an illuminated response key (a transparent plastic disc illuminated from behind, located on a wall of a test cubicle). Pecking the key resulted in the presentation of a few seconds access to mixed grain. Grain was presented according to two distinct schedules. In the presence of one schedule, grain was presented for the first key peck occurring after 15 min since the previous grain presentation (a fixed interval 15-min reinforcement schedule). All key pecks in the 15-min interval between food presentations were recorded, but only the one peck had a programed environmental consequence. In the presence of the second schedule, grain was presented after every 50th key peck (a fixed ratio 50 reinforcement schedule). The schedules alternated and each was in effect for a specified duration. After key pecking staiblized on each of these reinforcement schedules, several doses of pentobarbital were administered on different days.

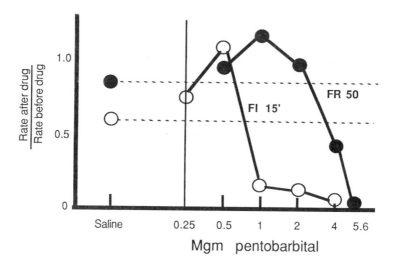

FIGURE 1.   Effects of pentobarbital on pecking behavior of pigeons. Each point represents the mean of the ratios for the same four birds at each dosage (dosages are expressed as mg/bird, rather than mg/kg). The rate of responding under the FI schedule is decreased at lower doses than those required to decrease rates under the FR schedule. (From Dews, P. B., J. *Pharmacol. Exp. Ther.*, 113, 393, 1955. With permission.)

Figure 1 summarizes the results from this study and clearly shows that the effect of the drug was a function of the reinforcement schedule. The effects were particularly interesting at doses of 1.0 and 2.0 mg, which increased the rate of key pecking in the presence of the fixed ratio schedule (FR) and decreased the rate in the presence of the fixed interval (FI) schedule. In both schedules, the response was the same (key peck) and responding had the same consequence (access to grain). Thus, whether the drug had stimulant or depressant properties was not only a function of the dose, but also of the scheduling of environmental events (the reinforcement schedules).

Dews' experiment demonstrated that drug effects could be altered by the scheduling of environmental events which follow responding (reinforcing events). Drug effects can also be affected by events which precede or are coincident with responding (discriminative events). For example, nonhumans responding in the presence of an FI reinforcement schedule generally display a reliable, temporally predictable pattern of responding in the interval between successive reinforcer presentations. The response pattern, generally called scalloping, begins with a response pause which follows reinforcement and has a duration of about one half of the interval. Responding begins at a very low rate and gradually increases in a positively accelerated fashion until very high rates of responding occur just prior to reinforcement. Amphetamine administration greatly increases the low response rates at the beginning of the interval and reduces the high rates near the end of the interval. However, if a ''clock'' is added to the reinforcement schedule in the form of a series of colored lights corresponding to different temporal segments of the interval, the rate-increasing effects of the drug are all but eliminated.[4] These results demonstrate how a drug effect can be moderated by environmental events (stimuli) which precede or are coincident with responding and which are related to important reinforcing stimuli. This role of antecedent and concurrent stimuli is the discriminative function of stimuli.

There are several points to be made about the general approach embodied in the examples cited above. First, behavior is measured repeatedly in the same subjects. In addition to more closely approximating human drug abuse, this methodological approach allows the behavior of a subject in a drugged state to be directly compared to its own undrugged behavior. Such

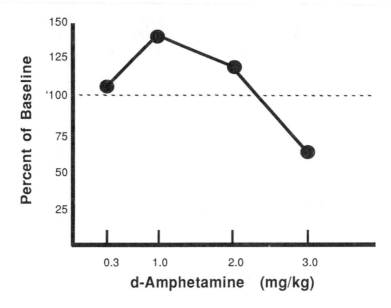

FIGURE 2.   Mean responses per minute for eight pigeons responding under an FI 60-sec schedule of reinforcement. Response rates are represented as a percentage of the baseline rate of responding. Low doses increase responding, while higher doses decrease responding, when compared to baseline rate.

repeated dosing also allows a within-subject reliability assessment. Second, repeated measurement places an extra burden on the experimenter to identify and control stimuli and events that affect behavior. Third, the effect of the drug is explained in terms of principals known to influence the behavior under study. This "mechanism of action approach" is well known in physiology and pharmacology. Finally, it should be clear that drugs not only modify the way in which environmental events control behavior, but also that the effect of a drug is malleable, subject to history and current stimulus conditions.

II. MECHANISMS OF ACTION: A NOTE ON BEHAVIORAL EXPLANATION

What effect a drug has on behavior may have two answers. First, we may simply describe the effect of a drug on topographically or functionally similar behaviors relative to a given stable baseline.[5] For instance, low to moderate doses of cocaine, as a stimulant-type drug, would be expected to increase the rate of occurrence of most behaviors and, indeed, this is what we find. Figure 2 is a typical stimulant dose-effect curve, with low doses increasing behavior and higher doses decreasing behavior. The effect of a drug may also be analyzed in terms of its "*mechanism of action*".[6,7] The locus of action of the behavioral effect of a drug is the specific topographical *unit of behavior* affected by the drug. Just as the neuromuscular junction is the locus of action for curare, the effect of a drug may also be described in relation to a specific *behavioral* locus of action. Examples of such behavioral units would be postreinforcement pause, overall response rate, or rate of response once responding resumes after pausing (run rate), response duration, interresponse time, temporal patterning, etc.

By *mechanism of action* Thompson and Schuster[6] meant the *process* which accounts for the behavioral effects of the drug. A *behavioral mechanism of action* is "a description of a drug's effect on a given behavioral system expressed in terms of some more general set of environmental principles regulating behavior".[7] Such factors as reinforcer magnitude, delay to reinforcement, deprivation (motivation), and changes in the discriminative stimuli that control responding are just a few of the candidates for such an explanation of drug effects. For example, moderate to high doses of methadone are known to reduce the response rate of a rat in a dose-dependent manner. The locus of action for this effect appears to be on the rate of responding after the subject finally begins to respond (i.e., run rate). The animal simply responds more slowly once responding begins, but does not take longer to get going after a pause. The *mechanism of action* for this decreased run rate has been attributed to a decrease in motivation. In the case of the rat, motivation transposes nicely into "level of food deprivation". That is, there is a relationship between motivation and level of deprivation; as we increase food deprivation we increase the motivation of the animal to respond for food reinforcers. The effect of methadone resembles the effects seen when deprivation is reduced and the animal is made less hungry. The change in run rate seen under methadone and under conditions of decreased deprivation or motivation is strikingly similar, suggesting that the mechanism of action for the decrease in response rate seen under methadone is a direct function of decreased motivation.

One of the problems for BP in the search for an understanding of drug dependence has been a lack of a conceptual framework by which we can compare the process of drug dependence across drugs and situations. Certainly, drug abuse does not have a single common cause nor is it controlled by a single set of circumstances or by the intrinsic nature of abused substances. However, conceptual frameworks like *mechanism of action* allow us the opportunity to evaluate drug abuse phenomenon behaviorally with the same metric, i.e., the general principles of behavior which control the phenomena under study.

III. DRUG DISCRIMINATIONS: MEASURING SUBJECTIVE EFFECTS

It is generally agreed that subjective effects of drugs play a role in their abuse. As such, it is important to develop procedures which reliably measure these subjective effects and bring them under experimental control. In humans, subjective effects are often measured by reports from subjects either under the influence of the drug or with considerable drug experience. Reports of subjective effects derived from different drugs (or different doses of the same drug) may then be compared. Such comparisons provide valuable indications of drug similarities and differences and may serve as a screening procedure, suggesting the abuse potential of new compounds. In addition to verbal reports, more rigorous procedures, such as questionnaires and inventories, have been developed to characterize subjective effects in humans.[8,9] Data from such procedures, when compared with data using nonhuman animal models, serve as a basis for the generality and validity of the nonhuman laboratory procedures. One such laboratory procedure, the drug discrimination paradigm, measures the subjective effect of a drug by establishing different responses in the presence of different drugs or drug doses. In the simplest drug discrimination procedure, subjects are trained to emit one response when drug is present and another response when it is not. With these procedures the stimulus properties of the drug are evaluated for their discriminative potential. Just as exteroceptive stimuli may aquire stimulus functions, so too may drug-produced interoceptive stimuli. Data from such procedures have demonstrated that the discriminative properties of drugs in laboratory animals are correlated with, and can serve as a model for, human interoceptive drug states. In addition, neurochemical questions, such as potential agonist/antagonist relations, may be addressed with these procedures. Colpaert[10] has recently written a comprehensive review of the drug discrimination literature as it relates to drugs of abuse.

The robust nature of drug-related stimuli has been demonstrated in a wide variety of species, procedures, and tasks. A typical drug discrimination experiment involves reinforcing an animal for responding on one manipulandum (e.g., lever) under one drug state and on another manipulandum (second lever) under another drug state. For example, a rat may be consistently reinforced with a food pellet after pressing the left lever when under the influence of cocaine, and reinforced on the right lever after receiving saline. In this situation, the interoceptive stimuli produced by the drug are the only cues as to which is the correct (reinforced) lever. If the animal responds on the incorrect lever (e.g., saline appropriate lever after receiving cocaine) a brief time-out may occur during which there is no opportunity for a reinforced response. The time-out period is followed by the start of the next trial with an opportunity to respond on either lever. Usually, a food reinforcer is delivered after a fixed number of responses occur on the correct lever (e.g., after 10 responses). If the training drug has strong discriminative properties, this procedure reliably produces subjects that respond almost exclusively on the appropriate lever after either saline or drug.

In the example described above, the presence of drug serves as a discriminative stimulus for responding on the drug-appropriate lever. As might be expected, animals typically respond with less accuracy when a lower dose of the training drug is given than when the training dose or a somewhat higher dose is administered.[11] This type of generalization curve is similar to one produced by varying some dimension of an exteroceptive stimulus that controls responding. After subjects have been trained to discriminate one drug from another, a new drug may be administered and the subject may then report the similarity of the interoceptive state of the new drug to either the training drug or saline, by choosing either of the two levers. In addition, drugs from a different class, producing substantially different subjective effects than the training drug, may be administered. Thus, a subject may be trained to discriminate morphine from cocaine and when new drugs are given, the behavior of a subject can "tell" the experimenter whether the new drug is more stimulant-like or more narcotic-like. Data from procedures like these show remarkable reliability and consistency across several species. In general, drugs pharmacologically similar to a training drug produce responding on the training drug-appropriate lever, while pharmacologically dissimilar drugs do not.[12] More complicated discriminations, involving more than two drugs, have also been successfully employed.[13]

Opioids were some of the first drugs of abuse to be evaluated for discriminative properties. Morphine was shown to function as a discriminative stimulus in the early 1970s.[14] Subsequently, a variety of opiates, from several different chemical subclasses, have been shown to have discriminative effects similar to each other and to morphine.[15] As a class, the opiates are also easily discriminable from other types of psychoactive drugs.[16] The subjective effects of narcotic agonists and antagonists appear particularly prognostic of their relative abuse liability, and it has been suggested that discriminative effects of opiates in animals are well correlated with subjective effects in man.[17]

Like other psychomotor stimulants, the subjective effects of cocaine are readily discriminable from saline.[18] Cocaine also serves as a good example of the use of these procedures to investigate neurochemical mechanisms by which one drug is discriminated from another. The discriminability of cocaine is probably based upon changes in catecholaminergic transmission.[19] Thus, subjects will respond on the cocaine manipulandum after receiving other drugs, such as d-amphetamine, that enhance catecholaminergic transmission.[20,21] Since dopamine blockers such as haloperidol interfere with the cocaine cue, evidence suggests that the specific neurotransmitter involved is dopamine,[22] but other researchers have argued that the interference produced by dopamine blockers involves more general changes rather than just disruption of the discriminability of subjective effects.[23]

Marijuana and related cannabinoid compounds are easily discriminable from vehicle under typical drug discrimination procedures such as those described above.[24] As with the opiates, the potency of cannabinoids in producing subjective effects in humans has correlated well with their discriminability under drug discrimination procedures.[25] Many of the hallucinogens, such as LSD and mescaline, are readily discriminable from vehicle and are indistinguishable from each other at comparable doses.[26] In general, the administration of other reputed hallucinogen-like drugs produces generalization to a hallucinogen training lever.[27] However, generalization also occurs for nonhallucinogenic serotonin agonists,[27] supporting the assumption that the mechanism of action for discriminability is primarily serotonergic, but may be unrelated to the ability of the drug to produce hallucinations. The data for hallucinogens other than marijuana are not quite as unambiguous as for opiates and CNS stimulants. For example, some known hallucinogens do not generalize to drugs with reportedly similar attributes. Colpaert[10] has argued that this inconsistency is due to qualitative differences in subjective effects produced by the various hallucinogens.

It would indeed be surprising if the subjective effects of commonly abused drugs were not discriminable from placebo and from drugs of different classes. The utility of the drug discrimination technique does not lie in these simple discriminations, but rather in opening these private and subjective effects to investigation. One of the most practical and productive aspects of this procedure is as a tool of pharmacology and neurochemistry. In this role it is used to infer mechanisms and test hypotheses about neurochemical phenomena, investigate receptor-mediated drug action, and test potency or efficacy of agonists and antagonists.[13,28] The procedure also allows investigation of environmental and pharmacological manipulations that may modify subjective effects of the drugs. For example, tolerance to the subjective effects of cocaine and cross tolerance to other amphetamine-like drugs has been convincingly demonstrated in the rat.[29] This study not only points out the similar subjective effects of drugs within the stimulant class, but also suggests similar mechanisms of tolerance development. An additional function of the procedure is as a screen for new compounds with high abuse potential. By comparing subjective effects of new compounds with those of known drugs of abuse, potentially dangerous drugs may be identified early in preclinical investigation.

IV. SELF-ADMINISTRATION OF DRUGS

Whereas the previous section was concerned with the discriminative properties of drugs, the present section is concerned with their reinforcing properties. With these procedures, drugs serve as reinforcers and increase behavior leading to the presentation of the drug. Identification of the circumstances under which the reinforcing properties of drugs can come to control behavior is the primary goal of these procedures. The paridigm has practical as well as theoretical implications. One practical implication is drug screening. Since abused substances are shown to have reinforcing functions in laboratory animals, it is possible to use animal models to screen new drugs for potential human abuse liability. From a theoretical perspective, the consideration of drugs as reinforcing stimuli has two implications. First, drugs can be analyzed, as are other reinforcers, for their shared and unique reinforcing properties. Second, "drug seeking behavior can be analyzed functionally in the same way as other operant behavior".[30]

One of the important considerations to keep in mind from the perspective of behavioral pharmacology is that the reinforcing properties of a drug, as with other stimuli, are not intrinsic to the drug, but can best be defined relative to the previous history of the organism and current circumstances under which the drug is taken. For example, Spealman[77] reported that monkeys would both work for cocaine injections and work for termination of those injection opportunities *at the same time*. Responding on one lever produced cocaine injections on the average of every 3 min (FI 3′); a response on the other lever produced a 1-min timeout from this injection schedule when the response occurred 3 min after the previous injection (FI 3′-termination). Thus, the same dose of cocaine was aversive and reinforcing at the same time, depending upon the contingency associated with presentation of the drug. These findings can be viewed in terms of an environmental method for reducing drug self-administration. When alternative behaviors that produce periods of abstinence from drug self-administration are made available under the proper circumstances, drug consumption, of even a powerfully reinforcing drug such as cocaine, can be reduced. The assertion that drug seeking and taking behavior is maintained by environmental and drug-related stimuli leads to solutions to the problems of drug abuse based on modifying or eliminating the conditions which maintain the behavior.

The number of research papers addressing the issue of drug reinforcing functions has grown dramatically in the past 25 years, and the size of the literature and the number of issues involved are beyond the scope of this chapter. The reader is referred to Johanson[31] and Young and Herling[32] for more general reviews.

The investigation of drug self-administration by animals can be traced to Shirley Spragg's[33] demonstration that a chimpanzee previously made physically dependent on morphine would choose one of two boxes concealing a syringe filled with morphine. A subsequent convincing demonstration of drug self-administration by Nichols et al.[34] showed that morphine-dependent rats would drink a morphine solution. However, the most significant contribution to the analysis of drug self-administration came with the development of procedures and technology to deliver i.v. injections of drugs to mobile or partially mobile animals.[35,36] These procedures allowed the programing of drug delivery and the arrangement of drug/behavior relations under rigorous experimental control. As such, it made possible the systematic analysis of the reinforcing properties of drugs. In one of the earliest studies to use these techniques, Weeks[35] showed that morphine-dependent rats would lever press for 10-mg/kg injections of morphine. Subsequently, Thompson and Schuster[7] extended these findings by demonstrating that monkeys would self-administer morphine injections if a series or chain of responses was required for each drug delivery. These early studies clearly demonstrated the reinforcing potential of drugs and the power of the research techniques.

Cocaine was first shown to have reinforcing properties by Pickens and Thompson.[37] This study showed that physical dependence was not a prerequisite for drug self-administration and included several controls which convincingly demonstrated that cocaine had reinforcing properties. Rats were prepared with i.v. catheters and placed in standard rodent operant chambers with levers. Each press on one of the levers was followed by the injection of 0.5 mg/kg cocaine. Under these conditions, lever pressing was maintained at a low, steady rate. To determine whether lever pressing was simply a function of increased activity resulting from the cocaine injection, cocaine was injected independently of the behavior of the rats. Under these conditions of noncontingent cocaine injections, lever pressing rates declined to zero. After cocaine-dependent lever pressing was reestablished, saline was substituted for the cocaine solution. A brief burst of early-session responding was followed by a decline to zero, similar to food-reinforced responding when the food is no longer presented. Under a third set of conditions, a light flash was presented with cocaine-reinforced lever presses and then the cocaine was discontinued while the light flash was continued. An early period of response bursts with the cessation of cocaine was followed by a decline in lever pressing. This indicates that the lever pressing was not maintained by stimuli related to cocaine injections, but rather by the drug itself. Finally, the response requirement was shifted to a second lever in the chamber and cocaine was no longer delivered for responding on the first lever. Lever pressing on the initial lever declined to zero, and responding on the second lever was maintained in a pattern similar to that originally established on the first lever. The conditions employed by Pickens and Thompson[37] clearly demonstrate that it was the cocaine/response contingency which was maintaining the lever pressing. Within a year, cocaine self-administration was demonstrated in monkeys,[38] and the reinforcing effects of cocaine were compared to those of morphine, *d*-amphetamine, pentobarbital, and ethanol. The same study showed that nalorphine, chlorpromazine, mescaline, and saline would not maintain behavior with the self-administration procedure.

These early studies convincingly demonstrated that the only environmental condition necessary for the self-administration of cocaine and many other abused substances is a simple reinforcing relation between a response and the presentation of the drug. The finding that these drugs themselves have properties which can maintain drug-seeking behavior, i.e., reinforcing functions, has resulted in a large number of studies designed to clarify the nature of the reinforcing function and, thus, compare the reinforcing properties of drugs with those of other, more conventional reinforcers.

One way of defining the reinforcing properties of a drug is to manipulate the drug/response relationship, i.e., the reinforcement schedule. The earliest self-administration studies used relatively simple reinforcement schedules. Basically, each response, or a small number of responses, was followed by an injection. This procedure generally results in very low response rates. There are, however, many ways of scheduling response/reinforcer relations. Reinforcement schedules may be based upon some property of behavior or upon a combination of behavior with some other event, e.g., time. Additionally, simple schedules may be combined and/or temporally alternated to result in very complex response/reinforcer relations.

In an FR reinforcement schedule, reinforcers are delivered after the completion of a specified number of responses. If the reinforcers were delivered after each tenth response, it would be an FR10 reinforcement schedule, etc. Hoffmeister and Schlichting[39] examined the self-administration of cocaine and several opioids in rhesus monkeys using an FR10 schedule. As with earlier studies, cocaine maintained very low rates of responding. The highest rate of responding was about seven responses per minute at 0.05 mg/kg cocaine injection. However, it would be a mistake to assume the low rates resulted from weak reinforcing properties of cocaine. In addition to having reinforcing properties, drugs can affect behavior directly. Other, more conventional reinforcers, like food pellets, have little if any direct effect on responding. As a consequence, procedures were developed to limit the frequency of drug presentation, thus, alleviating direct response-reducing drug effects.

By limiting session length and using reinforcement schedules which establish a minimum interval between injections, rates of drug-reinforced responding were increased to levels comparable to those maintained by food reinforcers under comparable conditions. Goldberg[40] and Goldberg and Kelleher[41] used squirrel monkeys responding on either a FR10 or FR20 reinforcement schedule. During 100-min sessions, food, i.v. cocaine or d-amphetamine were used as reinforcers. Additionally, there was a 60-sec time-out period after each reinforcement. During time-outs, responding had no programed consequences. An inverted-U dose-response relationship resulted, and at some doses, the rates of responding were comparable for cocaine and food. Additionally, the pattern of responding was similar for drug and food reinforcement.

A second basic reinforcement schedule is the FI schedule which generates a response pattern different than the FR. With the FI schedule, reinforcement is presented for the first response occurring after a specified time since the previous reinforcement. Nonhumans generate a characteristic scalloping pattern of responding in the presence of sufficiently long fixed intervals. As with the FR, FI reinforcement is followed by a pause. The pause duration is about one half the interval and is followed by a positively accelerated rate of responding which begins slowly and terminates with very high rates just prior to reinforcement. The reinforcing properties of cocaine and characteristic scalloping pattern using an FI schedule of self-administration have been observed for rats,[42] rhesus monkeys, [43] squirrel monkeys,[44] and baboons.[45]

The FI and FR schedules are fundamental and have provided much information about the reinforcing properties of various drugs. However, response/reinforcer relations in life are often complex and drug administration may maintain a large amount of drug-seeking behavior per fix or hit. Complex schedules are established in the laboratory by combining properties of more than one simple reinforcement schedule. One of the cleanest early demonstrations of complex schedule control and one of the most frequently referenced was Goldberg's[40] use of a "second order" FI-FR schedule. Squirrel monkeys responded on an FR schedule for the presentation of a 2-sec flash of yellow light. An i.v. cocaine injection was administered for the first FR completed after 5 min since the previous injection. The second-order schedule of cocaine administration resulted in higher rates of responding over a wider range of doses than those shown with comparable FI schedules. Subsequent work has shown that very long sequences of responding can be maintained using infrequent drug injections. In monkeys, responding has been maintained with second-order schedules with 60 min between cocaine or morphine injections.[46-48] These results show that under appropriate conditions of stimulus control, relatively infrequent administration of cocaine will maintain large amounts of drug-seeking behavior.

In summary, the self-administration research has shown that (1) nonhumans will self-administer cocaine when there is a reinforcing relation between responding and cocaine administration, (2) the reinforcing function of cocaine shares properties of schedule control with more conventional reinforcers, such as food, and (3) complex reinforcement schedules show that the reinforcing function of cocaine can combine with other stimulus control functions to generate a large amount of drug-seeking behavior for an occasional cocaine injection.

To this point, this section has been concerned exclusively with cocaine self-administration. However, a large number of substance have been found to have reinforcing properties when tested in self-administration studies. Additionally, there is a strong relation between substances which are self-administered in laboratory studies and those which are self-administered by humans in their natural environments. Although much of the research on self-administration concerns cocaine and the opiates, the list of self-administered substances is long indeed.[49] There are, however, substances which are abused by humans which have no, weak, or inconsistent reinforcing properties under animal procedures. For example, delta[9]-THC has been shown both to not maintain responding[50] and to maintain responding.[51] Harris et al.[50] found that rhesus monkeys would not self-administer delta[9]-THC. However, when cocaine was added to the injection solution, self-administration was established. When the cocaine was subsequently removed, self-administration declined. Pickens et al.[51] used monkeys that had self-administered phencyclidine prior to successful testing with THC. The critical procedural differences between the two studies remain to be elucidated.

Although the self-administration properties of THC are not yet clear in the animal literature, the evidence for cocaine and amphetamines has been amply demonstrated. In an extensive study of stimulant drugs, Wilson et al.[52] found that cocaine, methylphenidate, phenmetrazine, and pipraddrol all maintained responding during daily sessions. Additionally, Balster and Schuster[53] showed that *d*-amphetamine, *l*-amphetamine, and methamphetamine have reinforcing properties in self-administration tests.

Despite the fact that cocaine and other drugs can maintain responding through their reinforcing function, there currently exists no metric for comparing the relative reinforcing efficacy of a large number of compounds. Simply, a monkey will respond for either a food pellet or a raisin. However, if given a choice, the raisin would be found to be preferred under almost all conditions. In a study comparing the relative reinforcing efficacy of cocaine to diethylproprion and methylphenidate, Johanson and Schuster[54] used a two-choice procedure where monkeys would self-administer either cocaine or diethylproprion. In a second study, the same authors compared cocaine with methylphenidate.[55] Cocaine was preferred to diethylproprion at all doses tested. However, there was a dose-related effect for methylphenidate. As the dose of methylphenidate was increased, preference gradually shifted from cocaine to methylphenidate. Much more work of this nature needs to be done to clarify the relative reinforcing properties of drugs × dose × conditions relations. However, there is evidence that under certain conditions of *unlimited* access, cocaine and amphetamines can exert devastatingly strong control over behavior.

The studies reported to this point have used procedures which limit daily drug access. Under conditions of unlimited access, different pharmacological classes may result in different patterns of overall drug intake. The differences in the patterns of intake may be related to a large number of drug-related factors, e.g., toxic and direct effects on behavior, dose, kinetics, tolerance, etc. The pattern of intake for the opioids,[38,56] pentobarbital,[38,57] and phencyclidine[58] is one of relatively stable, cyclic daily injections of gradually increasing dose across time. Overall food intake is often maintained. In contrast, stimulants generate erratic and variable patterns of self-administration, often resulting in toxic side effects.[38]

Cocaine intake patterns may show 4- or 5-day periods of high intake followed by periods of no intake for up to 5 days. Periods of high drug intake may be accompanied by reduced food intake, convulsions, tremors, and death.[38] For example, Johanson et al.[59] tested rhesus monkeys under conditions of unlimited access to cocaine, *d*-amphetamine, and methamphetamine for 30 days. Few animals survived the study. The consistency of results like these with cocaine, some doses of amphetamines, and high doses of codeine indicates that under certain conditions of easy access, the reinforcing functions of a drug can be maintained despite the severity of its toxic effects.

The laboratory investigation of drug self-administration from a behavior analytic perspective using human subjects has a short history, perhaps dating from Mendelson and Mello.[60] Much of the work with human subjects has been related to alcohol and nicotine administration. For the substances and procedures investigated, there is a close correspondence between human and nonhuman self-administration behavior. In one human study Fischman and Schuster[61] showed the reinforcing potential of cocaine in humans. During daily 1-hr sessions, four subjects pressed one of two buttons for an injection of saline or one of two doses of cocaine (13 or 32 mg). By the end of the second day, cocaine was selected almost exclusively. Additionally, mood assessment and a variety of physiological measures were taken through each session. Mood tended to quickly elevate early in a session. This contrasted with a gradually increasing plasma level of cocaine. Although there are many interesting questions which remain about the nature of the reinforcing effects of cocaine, this study begins to narrow the gap between human and nonhuman behavioral pharmacology.

As with behavior maintained by nondrug reinforcers, the rate and pattern of drug-seeking behavior are dependent upon a large number of scheduling conditions which lie beyond the scope of this chapter. However, conceptualizing drug-seeking behavior as a form of behavior maintained by its consequences has implications for an analysis of drug abuse. First, to the extent that drugs maintain behavior through their reinforcing function, knowledge about the functional relationship between environmental circumstances and reinforcers in general may be applicable. Second, drug-seeking and administering behaviors may not constitute a "special" class of behavior, with its own unique properties, but rather these behaviors may be subject to the same types of controlling conditions as other operant behavior. As such, drug-related behavior must be analyzed in the context of other past and current reinforcing conditions in an individual's life. For example, it is possible that a drug abuser's life is deficient in other immediate, nondrug reinforcers. Additionally, a cycle may be established by the direct effects of a drug on behavior and discriminative performance. Thus, it becomes more difficult for an abuser to establish new response repertoires as other, previously adaptive, nondrug-related behaviors are reduced. These effects are compounded by other environmental and social reinforcers maintaining drug related behavior as an individual becomes socialized into a user's community.

V. PAVLOVIAN CONDITIONING IN DRUG DEPENDENCE

Imagine a situation in which a stimulus elicits a response of reliable strength and duration and is consistently paired with other stimuli over thousands of trials. This is precisely the situation we have in most drug abuse cases. Drugs of abuse are discriminable and reliably produce consistent physiological responses. In addition, drug taking often takes place in the same or similar environments, is accompanied by similar rituals, and involves standard paraphenalia. There is an overwhelming potential for Pavlovian conditioning to occur under these circumstances.

Indeed, Pavlovian or classical conditioning of drug effects has been shown both preclinically and in human studies. Preclinical studies probably start with Pavlov's[62] demonstration that dogs would begin to show what was called "morphine-like behavior" upon sight of the experimenter who had previously given the animals several injections of morphine. Subsequently, others have shown similar results.[63] Conditioned withdrawal has been produced by returning rats to the environment where they had previously experienced withdrawal.[64] In a study of the effect of withdrawal and addiction environments upon susceptibility to readdiction, Thompson and Ostlund[65] reported that rats orally addicted to morphine showed a more rapid rate of readdiction if they were given the opportunity to readdict in the same environment in which they went through withdrawal. This study suggests symptoms which were classically conditioned to the withdrawal environment produced an abstinence syndrome which in turn caused more rapid readdiction.

Several researchers have shown that "opposing processes" can be classically conditioned to opioid administration. Siegel[66] has convincingly demonstrated conditioning of tolerance and that this tolerance shows other classically conditioned properties such as extinction and recovery.[67] Siegel's work encompasses a series of experiments where stimuli associated with opioid drug administration produce responses opposite to opioid drug effects. Such work has evoked considerable debate as to the specific nature of the physiological response to opioid drugs and adaptive physiological responses to those drugs. While this argument goes beyond the scope of the current paper, Soloman and Corbit's[68] model of "opponent processes" shows promise for understanding many aspects of drug effects.

Humans have also shown classically conditioned responses associated with drug administration. Wikler[69] reported recovered addicts often showed withdrawal signs during conversations involving former drug use or when the addict returned to the environment where drugs were taken. These withdrawal symptoms sometimes resulted in relapse. O'Brien and associates[70] paired neutral stimuli with withdrawal signs (after naloxone injections) in methadone patients. The formerly neutral conditional stimulus plus a saline injection produced withdrawal symptoms similar to those produced by naloxone.[70] In this model of "conditioned abstinence" the formely neutral environmental stimuli (conditional stimulus) are repeatedly associated with withdrawal from the drug (unconditional response) and eventually come to elicit withdrawal-like responses even after months of abstinence. This type of classical conditioning process, combined with discriminative and reinforcing effects of drugs, facilitates drug-seeking and -taking behavior and has clinical implications for the planning of treatment programs for recovering addicts.

VI. BEHAVIOR-GENERATING SCHEDULES

Drugs can (1) enter into and modify established behavior/environment relations and (2) drugs themselves may become related to a behavior through their discriminative and reinforcing functions. Additionally, there remains a mechanism by which schedules of environmental events can increase or exaggerate the reinforcing properties of a drug. These "generator schedules"[71] are patterns of reinforcer presentation which increase the efficacy of *other* reinforcer classes and, thus, induce excessive patterns of responding. The earliest demonstration of such generator effects, schedule-induced polydipsia,[72] showed that the intermittent presentation of food pellets resulted in water intake many times in excess of normal or metabolically required levels of consumption. The excessive drinking induced by the food presentation schedule still has no adequate physiological or psychological explanation. Other patterns of activity have been shown to be sensitive to the programing of intermittent food presentation in the laboratory in a wide variety of species, including humans.[73]

The self-administration of drugs has been shown to be influenced by schedule generator effects. For example, under most conditions ethanol solutions are aversive or, at best, relatively weak reinforcers for laboratory rats. However, if ethanol solutions and water are concurrently available during periods of intermittent food pellet presentation, ethanol consumption and dependence develop.[74] When the temporal properties of the feeding schedule are arranged differently, preference for and consumption of ethanol declines to control levels. Many solutions, from drugs to sweetened condensed milk, may be substituted for the excessively consumed solution in this paridigm. The overindulgence in ethanol or its increased reinforcing efficacy resulted from the particular schedule of food presentation, independent of ethanol drinking. The classes of behavior induced by generator effects are related to the types of opportunities available while generator conditions are present. Thus, the complex, concurrently present tapestry of interwoven schedules present in a person's life may increase the reinforcing efficacy of work (i.e., workaholic), exercise, alcohol, cocaine, or any number of alternatives. The specific effects will depend upon the reinforcer classes available and operating in an individual's life.

VII. SUMMARY

Indulgence in commodities with reinforcing properties is to be expected. Overindulgence is of concern because of the individual and societal problems it creates. The results of research in BP lead to certain conclusions about the nature of drug overindulgence or abuse and how the problems may be profitably addressed. Under appropriate conditions drugs can have discriminative and reinforcing properties. Additionally, schedule generator effects can result in exaggerated and excessive patterns of behavior. As we are looking for the mechanisms for drug dependence, it is probably wise to consider the above stimulus functions in relation to the other reinforcers operating in a abuser's life.

There is probably nothing in a particular molecular structure or in the direct behavioral effects of a drug which makes it inherently and necessarily addictive. We need to look to the environmental events which initiate and maintain indulgence and overindulgence in drug-related behavior. The Robins et al.[75] now classic observation of Vietnam veterans shows the importance of a host of environmental factors in initiating and maintaining drug-taking behavior. Of Robins' sample, approximately 20% became narcotic addicts while in Vietnam. Upon return to the U.S., narcotic use fell to low, pre-Vietnam levels. Thus, easy access to cheap, high-quality drugs, in a new environment with new social and institutional reinforcement schedules (with strong aversive components), resulted in relatively high rates of drug use. Upon return home, the schedules present in a veteran's life prior to Vietnam were again in effect. Thus, previously adaptive behavior was once again adaptive and old social constraints and reinforcers were reinstated. Simply, the relative reinforcing efficacy of drugs was reduced in relation to the other simultaneously present contingencies in the returning veterans' lives.

We must look to a drug abuser's history and living conditions to understand why drugs are such relatively potent reinforcers for him/her. From a rehabilitation perspective, a person's genetic endowment and history cannot be changed, but his/her current and future living conditions are alterable. Sources of reinforcement initiating and maintaining drug-related behavior can be identified and reduced or eliminated. As important, response repertoires can be expanded to enrich the range of nondrug-related behavior. After all, "there are reinforcers sweeter than drugs"[71] if we can learn to use them.

REFERENCES

1. **Zavadskii, I. V.,** Experience with the application of the conditioned reflexes method to pharmacology toward the problem of the effects of certain drugs (alcohol, morphine, cocaine and caffeine) on the function of the higher regions of the central nervous system, *Truty Obschchestra Russkikh Vrachei, 1113 (St. Petersburg),* 75, 269, 1908.
2. **Dews, P. B.,** Studies on behavior. I. Differential sensitivity to pentobarbital of pecking performance in pigeons depending on the schedule of reward, *J. Pharmacol. Exp. Ther.,* 113, 393, 1955.
3. **Pickens, R.,** Behavioral pharmacology: a brief history, in *Advances in Behavioral Pharmacology* Vol. 1, Thompson, T. and Dews, P. B., Eds., Academic Press, New York, 1977, 230.
4. **Laties, V. G., and Weiss, B.,** Influence of drugs on behavior controlled by internal and external stimuli, *J. Pharmacol. Exp. Ther.,* 152, 388, 1966.
5. **Branch, M. N.,** Rate dependence, behavioral mechanisms, and behavioral pharmacology, *J. Exp. Anal. Behav.,* 42, 511, 1984.
6. **Thompson, T. and Schuster, C. R.,** *Behavioral Pharmacology,* Prentice Hall, Englewood Cliffs, N.J., 1968.
7. **Thompson, T. and Schuster, C. R.,** Morphine self-administration, food-reinforced and avoidance behaviors in rhesus monkeys, *Psychopharmacologia,* 5, 87, 1964.
8. **Fraser, H. F.,** Methods for assessing the addiction liability of opioids and opioid antagonists in man, *The Addictive States,* Winkler, A., Ed., Williams & Wilkins, Baltimore, 1968.
9. **Jasinski, D. R.,** Assessment of the abuse potentiality of morphine-like drugs (methods used in man), in *Handbook of Experimental Pharmacology,* Vol. 45, Martin, W. R. Ed., Springer-Verlag, Berlin, 1977.
10. **Colpaert, F. C.,** Drug discrimination: behavioral, pharmacological, and molecular mechanisms of discriminative drug effects, in *Behavioral Analysis of Drug Dependence,* Goldberg, S. R. and Stolerman, I. P., Eds., Academic Press, New York, 1986.
11. **Kuhn, D. B., Appel, J. B., and Greenberg, I.,** An analysis of some discriminative properties of d-amphetamine, *Psychopharmacologia,* 39, 57, 1974.
12. **Overton, D. A.,** Discriminable effects of antimuscarinics: dose response and substitution test studies, *Pharmacol. Biochem. Behav.,* 6, 656, 1977.
13. **France, C. P. and Woods, J. H.,** Opiate agonist-antagonist interactions: application of a three-key drug discrimination procedure, *J. Pharmacol. Exp. Ther.,* 234, 81, 1985.
14. **Hill, H. E., Jones, B. E., and Bell, E. C.,** State dependent control of discrimination by morphine and pentobarbital, *Psychopharmacologia,* 22, 305, 1971.
15. **Colpaert, F. C.,** Discriminative stimulus properties of narcotic analgesic drugs, *Pharmacol. Biochem. Behav.,* 9, 863, 1978.
16. **Shannon, H. E. and Holtzman, S. G.,** Evaluation of the discriminative effects of morphine in the rat, *J. Pharmacol. Exp. Ther.,* 198, 54, 1976.
17. **Schaefer, G. J. and Holtzman, S. G.,** Discriminative effects of cyclazocine in the squirrel monkey, *J. Pharmacol. Exp. Ther.,* 205, 291, 1976.
18. **Colpaert, F. C., Niemegeers, C. J. E., and Janssen, P A. J.,** Cocaine cue in rats as it relates to subjective drug effects: a preliminary report, *Eur. J. Pharmacol.,* 10, 195, 1976.
19. **Ho, B. T. and Silverman, P. B.,** Stimulants as discriminative stimuli, in *Stimulus Properties of Drugs: Ten Years of Progress,* Colpaert, F. C. and Rosecrans, J. A., Eds., Elsevier/North-Holland, Amsterdam, 1978, 53.
20. **Colpaert, F. C., Niemegeers, C. J. E., and Janssen, P. A. J.,** Discriminative stimulus properties of cocaine and d-amphetamine, and antagonism by haloperidol: a comparative study, *Neuropharmacology,* 17, 937, 1978.
21. **D'Mello, G. D. and Stolerman, I. P.,** Comparison of the discriminative stimulus properties of cocaine and amphetamine in rats, *Br. J. Pharmacol.,* 61, 415, 1977.
22. **Jarbe, T. U. C.,** Cocaine as a discriminative cue in rats: interaction with neuroleptics and other drugs, *Psychopharmacology,* 59, 183, 1978.
23. **Cunningham, K. A. and Appel, J. B.,** Discriminative stimulus properties of cocaine and phencyclidine: similarities in the mechanism of action, in *Drug Discrimination: Applications in CNS Pharmacology,* Colpaert, F. C. and Slangen, J. L., Eds., Elsevier, Amsterdam, 1982.
24. **Balster, R. L. and Ford, R. D.,** The discriminative stimulus properties of cannabinoids: a review, in *Drug Discrimination and State Dependent Learning,* Ho, B. T., Richards, D. W., and Chute, D. L., Eds., Academic Press, New York, 1978.
25. **Weissman, A.,** Generalization of the discriminative stimulus properties of delta-9-tetrahydrocannabinol to cannabinoids with therapeutic potential, in *Stimulus Properties of Drugs: Ten Years of Progress,* Colpaert, F. C. and Rosecrans, J. A., Eds., Elsevier/North-Holland, Amsterdam, 1978.
26. **Hirschhorn, I. D. and Winter, J. C.,** Mescaline and lysergic acid diethylamide (LSD) as discriminative stimuli, *Psychopharmacologia,* 22, 64, 1971.

27. **Apple, J. B., White, F. J., and Holohean, A. M.,** Analyzing mechanisms of hallucinogenic drug action with drug discrimination procedures, *Neurosci. Biobehav. Rev.,* 6, 529, 1982.

28. **Herling, S. and Woods, J. H.,** Mini symposium IV. Discriminative stimulus effects of narcotics: evidence for multiple receptor-mediated actions, *Life Sci.,* 28, 571, 1981.

29. **Wood, D. M., Lal, H., and Emmett-Dylesby, M.,** Acquisition and recovery of tolerance to the discriminative stimulus properties of cocaine, *Neuropharmacology,* 23, 1419, 1984.

30. **Kelleher, R. T. and Goldberg, S. R.,** General introduction: control of drug-taking behavior by schedules of reinforcement, *Pharmacol. Rev.,* 27, 291, 1976.

31. **Johanson, C. E.,** Drugs as reinforcers, in *Contemporary Research in Behavioral Pharmacology,* Blackman, D. E. and Sanger, D. J., Eds., Plenum Press, New York, 1978.

32. **Young, A. M. and Herling, S.,** Drugs as reinforcers: studies in laboratory animals, in *Behavioral Analysis of Drug Dependence,* Goldberg, S. R. and Stolerman, I. P., Eds., Academic Press, New York, 1986.

33. **Spragg, S. D. S.,** Morphine addiction in chimpanzees, *Comp. Psychol. Monogr.,* 15, 79, 1940.

34. **Nichols, J. R., Headlee, C. P., and Coppock, H. W.,** Drug Addiction. I. Addiction by escape training, *J. Am. Pharm. Assoc.,* 45, 788, 1956.

35. **Weeks, J. R.,** Experimental morphine addiction: method for automatic intervenous injections in unrestrained rats, *Science,* 138, 143, 1962.

36. **Schuster, C. R. and Thompson, T.,** Self-Administration of Morphine in Physically-Dependent Monkeys, *Tech. Rep. 62-69. University of Maryland Laboratory of Psychopharmacology,* College Park, Md., 1962.

37. **Pickens, R. and Thompson, T.,** Cocaine-reinforced behavior in rats: effects of reinforcement magnitude and fixed ratio size, *J. Pharmacol. Exp. Ther.,* 161, 122, 1968.

38. **Deneau, G. A., Yanagita, T., and Seevers, M. H.,** Self-administration of psychoactive substances by the monkey, *Psychopharmacologia,* 16, 30, 1969.

39. **Hoffmeister, R. F. and Schlichting, U. U.,** Reinforcing properties of some opiates and opioids in rhesus monkeys with histories of cocaine and cocaine administration, *Psychopharmacologia,* 23, 55, 1972.

40. **Goldberg, S. R.,** Comparable behavior reinforced under fixed-ratio and second order schedules of food presentation, cocaine injection, or d-amphetamine injection, in the squirrel monkey, *J. Pharmacol. Exp. Ther.,* 186, 18, 1973.

41. **Goldberg, J. R. and Kelleher, R. T.,** Behavior controlled by scheduled injections of cocaine in squirrel and rhesus monkeys, *J. Exp. Anal. Behav.,* 25, 93, 1976.

42. **Dougherty, J. and Pickens, R.,** Fixed interval schedule of intravenous cocaine presentation in rats, *J. Exp. Anal. Behav.,* 20, 111, 1973.

43. **Balster, R. L. and Schuster, C. R.,** Fixed-lateral schedules of cocaine reinforcement: effect of dose and infusion duration, *J. Exp. Anal. Behav.,* 20, 119, 1973.

44. **Kelleher, R. T. and Goldberg, S. R.,** Fixed-interval responding under second order schedules of food presentation or cocaine injection, *J. Exp. Anal. Behav.,* 28, 221, 1977.

45. **Bradford, L. D. and Griffiths, R. R.,** Responding reinforced by cocaine of d-amphetamine under fixed-interval schedules in baboons, *Drug Alcohol Depend.,* 5, 393, 1980.

46. **Goldberg, S. R.,** The behavior analysis of drug addiction, in *Behavioral Pharmacology,* Glick, S. D. and Goldfarb, J., Eds., C. V. Mosby, St. Louis, 1976, 282.

47. **Goldberg, S. R., Morse, W. H., and Goldberg, D. M.,** Behavior maintained under a second order schedule by intramuscular injection of morphine or cocaine in rhesus monkeys, *J. Pharmacol. Exp. Ther.,* 199, 278, 1976.

48. **Katz, J. L.,** A comparison of responding reinforced under second order schedules of intramuscular cocaine injection or food presentation in squirrel monkeys, *J. Exp. Anal. Behav.,* 32, 419, 1979.

48b. **Katz, J. L.,** Second order schedule of intramuscular cocaine injection in the squirrel monkey: comparisons with food presentation and effects of d-amphetamine and promezine, *J. Pharmacol. Exp. Ther.,* 212, 405, 1980.

49. **Schuster, C. R. and Johanson, C. E.,** The use of animal models for the study of drug abuse, in *Research Advances in Alcohol and Drug Abuse,* Vol. 1, Gibbins, R. J., Israel, K., Kalant, H., Popham, R. E., Schmidt, W., and Sment, R., Eds., John Wiley & Sons, New York, 1974.

50. **Harris, R. T., Water, W., and McLendon, D.,** Reduction of reinforcing capability of delta-9-tetrahydrocannabinol in rhesus monkeys, *Psychopharmacologia,* 37, 23, 1974.

51. **Pickens, R., Thompson, T., and Muchow, D. C.,** Cannabis and phencyclidine self administration in animals, in *Psychic Dependence,* Goldberg, L. and Hoffmeister, F., Eds., Springer-Verlag, Berlin, 1973, 70.

52. **Wilson, M. C., Hitomi, M., and Schuster, C. R.,** Psychomotor stimulant self administration as a function of dosage per injection in the rhesus monkey, *Psychopharmacologia,* 22, 271, 1971.

53. **Balster, R. L. and Schuster, C. R.,** A comparison of d-amphetamine, 1-amphetamine, and methamphetamine self-administration in rhesus monkeys, *Pharmacol. Biochem. Behav.,* 1, 67, 1973.

54. **Johanson, C. B. and Schuster, C. R.,** A comparison of cocaine and diethylpropion under two different schedules of drug presentation, in *Cocaine and Other Stimulants,* Ellinwood, B. H. and Kilbey, M. M., Eds., Plenum Press, New York, 1977, 545.

55. **Johanson, C. B. and Schuster, C. R.,** A choice procedure for drug reinforcers: cocaine and methylphenidate in the rhesus monkey, *J. Pharmacol. Exp. Ther.,* 193, 676, 1975.

56. **Hoffmeister, F.,** Self administration of codeine plus acetylsalicylic acid in rhesus monkeys with unlimited access to the drugs, *Pharmacol. Biochem. Behav.,* 6, 179, 1977.

57. **Yanagita, T. and Takahashi, S.,** Development of tolerance to and physical dependence on barbiturates in rhesus monkeys, *J. Pharmacol. Exp. Ther.,* 172, 163, 1970.

58. **Balster, R. L. and Woolverton, W. L.,** Continuous-access phencyclidine self-administration by rhesus monkeys leading to physical dependence, *Psychopharmacology,* 70, 5, 1980.

59. **Johanson, C. E., Balster, R. L., and Bonese, K.,** Self-administration of psychomotor stimulant drugs: the effects of unlimited access, *Pharmacol. Biochem. Behav.,* 4, 45, 1976.

60. **Mendelson, J. H. and Mello, N. K.,** Experimental analysis of drinking behavior of chronic alcoholics, *Ann. N.Y. Acad. Sci.,* 133, 828, 1966.

61. **Fischman, M. and Schuster, C. R.,** Cocaine self-administration in humans, *Fed. Proc. Fed. Am. Soc. Exp. Biol.,* 44, 241, 1982.

62. **Pavlov, I. P.,** *Conditioned Reflexes,* Anrep, G., Ed., Oxford University Press, London.

63. **Eikelboom, R. and Stewart, C. R.,** The conditioning of drug-induced physiological responses, *Psychol. Rev.,* 89, 507, 1982.

64. **Wikle, A. and Pescor, F. T.,** Classical conditioning of a morphine abstinence phenomenon, reinforcement of opioid drinking behavior and "relapse" in morphine addicted rats, *Psychopharmacologia,* 10, 255, 1967.

65. **Thompson, T. and Ostlund, N. J.,** Susceptibility to readdiction as a function of the addition and withdrawal environments, *J. Comp. Physiol. Psychol.,* 60, 388, 1968.

66. **Seigel, S.,** Evidence from rats that morphine tolerance is a learned response, *J. Compet. Physiol. Psychol.,* 89, 498, 1975.

67. **Poulos, C. X., Hinson, R. E., and Siegel, S.,** The role of Pavlovian processes in drug tolerance and dependence: Implications for treatment, *Addict. Behav.,* 6, 205, 1981.

68. **Solomon, R. L. and Corbit, J. D.,** An opponent-process theory of motivation, *Psychol. Rev.,* 91, 251, 1974.

69. **Wickler, A.,** Conditioning factors in opiate addiction and relapse, in *Narcotics,* Wiher, D. I. and Kasseboun, G., Eds., McGraw Hill, New York, 1965.

70. **O'Brien, C. P., O'Brien, T. J., Mintz, J., and Brady, J. R.,** Conditioning of narcotic abstinence in human subjects, *Drug Alcohol Depend.,* 1, 115, 1975.

71. **Falk, J. L.,** Drug dependence: myth or motive, *Pharmacol. Biochem. Behav.,* 19, 385, 1983.

72. **Falk, J. L.,** Control of schedule-induced polydipsia, *J. Exp. Anal. Behav.,* 10, 199, 1967.

73. **Falk, J. L.,** The environmental generation of excessive behavior, in *Behavior in Excess: An Examination of Volitional Disorders,* Mule, S. J., Ed., Free Press, New York, 1981, 313.

74. **Falk, J. L. and Samson, H. H.,** Schedule induced physical dependence on ethanol, *Pharmacol. Rev.,* 27, 449, 1975.

75. **Robins, L. N., Helzer, J. E., and Davis, D. H.,** Narcotic use in Southeast Asian and aftermath, *Arch. Gen. Psychiat.,* 32, 955, 1975.

76. **Belleville, R. E.,** Control of behavior by drug-produced internal stimuli, *Psychopharmacologia,* 5, 95, 1964.

77. **Spealman, R. D.,** Behavior maintained by termination of a schedule of self-administration of cocaine, *Science,* 204, 1231, 1979.

Chapter 4

GETTING INVOLVED IN DRUG ABUSE EDUCATION AND PREVENTION

Carol Bohach

TABLE OF CONTENTS

I. INTRODUCTION

Pharmacists have both a moral and a professional responsibility to become active in the fight against drug abuse. In view of the fact that legislation and law enforcement activities have generally failed to contain the drug problem, the involvement of medical specialists in the prevention effort may well be the missing link needed for solving our national drug abuse crisis. As stated so well by Mobile (Ala.) pharmacist James Vann at a 1984 drug abuse conference for physicians, "We aren't going to do it alone. It's going to take everyone in our professions working together."[1]

We, as pharmacists, are in an especially good position for getting involved in substance abuse education and prevention activities. Although many pharmacists are not familiar with the terminology used by street drug users, a basic knowledge of pharmacy provides virtually all the background information necessary to allow you to become an expert on drug abuse topics in a very short period of time.

Deciding how and where to begin, however, may be quite another matter. Sitting at home reading about the drugs of abuse is a nice way to introduce yourself to the problem, as would be attending a continuing education event on the subject. But, if you really want to take an active role in helping to stem the ever-growing problem of drug abuse, you will need to learn more about the complexities of the addictive process. Furthermore, you will also need to decide what you can personally do to become involved in positive, productive, and, most importantly, practical measures for educating others about the drug abuse problem.

This paper is divided into three sections and is designed to

1. Provide pharmacists with basic information about addiction so they may better understand how a person becomes an addict.
2. Acquaint pharmacists with informational resources that will prove useful for acquiring basic and timely information about drug abuse on an ongoing basis.
3. Offer practical suggestions for incorporating drug abuse education and prevention activities into everyday community pharmacy practice.

II. WHAT IS ADDICTION?

Over the past 20 years the use of legal and illegal substances for intoxicating purposes has mushroomed. According to Edward Senay, a University of Chicago psychiatrist, "This increase has been accompanied by an increase in the frequency of intoxicant-related problems such as disruptions of family life, accidents, fires, homicides, suicides, drownings, psychoses, loss of productivity, severe medical problems, and syndromes of dependence".[2]

Although many people are well aware of the problems caused by drug abuse and the fact that few of us have remained untouched by these problems, most individuals haven't an inkling of what really happens to the person who develops an adverse dependency to a drug.

First, consider what is meant by the term "substances of abuse". "All substances of abuse", says pharmacologist Kenneth Blum, "either raise or lower consciousness and enhance or depress mood. The varieties of changes range from a complete obliteration of consciousness, such as large doses of central nervous system (CNS) depressants can bring, to a vast intensification of awareness, such as experienced in the LSD state".[3]

However, while it is fairly easy to talk about the drugs of abuse and objective considerations, such as their pharmacology, legal control, and adverse physical and mental risks to their users, confusion often results when we try to discuss drug abuse and addiction.

Surely, not all drug abusers are addicts. As Blum most aptly points out, "Far fewer persons are actually dependent on drugs than abuse them, especially if a legal definition of abuse, with all of its limitations is adopted".[3]

In fact, the American Medical Association's guide on drug abuse suggests that "drug users" can be divided into two general groups. The first group uses drugs occasionally and control their intake of these agents much the same way others drink alcohol in a "responsible" manner. People in the second category use drugs fairly regularly, but are not physically or psychologically dependent on them. The AMA says that, "In defining drug *use* as opposed to *abuse,* it becomes crucial to consider not only the nature and amount of the drug used, but also the situation in which the drug is used, the personality, experience and expectations of the person using it, and the prevailing attitudes of society".[4]

So, what does the term "addiction" really mean? What actually comprises the disease called addiction?

The following general definition, as offered by David E. Smith, M.D., of the Haight-Ashbury Free Medical Clinic in San Francisco, highlights the major aspects of the disease known as "drug addiction":

"Addictive disease is diagnosed as the abuse of psychoactive drugs, including alcohol, which interferes with health, economic or social functioning, characterized by compulsion, loss of control and continued use despite adverse consequences. Addictive disease is diagnosed as a pathological state with characteristic signs and symptoms and a predictable prognosis if untreated. Addictive disease is a progressive and potentially fatal illness unless properly treated".[5]

For the individual who experiences the compulsion and loss of control and who continues to use an abusable drug despite adverse consequences (i.e., loss of job, break-up of marriage, loss of health, DUI arrests, depletion of personal assets, etc.), the disease of addiction is not only serious, but life threatening. If allowed to progress, drug addiction kills. Fortunately, treatment and rehabilitation are possible and hope does exist for recovery.

Like any other progressive, life-threatening disease, it is always desirable to intervene as early as possible when symptoms become apparent. What then are the signs and symptoms of drug addiction, and how do they fit into a recognizable progression?

III. THE JOHNSON INSTITUTE MODEL (JIM)

In his book, *Drugs, Drinking and Adolescents,*[6] pediatrician Ian MacDonald (formerly the Administrator of ADAMHA, the Alcohol, Drug Abuse and Mental Health Administration) reminds us that, "Drug and alcohol users do not begin with the goal of becoming addicted or alcoholic." They do however, embark on a course, "that for many is a downward trail." MacDonald, as do many other specialists, refers to the Johnson Institute Model (JIM) when describing the progression of drug addiction.

Table 1 is an adaptation of the JIM, a device originally designed to describe the progression of alcoholics through the addictive disease process. The important thing to remember when studying the table is that the time needed to progress through the stages of drug use will vary with each individual. Further, the stages may occur in rapid sequence, as typically seen in cocaine free base addicts who may take only 3 or 4 months to go from Stage 1 to Stage 4. For the alcoholic, however, it ordinarily takes 15 or more years of alcohol abuse to progress through all four stages.

Note also that although a person's problems with drug abuse worsen as the individual progresses through the stages, acute reactions to drug use can occur anytime a drug is used. While overdoses, for example, occur more frequently in Stage 4, a fatal overdose can just as easily occur in Stage 1.

IV. DRUG ABUSE INFORMATION RESOURCES
AND LOCAL KNOWLEDGE

In an earlier paper, this writer reviewed a number of informational resources suitable for

Table 1
HELPING PATIENTS AND FAMILIES IN TROUBLE WITH DRUGS

Stages of drug use	Mood changes	Feelings	Sources	Behavior	Frequency	Intervention/therapy	
						Physician	Pharmacist
Learning to use the drug	Learning the mood swing	User feels good; few adverse consequences to health or mental functioning	Drug is usually obtained from friends and used in social setting	Few detectable changes; moderate lying about drug use	Occasional use; may limit use to weekends	Counseling by family physician; discuss adverse aspects of experimental use; determine why the drug was used; general emphasis on preventive support	Discuss adverse effects of drug(s) being used; offer written information to family/intimate others; preventive support
Seeking the drug for its pleasurable effects	Seeking the mood swing	Use of drug produces excitement early; guilt feelings may be present	User begins to buy the drugs and may limit social activities to other drug users	Pronounced mood swings and changes in daily routine; denial of drug abuse problem	Weekend use progresses to 4—5 times a week; some solo drug use	Counseling by family physician plus referral to outpatient treatment and family therapy if appropriate; periodic urine testing may be helpful	Offer names of support groups/treatment facilities as appropriate; explain dangers of regular drug use/abuse; identify possible interactions w/drug used for therapeutic purposes

EUPHORIA

NORMAL

PAIN

1

EUPHORIA

NORMAL

PAIN

2

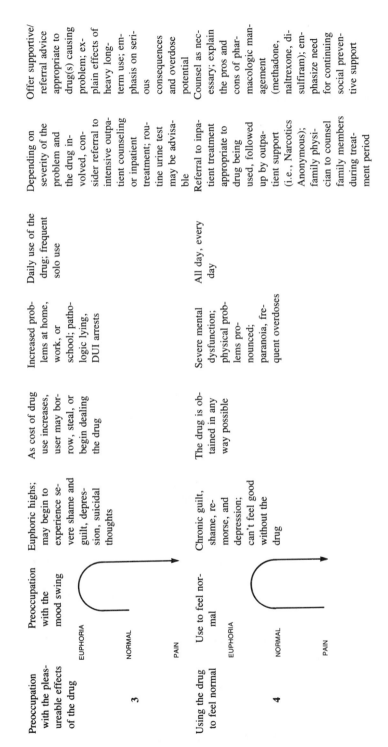

Preoccupation with the pleasureable effects of the drug	Preoccupation with the mood swing EUPHORIA **3** NORMAL PAIN	Euphoric highs; may begin to experience severe shame and guilt, depression, suicidal thoughts	As cost of drug use increases, user may borrow, steal, or begin dealing the drug	Increased problems at home, work, or school; pathologic lying; DUI arrests	Daily use of the drug; frequent solo use	Depending on severity of the problem and the drug involved, consider referral to intensive outpatient counseling or inpatient treatment; routine urine test may be advisable	Offer supportive/referral advice appropriate to drug(s) causing problem; explain effects of heavy long-term use; emphasis on serious consequences and overdose potential
Using the drug to feel normal	Use to feel normal EUPHORIA **4** NORMAL PAIN	Chronic guilt, shame, remorse, and depression; can't feel good without the drug	The drug is obtained in any way possible	Severe mental dysfunction; physical problems pronounced; paranoia, frequent overdoses	All day, every day	Referral to inpatient treatment appropriate to drug being used, followed up by outpatient support (i.e., Narcotics Anonymous); family physician to counsel family members during treatment period	Counsel as necessary; explain the pros and cons of pharmacologic management (methadone, naltrexone, disulfiram); emphasize need for continuing social preventive support

Adpated from MacDonald, D. I., *Drugs, Drinking and Adolescents*, Year Book Medical, Chicago, 1984, 16.

Table 2

SUGGESTIONS FOR A PHARMACIST'S DRUG ABUSE EDUCATION LIBRARY

Reference Texts

The Pharmacological Basis of Therapeutics (Goodman & Gilman) — MacMillan, New York
Psychotropic Drugs: Manual for Emergency Management of Overdoses (Kline & Lindmayer) — Medical Economics, Oradell, N.J.
Drugs, Drinking and Adolescents (MacDonald) — Year Book Medical, Chicago
Handbook of Abusable Drugs (Blum) — Gardner Press, New York

Curriculum Guides

Teaching About Drugs, A Curriculum Guide, K—12 (Pharmaceutical Manufacturers Assoc. & American School Health Assoc.) — Tichenor, Bloomingdale, Ind.
Family Medicine Curriculum Guide to Substance Abuse (Leipman, Anderson, & Fisher) — Society of Teachers of Family Medicine, Kansas City, Mo.

Newsletters

PharmChem Newsletter, Bohannon Drive, Menlo Park, Calif. 94025
Street Pharmacologist, c/o Up Front Drug Information, 5701 Biscayne Blvd., Suite #602 Miami, Fla. 33137
Substance Abuse Report, c/o Pace Publications, 443 Park Avenue South, New York, N.Y. 10016

Brochures

Two excellent brochures for drug abuse education are available from the Pharmaceutical Manufacturers Association:
　Signs and Symptoms of Drug Abuse
　Lists physical signs and behavioral characteristics associated with the abuse of various drugs
　Substance Abuse, Drug and Chemical Chart
　A complete chart of information in commonly used street drugs

For sample copies write: PMA, 1100 15 St. N.W., Washington, D.C. 20005

pharmacists.[7] Since then, a number of other publications have become available. These publications, thought likely to be useful to pharmacists who are interested in becoming active in the education and preventive aspects of the drug abuse problem, are listed in Table 2.

Remember, however, that the use of printed resource materials needs to be teamed with information gleaned from local community resources. In order for an individual pharmacist's efforts to be most effective, it is necessary to know what drugs are causing the greatest problems in the practitioner's community.

Talk to a high school teacher, an emergency room nurse, and a number of drug abuse rehabilitation counselors with regard to the local situation. Find out what they consider to be the most troublesome drug problems locally and then go about learning more about those particular agents and the consequences of their use.

Armed with this type of information and a sound collection of published resources, the pharmacist is then finally prepared to get to work on an active, effective plan to fight the drug abuse problem in his or her own backyard!

V. DOING YOUR PART

As concerned professionals, pharmacists need to play an active professional role in promoting good attitudes toward medicines. We need to discourage the misuse and abuse of drugs of all kinds. As stated in *A Pharmacist's Guide To Drug Abuse,*[8] a pharmacist possesses a special ability for understanding the scientific dimensions of the drug abuse problem and its implications for all segments of the community. This makes it possible for you "to speak out authoritatively, and more important, to be heard. You are, in a word, credible".[8]

One of the first things you can do is provide printed information on the drug abuse problem to the people who come into your pharmacy. Suitable brochures are widely available and many can be obtained for free. Some pharmacies, particularly the stores in retail chains, already have such brochures available. Make it a point to see that the rack for brochures is in plain sight.

Next, come out against the sale of tobacco products in pharmacies and hospitals. The American Pharmaceutical Association can provide you with signs to announce why tobacco products are not sold in your store. Also make sure that your candy department doesn't stock candy cigarettes and shredded chewing gum packaged in pouches like those used for chewing tobacco.

If the pharmacy in which you work carries nonhealth related items, walk through the isles every once and a while to check the shelves and display racks for products with prodrug abuse messages. This author once found a large bin filled with marijuana "power-hitters" in a chain pharmacy located in Miami. A letter to the Florida Board of Pharmacy resulted in an investigation that caused the removal of these offensive items not only from one store, but from the warehouse of that chain and other local stores as well. T-shirts, posters, and other novelties need to be checked for similar drug culture messages.

If public speaking appeals to you, be sure to let neighborhood groups know of your willingness to present lectures on the drug abuse problem. Contact schools, civic and church groups, and parent's groups interested in the drug abuse problem to let them know of your availability.

Finally, be ready to discuss the proper use of medicines with patients and customers. Never forget that drug interaction problems may also occur between prescription products and commonly used or abused drugs. A simple but effective way of dealing with this possibility is to use the statement, "I realize that this may not be a problem for you, but this medicine should not be used along with alcohol, marijuana or other drugs causing drowsiness." Try incorporating such statements into your patient counseling routine. Obviously, offering this type of information to patients who are pregnant or nursing is of very critical importance.

By making recognition of the problem of our society with drug abuse part of your practice of pharmacy, you too can actively promote healthy attitudes towards all the drugs and chemicals in our lives.

REFERENCES

1. **Vann, J. F.,** Prescription drug abuse and misuse, *Am. Pharm.,* NS24 (8), 493, 1984.
2. **Senay, E. C.,** *Substance Abuse Disorders in Clinical Practice,* John Wright-PSG, Littleton, Mass., 1983, vii.
3. **Blum, K.,** *Handbook of Abusable Drugs,* Gardner Press, New York, 1984, 2.
4. **Wilford, B. B.,** *Drug Abuse, A Guide for the Primary Care Physician,* American Medical Association, Chicago, 1981, 4.
5. **Smith, D. E.,** *On file, Up Front Drug Information, Miami, Fla. 1985.*
6. **MacDonald, D. I.,** *Drugs, Drinking and Adolescents,* Year Book Medical, Chicago, 1984, 13.
7. **Bohach, C.,** Resources on substance abuse, *Am. Pharm.,* NS23 (12), 663, 1983.
8. **Pharmacists Against Drug Abuse,** *A Pharmacist's Guide to Drug Abuse,* McNeil Pharmaceutical, Spring House, Pa., 1983, 35.

Chapter 5

PHARMACOLOGY OF COCAINE ABUSE

Roger M. Brown

TABLE OF CONTENTS

I. A BRIEF HISTORY OF COCAINE

At various times in its history, the medical community has both praised cocaine as a cure-all, some sort of miracle drug, as well as cursed it as a scourge to humanity. The history of cocaine certainly bears witness to man's attraction to the drug. The following few paragraphs aim to highlight some of the historical aspects of cocaine, and for further detail the reader is referred to Ray,[1] Denzler,[2] and Van Dyke and Byck.[3]

The earliest documentation of cocaine use goes back at least as far as 500 A.D. A grave in Peru was discovered which contained several bags of cocaine, as well as other things, for the occupant to take into the afterlife. Apparently the individual enjoyed coca so much that he wanted it with him forever, or perhaps he was afraid to be eternally without it! During the 16th century, the Spanish entrepreneurs in South America noted the power of the influence of coca and they used the leaves to recruit Indians for labor. The conquistadors brought reports to Europe of the invigorating properties of coca and how it improved the stamina of the Peruvians working at high altitudes. The Europeans, however, weren't much impressed with coca leaves; this was probably due to an inactivation of the alkaloid during the long boat trip from South America. It wasn't until about 1750 that the plant itself reached the continent.

By the mid 1800s, cocaine was being recommended among other things for toothache, digestive disorders, and even as a "balm for young people suffering from timidity." In 1846 Johan Jakob von Tschudi wrote, "I am clearly of the opinion that moderate use of coca is not merely innocuous, but that it may even be conducive to health," and in 1859 Paolo Mantegazzi, a neurologist famed at the time, wrote, "I prefer a life of ten years with coca to one hundred thousand without it." The widespread use of coca was facilitated in 1863 by Angelo Mariana's concoction, Vin Mariani, a mixture of Bordeaux wine, a small amount of alkali, and fragments of coca leaf sufficient to yield 30 grains per wine glass. Mariana's wine was advertised as a tonic to "aid digestion, strengthen the system, and prevent malaria, influenza, and wasting disease." The tonic received testimonials from popes, kings, and czars; even Thomas Edison appeared among the notables who enthusiastically supported the mixture. Thus, cocaine was available not only to professional and so-called "intellectual" circles, but also to the general public through various nostrums. Another way cocaine became generally available was through the drug store soda fountain. John Styth Pemberton, a pharmacist, formulated a product in 1885 which he called "French Wine of Coca, Ideal Tonic". This mixture was so popular that he sought to improve on it. He combined coca with kola nut, aromatized it, added syrup, and therewith gave birth to Coca-Cola®, "the brain tonic and intellectual soda fountain beverage." The soda fountain at Jacobs Pharmacy in Atlanta where Coca-Cola® was introduced rapidly became one of the most popular places in the city.

Cocaine also received more serious medical considerations. In 1880 an article appeared in the *Therapeutic Gazette* by W. H. Bently in which the rationale was set forth for its use in the treatment of opiate and alcohol addiction. Cocaine was seen as a means of providing the customary "stimulus" to the opiate or alcohol addict without leaving a feeling of depression. In this way, the victim of drugs could walk away from his vice with little effort. Numerous articles appeared about this time testifying to the treatment of opiate addiction with cocaine. Among them was a statement in the *Louisville Medical News:* "One feels like trying coca with or without the opium habit. A harmless remedy for the blues is imperial. And so say we." Among the many proponents of the use of cocaine in the treatment of addiction was Sigmund Freud, whose experience with cocaine treatment is well-known. Freud was initially so enthused with cocaine that he spoke of administering an "offering" rather than a dose, and he described all attacks on cocaine as "slander". His enthusiasm greatly diminished, however, after he nursed a close friend through a bout of cocaine psychosis. After that he was very much disenchanted with the drug.

Cocaine was found to have beneficial properties and Karl Koller is given the credit for recommending cocaine as a local anesthetic in 1884. The drug was known to produce numbness, but it took Koller to suggest its use in surgery. Soon it was being recommended for surgery of eye, ear, nose, and throat, not to mention its use as a nerve block for hernia operations and amputations.

By the late 1800s the enthusiam for cocaine diminished as negative experiences with the drug started to make an impact. There were reports of "substituting one addiction for another," cocaine psychosis, and other consequences such as "cocaine bugs". Even as early as 1836, Edvard Poppig said that the cocaine user is, "a slave of his passion even more so than the drunk." As a result of excessive use and negative outcome, legislation was initiated to control cocaine. First, the Pure Food and Drug Act of 1906 attempted to limit the import of cocaine to medical purposes only. Later, legislators involved in formulating the Harrison Narcotic Act of 1914 were so enthusiastic that they labeled cocaine as a narcotic. Even today confusion still exists over the legal vs. pharmacological definition of a narcotic! Finally, the Controlled Substances Act of 1970 was the first act in which illegal possession of cocaine was made a Federal crime. Hence, the history of cocaine is very much like that of many psychoactive drugs, LSD and opiates, for example. First there were fantastic claims for its pharmacological properties, followed by widespread use in professional and nonprofessional circles, and finally all the promise of a new and beneficial drug has been replaced by abuse and legislation.

II. PHARMACOLOGY OF COCAINE

A. Major Actions

Cocaine has two major pharmacological actions. It is (1) a local anesthetic and (2) an indirect acting sympathomimetic which potently enhances the effect of neural transmission.

1. Cocaine is a Local Anesthetic

Cocaine prevents conduction of sensory impulses by reacting with the neuron membrane to block ion channels. As a result of this block, the ion exchange which is normally responsible for the electrical signals cannot be propagated along the axon and so sensory messages are not received in the central nervous system. This is the basis for the early application of cocaine in eye surgery. Problems with abuse, however, led to a search for other local anesthetics and, as a result, novocaine (Procaine®) was synthesized in 1905 followed by xylocaine (Lidocaine®) about 1906. The local anesthetic action is important in and of itself. In addition, the role of a local anesthetic action in the subjective psychotropic response to cocaine is presently being debated with respect to its contribution to the abuse liability of cocaine.[4,5]

2. Cocaine is a Sympathomimetic

The second major action of cocaine is its ability to potentiate neurotransmission in neurons that use one of the monoamines, norepinephrine (NE), dopamine (DA), or serotonin (5-HT), as a neurotransmitter. In the periphery this occurs mainly at the noradrenergic terminals of the sympathetic component of the autonomic nervous system, and in the brain at monoaminergic terminals (i.e., those that utilize NE, DA, or 5-HT), for which there are many fiber networks. Neurons normally transmit or modulate electrical signals across the synaptic gap by releasing a chemical which induces a change in ion permeability in the receiving tissue (a neuron in the brain, the innervated tissue in the periphery); this allows further conduction to take place. Normally monoamine neurons terminate the transmission process and then recycle their transmitter by actively taking the chemical back up into the terminal from which it was released. When this process is blocked, the effect of nervous system activity is greatly enhanced. In the peripheral nervous system, one of the effects of sympathetic nervous system activation is vasoconstriction. This is why cocaine was originally recommended so highly for eye surgery — this is a drug with local anesthetic properties in addition to a vasoconstrictor action which limits hemorrhage. (Cocaine is no longer an agent of choice for this purpose because of ischemic injury to the eye, but it is still used in the surgery of ear, nose, and throat.)

The effects of cocaine on the nervous system are dose-dependent. At low doses it increases arousal and motor activity. At moderate doses, heart rate increases. Hypertension results from the increased peripheral resistance (due to vasoconstriction) plus the increase in heart rate. Body temperature is increased and dilation of the pupils may occur as well. At high doses, cocaine can induce convulsions. Cardiac arrest is not uncommon due to a direct action of the drug on the heart muscle.

B. Illicit Use of Cocaine

1. Pharmacokinetics

The main objective of abusing cocaine is to get "high" or "euphoric". The intensity and duration of the high are dependent on dose and route of administration. The duration of the high is greatest when cocaine is taken by a route which gives slow absorption; on the other hand, the intensity of the effect is low. In contrast, when cocaine is taken by routes which give rapid absorption, the resulting high is intense, but its duration is brief.[4,6,7]

2. Routes of Administration

Various routes of administration have been tried by the cocaine user, and each produces its own characteristic absorption pattern and associated problems.

Topical — This route is mentioned only for the sake of completeness. It is the only licit route of administration and is used for local application of anesthetic. There is insufficient absorption from the cutaneous route to cause a psychotropic response.

Oral (chewing leaves) — The natives of South America chew coca leaves by mixing them with alkali (ashes) and then chewing the mixture into a quid which is then placed between the cheek and gum. There is no or little high produced by chewing, probably due to the relatively slow absorption and the low concentration of cocaine in the blood which is only half that obtained by snorting. Cocaine can also be absorbed by the gastrointestinal tract, but the absorption is too slow to produce any profound subjective effect.[7]

Nasal inhalation (snorting) — Cocaine is readily absorbed from the nasal mucosa. By snorting, the powder is forced high into the mucosa where it is rapidly absorbed. If the abuser can minimize the amount of drug which makes contact with the septum, it is less likely that ischemic nasal damage will occur. Nevertheless, there is still a great likelihood that inhalation will result in the hallmark of a snorter — a perpetual runny nose! How the effect of snorting was discovered can only be guessed. The high induced by inhaled cocaine may have been first noticed by an allergy sufferer since cocaine was once used as a decongestant and for a time was the official remedy of the Hay Fever Association.[3]

Intravenous administration — When cocaine is taken parenterally, the rapid onset produces an intense high which is similar to that following inhalation (see freebasing, below). This is not a popular method of administration, however, because of problems associated with needles such as hepatitis and AIDS. Hence, snorting the hydrochloride salt or smoking the alkaloid as the freebase are more common methods of self-administration.

Smoking (freebasing) — This is done by placing the pure alkaloidal cocaine in a pipe, smoking a mixture of the alkaloid and parsley, tobacco, or marijuana, or by mixing a paste into cigarettes.

Cocaine is an alkaloid, i.e., a nitrogenous plant base, and it exists in this form in coca leaves. Because cocaine alkaloid is not stable, practically all isolated cocaine is converted to the form of the stable hydrochloride salt.

The high from cocaine base is said to be more intense. This probably depends more on the route of administration than the form of cocaine per se. Alkaloidal cocaine, but not the salt, is volatile and so can be smoked. It is, no doubt, the extremely rapid absorption from the lung which is responsible for the enhanced subjective effects from smoking.

Because of the intense high and the ease of self-administration, methods have been devised to free the cocaine from its hydrochloride salt. This is usually done by neutralizing the salt with aqueous bicarbonate, followed by an extraction of the alkaloid in ether which is then evaporated to yield a very pure cocaine alkaloid. As witnessed by several recent tragic outcomes from careless freebasing, this is a very hazardous procedure due to the explosiveness of the ether.

"Crack" or "Rock" is a form of free base cocaine processed from the salt using baking soda (sodium bicarbonate). The product still contains filler and other impurities found in the original material along with some excess bicarbonate from the processing. It's the bicarbonate in the resulting chunks of cocaine which causes the crackling sound when the mixture is heated — hence, the street name.

Coca Paste is a form of free base cocaine. It is more common in South America where coca leaves are readily available and has not been found in any appreciable extent in the U.S. The paste is a partially purified extract of the leaf and it contains anywhere from 20 to 90% cocaine sulfate. A precipitate leaf material is extracted in kerosene and the mixture is filtered and dried to produce a preparation which is essentially an impure form of free base. The paste may contain trapped kerosene and/or other solvents used in the processing, the smoking of which might have pathological effects on the lung and liver in addition to the potential toxicity of cocaine itself.

3. Effects of Cocaine

The *"high"* is the action of interest to the cocaine abuser. This is an intense rush of feelings of energy, power, and competency. It soon subsides and is replaced by a phase of *restless irritability*. Sleep is not possible during a binge of freebasing, but exhaustion can overcome the resulting restlessness. During the phase of direct cocaine action, there is autonomic and central activation such as *tachycardia*. *Cardiac Arrhythmia* is not uncommon at high doses or even at low doses in the inexperienced user.

On prolonged use of cocaine, there is considerable *weight loss* due to an anorectic action. *"Cocaine bugs"* might develop in which the user feels like there are insects crawling under the skin (medically, called formication). The sensation may be so great that the user will use a knife in an attempt to cut them out. Unless restrained, laboratory monkeys on cocaine often exhibit skin ulcerations from picking, scratching, and biting the "bugs". The basis of this is unknown. It could be related to a stimulation of nerve endings in the skin, to an action of cocaine on the enriched noradrenergic innervation of the primate somatosensory cortex,[8] or to drug-induced degeneration of pyramidal cells in sensory motor cortex.[9]

Long-term use may also result in *cocaine psychosis*. This is usually in the form of paranoia, although hallucinations can occur and these can be misperceptions in any sensory modality, but touch is most frequently affected. Manic behavior is expressed as hyperactivity and distractibility. Violence has resulted from the hyperactivity when accompanied by paranoia. Delirium which may also develop, includes disorientation and confusion.

Liver damage has been found in cocaine addicts, but it is unclear whether this is directly due to cocaine or whether it is a result of viral hepatitis. In experimental animals, there is evidence to suggest that under proper conditions, cocaine is metabolized to hepatotoxic intermediates. Following chronic barbiturate use, which induces cytochrome P450, or under conditions of genetic or drug-induced low-cholinerestase activity, cocaine is N-demethylated to norcocaine. A hepatotoxin is then formed from norcocaine either through N-hydroxylation to N-hydroxynorcocaine or through oxidation to norcocaine nitroxide.[10] *Pulmonary damage* may result as well. The most likely cause of lung pathology is through cocaine-induced ischemic injury. In addition, damage due to inhalation of kerosene and other solvents and impurities from freebasing procedures might contribute to the direct cocaine-induced insult, if not directly exerting damage.

The extent of *birth defects* that may result from cocaine use is of appropriate concern because a mother taking cocaine during pregnancy could harm her baby in two ways. First, cocaine passes the placental barrier to exert a direct action on the fetus. Second, the drug may act indirectly by causing maternal vasoconstriction thereby compromising the amount of oxygen reaching the fetus. To date there is little information about the perinatal effects of cocaine, either from clinical experience with human births or from animal studies. According to a recent report, however, cocaine use can cause a high incidence of *miscarriage* (38%) and *behavioral deficits* in those infants normally delivered. Infants born to mothers who admitted using cocaine showed a reduced ability to interact with environmental stimuli.[11]

C. Is Cocaine Addicting?

There is a general misconception that cocaine is a safe recreational drug. This idea might be due, at least in part, to statements in literature that cocaine is not addicting. The term "drug addiction" (or "drug dependency") generally refers to a drug response which involves *tolerance* and *physical dependence*. Tolerance refers to the process whereby higher and higher doses are needed to produce the initial drug effect. In drug dependency, which develops along with tolerance, repeated dosing occurs to prevent the physiological withdrawal syndrome. These processes, i.e., the need to take larger doses, the development of physical dependence, and repeated self-administration, match the events seen with opiates, barbiturates, and alcohol. However, abrupt discontinuation of the use of cocaine does not cause the degree of physiological disruption that necessitates a gradual withdrawal. Therefore, there is a general reluctance to accept cocaine as a physiologically addicting drug.

1. Criteria for Physical Addiction and Cocaine

Cocaine does have certain elements which fit the criteria for physical dependence, as discussed below.

a. Tolerance

In general, cocaine users can take the same dose every day and get the same effects. However, there does appear to be an *acute tolerance* to the action of cocaine. Fischman[4] reported a tachyphylaxis to the cardiovascular and subjective effects of intravenous cocaine. When subjects were allowed to self-administer cocaine every 6 to 10 min. for 1 hr, the initial effects were noted higher than the effects toward the end of the hour. Similar results were observed when a "snorted" dose was taken 1 hr after an intravenous dose, i.e., the "high" was less from the inhaled cocaine when it was preceeded by an intravenous dose.

b. Withdrawal

Posthigh down ("anguish") — The restless irritability referred to above is so aversive that it has been termed *"anguish"*; to prevent it, the user may repeatedly administer cocaine — at least until the supplies are gone. Another way the intravenous user attempts to suppress "anguish" is to administer *"speedballs"*, a combination of heroin and cocaine, to take the edge off the "down". It's interesting to note that in the late 1800s cocaine was being recommended for the relief of opiate addiction. Contemporary drugs users have now reversed the situation: opiate is being used to alleviate the cocaine habit.

Use pattern and drug seeking — Drug-seeking liability is greater with intravenous self-administration or smoking than after snorting. Snorting may result in continued use as long as supplies are available, but there is total abstinence when supplies are gone. On the other hand, intravenous use or smoking leads to continual consumption and, when the supply is gone, drug-seeking behavior is initiated.

Other symptoms — Cocaine use induces alterations in normal neurophysiology and these can be seen as changes in EEG patterns and disrupted sleep cycles when cocaine use is terminated.

Overall, the above symptoms indicate that normal neurophysiology is indeed disrupted as a result of cocaine use. However, the symptoms are considered to be "minor" compared to the so-called "true" addiction syndrome. On the other hand, the question of "drug addiction" may not be appropriate. Physical dependence has nothing to do with the initiation of drug seeking in the first place. It's the rewarding impact of drugs, not their dependence liability, which poses the danger!

III. THE BRAIN REWARD SYSTEM AND THE ACTION OF COCAINE

A. The Brain Reward Model for Drug-Seeking Behavior

One of the most exciting areas of neuroscience research relevant to drug-seeking behavior is the neuropsychopharmacology of reward. In the 1950s, Olds and Milner[12,13] discovered that animals would press a lever to obtain electrical stimulation via an electrode implanted in certain regions of their brain, but not in others. This finding gave rise to the concept that there are systems or networks of neurons in the brain which are responsible for pleasure, and these pathways became known, as "pleasure" or "reward" centers. Presumably, this system is activated physiologically when an event, activity, or stimulus (such as eating, praise, sex, music, etc.) is perceived as pleasurable. In the experiments of Olds, rats would press a lever for stimulation rather than seek food or water and, unless they were "unplugged", the animals would die. The presumed reason why the animals would "self-stimulate to death" is that direct activation of the "reward system" is so powerful that natural rewards (eating and drinking, in this case) seem less rewarding in contrast.

Since the time of Olds' report in 1954, neuroscientists have been trying to identify the neuroanatomical and neurochemical basis of these reward circuits. As a result of such investigations, it has been discovered that animals will work not only for electrical stimulation of certain areas of their brain, but also for direct intracerebral drug injections. From the finding that the reward circuitry can be directly activated by drugs has developed a *model for drug-seeking behavior:* drugs of abuse are those that activate the synapses of the reward system of the brain and thereby produce an intense sensation of "euphoria" or "pleasure". That is, whether taken systemically (as on the street) or directly administered (experimentally), they produce a "high" which is the result of intense activation of the reward circuits which are normally activated by natural pleasurable stimuli.

B. Heroin and Cocaine Act on the Same Substrate in the Brain

The chemical neuroanatomy of the reward system is gradually being elucidated. An important discovery from this research is that a dopaminergic region known as the ventral tegmental area (VTA) is an integral part of the system(s) involved in the brain reward phenomenon. This system has its cell bodies, which contains opiate receptors, in the midbrain, and its projections innervate the cortex, nucleus accumbens, and other areas of the limbic system. This is consistent with evidence for the involvement of a dopaminergic system in drug-induced reward: (1) mapping studies have shown overlap between neurons of the dopaminergic VTA and those that support ICSS behavior, (2) drugs that inhibit catecholamine biosynthesis have been shown to prevent alcohol-induced euphoria,[14] as well as stimulation due to amphetamine,[15] and (3) dopamine receptor-blocking drugs (i.e., neuroleptics) attenuate the intracranial or systemic self-administration of a variety of drug classes including cocaine, amphetamine, opiates (morphine and heroin, among others), barbiturates, and alcohol.[16] A common basis of action among drugs of abuse is further substantiated by the finding that, with few exceptions, drugs of abuse lower the threshold for intracranial self-stimulation.[17] These findings are important because they implicate the VTA and its projections as a locus which determines the abuse liability of a drug. At what point along this particular pathway various drugs act, whether there is one or several pathways, and the degree of overlap between physiological and drug reinforcers are points in contemporary neuropsychopharmacological research.[18-29]

C. Dissociation of Brain Reward and Physical Addiction

Heroin and other opiates have generally been considered to be more dangerous than cocaine because opiates produce physical dependence. This assumption is a bad one, however. Both heroin and cocaine act on the reward circuitry of the VTA, and according to the model, different classes of drugs are sought because they activate this system. The ability of a drug to induce physical dependence has nothing to do with its desirability. Cocaine is sought and is dangerous because it is rewarding, not because it lacks physical-dependence liability. Heroin, as well as other opiates, are dangerous because they are rewarding and, in addition, they have the ability to produce physical dependence. Once a user gets "hooked" on narcotics, he may have to continuously use a drug in order to avoid the distress of withdrawal, but the alleviation of abstinence symptoms is not the reason the drug is taken in the first place.

To take this a step further, the brain site responsible for reward has been dissociated from the brain site responsible for opiate physical dependence. As with cocaine, animals will self-administer opiates into the VTA; they will not self-administer into the periaqueductal gray (PAG), which is an important anatomical locus in the production of analgesia and which, like the VTA, is populated with opiate receptors. This demonstrates that it is the VTA which is responsible for mediating opiate drug-seeking behavior. On the other hand, when opiates are continuously infused into the PAG over a 24- to 48-hr period, an abstinence syndrome is observed when naloxone is administered. In contrast, infusions of opiate into the VTA does not result in a precipitated abstinence syndrome following administration of narcotic antagonist.[30] Thus, the PAG is responsible for physical dependence while the VTA mediates drug self-administration.

D. Reinforcing Efficacy of Cocaine

How desirable is cocaine? All indications are that its reinforcing magnitude (or rewarding efficacy) is very powerful.[31] First, cocaine maintains responding regardless of its route of administration — intravenous, intragastric, smoking, intramuscular, intracerebral, etc. Second, it is inherently reinforcing as shown by the fact that no priming is needed to get animals to self-administer cocaine. In fact, cocaine is often used as the training drug in abuse liability studies to shape drug-taking behavior. Animals won't self-administer morphine, but they will if first trained on cocaine and then switched to morphine. Cocaine is not altogether unique in this respect, however. Heroin, too, is inherently reinforcing and requires no manipulations to set the occasion for drug self-administration to occur. Thus, cocaine is at least as powerful as heroin as a reinforcer!

Third, breaking-point studies, using a progressive ratio schedule, can demonstrate how much work output can be obtained for a small amount of cocaine. Amphetamines and cocaine produce similar patterns of self-administration behavior, but when breaking point tests are conducted, cocaine is by far the stronger reinforcer. Rats will press a lever over 12,000 times for a single cocaine dose of 0.5 mg/kg.[32] Among drugs tested, the breaking point of cocaine exceeds that of methylphenidate, fenfluramine, amphetamine, methamphetamine, nicotine, and local anesthetics. No direct comparison has yet been made between the breaking point for narcotics and cocaine, since it is difficult to make such a direct comparison. For example, there is no way to determine how much of the rewarding impact of opiates is partitioned between "reward" and alleviation of withdrawal symptoms.

Finally, the rewarding efficacy of cocaine is dramatically illustrated with the finding that, unlike heroin, cocaine is self-administered to death. When given unlimited access, animals were found to self-administer cocaine erratically over a 2-week period with a consequent loss of grooming behavior, loss of body weight, and finally death. In contrast, heroin intake was evenly distributed over time, animals showed normal grooming activity, and there was no weight loss. Furthermore, minimal mortality occurred from heroin self-administration. Cocaine is not unique in this respect, however. Alcohol and amphetamine are also self-administered to the point of toxicity. It might be said that given an abundant amount of drug, cocaine is "craved" in a manner similar to alcohol.[36]

Thus, the answer to the question of whether cocaine is a mere recreational drug is an emphatic no! Cocaine is as dangerous as are the hard drugs and, in some respects, even more so. Cocaine is inherently reinforcing, whereas most narcotics are not, an exception being heroin. Cocaine is self-administered to the point of toxicity, whereas opiates are not. Thus, even though cocaine has minimal physical-dependence liability, it is as dangerous to an individual's well-being as are the hard drugs. This is because of the rewarding impact of the drug. In spite of the fact that cocaine can be placed alongside heroin as a highly dangerous drug, cocaine is not truly "addicting", at least according to the classic definition of addiction. But, because of inadequacies in the definition of "addiction", Cohen[6] has pointed out the need to define addiction in behavioral terms and has suggested "the loss of control over the intake of a drug that leads to its compulsive use despite harmful effects in some area of the person's functioning." Cocaine certainly falls into this category!

IV. IMPLICATIONS AND SUMMARY

Neuroscientists who have been examining the biological basis of drug abuse have made important advances in the past few years in understanding the neuropsychological basis of drug seeking. Because of this diligent work, there is a new appreciation for the "why" of drug abuse and with it are important implications for the design of new drugs, or at least the preparation of dosage forms, to attenuate the abuse potential of a drug. For example, the existence of multiple drug/transmitter receptors, with their inherent neuropharmacological properties, opens up the possibility of manufacturing drugs with highly selective actions which by-pass VTA agonism. Another possibility is the development of specific VTA antagonists which would limit the dopaminergic action of the VTA without influencing other receptor functions. Such "antieuphoriants" might be added to the dosage form of those drugs possessing significant abuse potential.

Understanding the basis for drug seeking also has implications in drug abuse treatment. There are at least three consequences of cocaine use which must be "neutralized" in any pharmacological approach to treatment.

A. Acute Toxicity
Medical attention is usually sought in the first place because the user is experiencing acute toxic symptoms such as convulsions, tremor, arrhythmia, sweating, chest pain and palpitations, and dizziness. *Diazepam* is the drug of choice in treating convulsions, while *propanolol* is called for in treating arrhythmia. Sympatholytics can be used to treat the other general autonomic effects, and *chlorpromazine* is quite effective for this purpose.

B. "Withdrawal" and Other Autonomic Symptoms
Following chronic use, a user may develop certain "abstinence" symptoms. It is important

to realize that cocaine acts neurochemically, and as a result, neural adaptations occur to compensate for the presence of the drug. Pharmacological treatment is therefore probably essential to counteract neurochemical imbalances resulting from cocaine use. While the precise mechanism underlying these symptoms are not all understood, a variety of rationales for drug treatment have been developed around long-term consequences with some methods being more successful than others.[37]

Tricyclic antidepressants — Desmethylimipramine (DMI), has been used successfully in treating the cocaine user. Animal studies of receptor changes in the brain following chronic cocaine administration have shown increased noradrenergic, as well as dopaminergic, receptor sites. Thus, drug-induced receptor supersensitivity could be the basis for post-cocaine dysphoria or craving. The course of DMI treatment parallels that of the neurochemical readjustment that is seen in the treatment of depression. It should be emphasized that treatment with DMI, or any tricyclic antidepressant for that matter, should be done while the patient is stimulant free. DMI, like cocaine, blocks the reuptake of neurotransmitters and for this reason if cocaine were taken concomitantly there would be a potentiation of its action.

Lithium — Lithium has been advocated for stimulant abuse because it dampens the large swings in the dynamics of neural synaptic activity which is believed to occur in manic/depressive states. Those individuals which show a mania in response to cocaine are usually targeted for lithium treatment, although some patients with "the blues" also profit from this agent.

Bromocriptine — This direct-acting dopamine agonist is claimed to be beneficial in treating cocaine craving.[38] In spite of any evidence whatsoever that cocaine causes a dopamine depletion, the rationale for the use of bromocriptine is a purported reinstatement of dopamine receptor integrity following dopamine loss. In view of the dopamine theory of reward, treating cocaine use with a dopamine agonist is irrational, particularly since animals will self-administer dopamine agonists including bromocriptine.[39]

Tyrosine — Tyrosine, too, is being recommended as a treatment for a presumed cocaine-induced dopamine depletion.[40] Even if dopamine were depleted, excessive tyrosine would be shunted off into routes other than dopamine synthesis. It is well-known that the enzyme which places tyrosine in the dopamine synthetic pathway (i.e., tyrosine hydroxylase) is fully saturated so that tyrosine administration does not result in an enhanced catecholamine synthesis rate.

Tryptophan — Since serotoninergic activity counteracts nonadrenergic influences,[41,42] treatment of tryptophan, the amino acid precursor of serotonin, might be preferable to tyrosine. Because tryptophan hydroxylase is not fully saturated, this amino acid is readily converted to serotonin following dietary ingestion. Hence, tryptophan treatment would seem to be a good approach in the treatment of stimulant abuse, particularly if there is any chance that the patient is still taking such drugs.

C. Rewarding Impact of the Drug

Another aspect of drug abuse which must be attended to is the rewarding efficacy of the drug. According to the model just presented, this is the basic feature which perpetuates drug use. There are at least two methods which might be attempted to attenuate drug-induced reward:

1. Dopamine-blocking drugs (neuroleptics) reduce drug self-administration in animal studies, and should be effective in the clinical situation as well. Since the dopaminergic VTA plays such an important role in drug-seeking behavior, it would be anticipated that dopamine-blocking drugs would be an effective treatment. However, there have been reports of difficulty with neuroleptic treatment which seem to focus around compliance problems. It isn't clear whether patients refuse to take medication due to

physical side effects or a blunted reward process. The appropriate antagonist might be one which has a selective action on the VTA system. The purported success of bromocriptine in alleviating cocaine craving might be its dopamine antagonist activity. Through autoreceptor mechanisms, an antagonist can exert feedback control and modulate transmitter release.[43]

2.   There is some evidence that the cocaine "high" is due to the degree of change in cocaine brain levels. For example, cocaine blues begin at a time when the plasma cocaine concentration, and presumably brain cocaine concentration, is identical to that during the high. From this finding, the idea developed that the degree of "high" depends on the amount of change in drug concentration at receptor sites rather than from a critical drug concentration. Further, it has been suggested that increases in plasma cocaine concentration in subjects with preexistent stimulant concentration may produce less euphoria than the same increase in a stimulant-free individual. This is why methylphenidate is used in treating cocaine craving. This treatment approach is essentially based on the concept of acute tolerance. It should also be worth noting that it has been estimated that about 10% of cocaine abusers have attention deficit disorder (ADD), and these individuals self-medicate with cocaine. If these individuals are given methylphenidate, the usual treatment of ADD, there will be an apparent success in treating their cocaine habit.

Hence, there are at least three aspects of cocaine which need to be neutralized: the acute toxicity, the "withdrawal", and the rewarding impact. Probably many other consequences and actions will become known in the future. Even though it has been almost 100 years since cocaine was first used in medicine, and it might be assumed that scientific knowledge concerning cocaine is relatively complete, this is not the case. There is still alot of information lacking concerning the actions and consequences of cocaine abuse. Much of what is known about cocaine, its local anesthetic properties, central nervous system-stimulating actions, and general subjective and cardiovascular effects when ingested by a variety of routes, was described 50 to 100 years ago. Most of the newer information regarding the clinical pharmacology of cocaine has been recently collected from reports since 1975, when the National Institute on Drug Abuse funded a series of research grants and contracts to study the pharmacology of cocaine in humans. Those studies and ones evolving from them provide detailed descriptions of the relationship between dose, route of administration, blood levels, and limited physiological or psychological effects.[7,44-49] As for basic mechanisms, much more information is needed. For example, the major mechanism of action of cocaine, monoamine reuptake block, can't account for the abuse liability of cocaine since other reuptake blockers (such as amphetamine, DMI, etc.) aren't abused to the extent that cocaine is. Situational effects must also be taken into account in treating cocaine abuse. Virtually nothing is known regarding the role and mechanisms of so-called situational factors or "setting conditions" in determining the impact of the subjective effects of the drug, and these can be powerful influences.[50,51] Clearly, basic research must continue to uncover the secrets of the psychotropic action of cocaine.

REFERENCES

1. **Ray, O.,** *Drugs, Society, and Human Behavior,* 3rd ed., C. V. Mosby, St. Louis, 1983.
2. **Denzler, J. W.,** Cocaine: origins as a medicinal agent and abused drug, *Minn. Pharm.,* October, 22, 1985.
3. **Van Dyke, C. and Byck, R.,** Cocaine use in man, *Adv. Subst. Abuse,* 3, 1, 1983.

4. **Fischman, M. W.,** The behavioral pharmacology of cocaine in humans, in Cocaine: Pharmacology, Effects, and Treatment of Abuse, Grabowski, J., Ed., NIDA Res. Monogr. No. 50, DHHS Publ. No. (ADM) 84-1326, Department of Health and Human Services, Washington, D.C., 1984, 72.

5. **Johanson, C. E. and Aigner, T.,** Comparison of the reinforcing properties of cocaine and procaine in rhesus monkeys, *Pharmacol. Biochem. Behav.,* 15, 49, 1981.

6. **Cohen, S.,** Cocaine: The Bottom Line, American Council for Drug Education, Rockville, Md., 1985.

7. **Resnick, R. B., Kestenbaum, R. S., and Schwartz, L. K.,** Acute systemic effects of cocaine in man: a controlled study by intranasal and intravenous routes, *Science,* 195, 696, 1977.

8. **Brown, R. M., Craine, A. M., and Goldman, P. S.,** Regional distribution of monoamines in the cerebral cortex and subcortical structures of the rhesus monkey: concentrations and in vivo synthesis rates, *Brain Res.,* 168, 133, 1979.

9. **Seiden, L. S.,** Methamphetamine: toxicity to dopaminergic neurons, in Neuroscience Methods in Drug Abuse Research, Brown, R. M., Friedman, D. P., and Nimit, Y. N., Eds., NIDA Monogr. No. 62, DHHS Publ. No. (ADM) 85-1415, Department of Health and Human Services, Washington, D.C., 1985, 100.

10. **Thompson, M. L., Shuster, L., and Shaw, K.,** Cocaine-induced hepatic necrosis in mice: the role of cocaine metabolism, *Biochem. Pharmacol.,* 28, 2389, 1979.

11. **Chasnoff, I. J., Burns, W. J., Schnell, S. H., and Burns, K. A.,** Cocaine use in pregnancy, *N. Engl. J. Med.,* 313, 15, 1985.

12. **Olds, J. and Milner, P.,** Positive reinforcement produced by electrical stimulation of the septal area and other regions of the rat brain, *J. Comp. Physiol. Psychol.,* 47, 419, 1954.

13. **Olds, J.,** Self-stimulation of the brain, *Science,* 127, 315, 1958.

14. **Ahlenius, S., Carlsson, A., Engel, J., Svensson, T. H., and Sodersten, P.,** Antagonism by alpha-methyltyrosine of the ethanol-induced stimulation and euphoria in man, *Clin. Pharmacol. Ther.,* 14, 586, 1973.

15. **Jonsson, L., Anggard, E., and Gunne, L.,** Blockade of intravenous amphetamine euphoria in man, *Clin. Pharmacol. Ther.,* 12, 889, 1971.

16. **Wise, R. A. and Bozarth, M. A.,** Brain substrates for reinforcement and drug self-administration, *Prog. Neuropsychopharmacol.,* 5, 467, 1981.

17. **Kornetsky, C.,** Brain-stimulation reward: a model for the neuronal basis for drug-induced euphoria, in Neuroscience Methods in Drug Abuse Research, Brown, R. M., Friedman, D. P., and Nimit, Y., Eds., NIDA Res. Monogr. No. 62, DHHS Publ. No. (ADM) 85-11415, Department of Health and Human Services, Washington, D.C., 1985.

18. **Goeders, N. E. and Smith, J. E.,** Cortical dopaminergic involvement in cocaine reinforcement, *Science,* 221, 773, 1983.

19. **Goeders, N. E., Lane, J. D., and Smith, J. E.,** Self-administration of methionine enkephalin into the nucleus accumbens, *Pharmacol. Biochem. Behav.,* 20, 451, 1984.

20. **Dworkin, S. I., Guerin, G. F., Goeders, N. E., Cherek, D. R., Lane, J. D., and Smith, J. E.,** Reinforcer interactions under concurrent schedules of food, water, and intravenous morphine, *Psychopharmacology,* 82, 282, 1984.

21. **Smith, J. E. and Lane, J. D.,** Brain neurotransmitter turnover correlated with morphine self-administration, in *The Neurobiology of Opiate Reward Process,* Smith, J. E. and Lane, J. D., Eds., Elsevier, New York, 1983, 361.

22. **Vaccarino, F. J., Bloom, F. E., and Koob, G. F.,** Blockade of nucleus accumbens opiate receptors attenuates intravenous heroin reward in the rat, *Psychopharmacology,* 86, 37, 1985.

23. **Pettit, H. O., Ettenberg, A., Bloom, F. E., and Koob, G. F.,** Destruction of dopamine in the nucleus accumbens selectively attenuates cocaine but not heroin self-administration in rats, *Psychopharmacology,* 84, 167, 1984.

24. **Wise, R. A.,** Brain neuronal systems mediating reward processes, in *The Neurobiology of Opiate Reward Process,* Smith, J. E. and Lane, J. D., Eds., Elsevier, New York, 1983, 405.

25. **Bozarth, M. A. and Wise, R. A.,** Neural substrates of opiate reinforcement, *Prog. Neuropsychopharmacol.,* 7, 569, 1983.

26. **Wise, R. A. and Bozarth, M. A.,** Brain reward circuitry: four circuit elements "wired" in apparent series, *Brain Res. Bull.,* 12, 203, 1984.

27. **Kornetsky, C., Esposito, R. U., McLean, S., and Jacobson, J. O.,** Intracranial self-stimulation thresholds, *Arch. Gen. Psychiatry,* 36, 289, 1979.

28. **Kornetsky, C. and Bain, G.,** Effects of opiates on rewarding brain stimulation, in *The Neurobiology of Opiate Reward Processes,* Smith, J. E., and Lane, J. D., Eds., Elsevier, New York, 1983, 237.

29. **Unterwald, E. M. and Kornetsky, C.,** Effects of concomitant pentazocine and tripelennamine on brain-stimulation reward, *Pharmacol. Biochem. Behav.,* 21, 961, 1984.

30. **Bozarth, M. A. and Wise, R. A.,** Anatomically distinct receptor fields mediate reward and physical dependence, *Science,* 224, 516, 1984.

31. **Johanson, C. E.,** Assessment of the dependence potential of cocaine in animals, in Cocaine: Pharmacology, Effects, and Treatment of Abuse, Grabowski, J., Ed., NIDA Res. Monogr. No. 50, DHHS Publ. No. (ADM) 84-1326, Department of Health and Human Services, Washington, D.C. 1984, 54.

32. **Yanagita, T.,** An experimental framework for evaluation of dependence liability in various types of drugs in monkeys, *Bull. Narcot.,* 25, 57, 1973.

33. **Griffiths, R. R., Findley, J. D., Brady, J. V., Dolan-Gutcher, K., and Robinson, W. W.,** Comparison of progressive-ratio performance maintained by cocaine, methylphenidate and secobarbital *Psychopharmacologia,* 43, 81, 1975.

34. **Griffiths, R. R., Brady, J. V., and Snell, J. D.,** Progressive-ratio performance maintained by drug infusions: comparison of cocaine, diethylpropion, chlorphentermine, and fenfluramine, *Psychopharmacology,* 53, 5, 1978.

35. **Johanson, C. E., Balster, R. L., and Bonese, K.,** Self-administration of psychomotor stimulant drugs: the effects of unlimited access, *Pharmacol. Biochem. Behav.* 4, 45, 1976.

36. **Bozarth, M. A. and Wise, R. A.,** Toxicity associated with long-term intravenous heroin and cocaine self-administration in the rat, *JAMA,* 254 (1), 16, 1985.

37. **Kleber, H. D. and Gawin, F. H.,** Cocaine abuse: a review of current and experimental treatments, in Cocaine: Pharmacology, Effects, and Treatment of Abuse, Grabowski, J., Ed., NIDA Res. Monogr. No. 50, DHHS Publ. No. (ADM) 84-1326, Department of Health and Human Services, Washington, D.C., 1984, 111.

38. **Dakis, C. A. and Gold, M. S.,** Bromocriptine as a treatment of cocaine abuse, *Lancet,* 8438 (May 18), 1151, 1985.

39. **Woolverton, W., Goldberg, L. I., and Giros, J. Z.,** Intravenous self-administration of dopamine receptor agonists by rhesus monkeys, *J. Pharmacol. Exp. Ther.,* 230, 678, 1984.

40. **Gold, M. S., Pottash, A. L. C., Annitto, W. J., Vereby, K., and Sweeny, D. R.,** Cocaine withdrawal: efficacy of tyrosine, *Soc. Neurosci. Abstr.,* 9, 157, 1983.

41. **Green, T. K. and Harvey, J. A.,** Enhancement of amphetamine action after interruption of ascending serotonergic pathways, *J. Pharmacol. Exp. Ther.,* 190, 109, 1974.

42. **Mabry, P. D. and Campbell, B. A.,** Serotonergic inhibition of catecholamine-induced behavioral arousal, *Brain Res.,* 49, 381,

43. **Carlsson, A.,** Dopaminergic autoreceptors: background and implications, in *Nonstriatal Dopaminergic Neurons,* Costa, E. and Gessa, G. L., Eds., Raven Press, New York, 1977, 439.

44. **Fishman, M. W., Schuster, C. R., and Hatano, Y.,** A comparison of the subjective and cardiovascular effects of cocaine and lidocaine in humans, *Pharmacol. Biochem. Behav.,* 18, 123, 1976.

45. **Van Dyke, C., Jatlow, P., Ungerer, J., Barash, P. G., and Byck, R.,** Oral cocaine: plasma concentrations and central effects, *Science,* 200, 211, 1978.

46. **Fishman, M. W. and Schuster, C. R.,** Cocaine effects in sleep-deprived humans, *Psychopharmacology,* 72, 1, 1980.

47. **Fishman, M. W. and Schuster, C. R.,** Acute tolerance to cocaine in humans, in Problems of Drug Dependence, 1980, Harris, L. S., Ed., NIDA Res. Monogr. No. 34, DHHS Publ. No. (ADM) 81-1058, Department of Health and Human Services, Washington, D.C., 1981, 241.

48. **Fishman, M. W. and Schuster, C. R.,** Cocaine self-administration in humans, *Fed. Proc. Fed. Am. Soc. Exp. Biol.,* 41, 241, 1982.

49. **Van Dyke, C., Ungerer, J., Jatlow, P., Barash, P., and Byck, R.,** Intranasal cocaine: dose relationships of psychological effects and plasma levels, *Int. J. Psychiat. Med.,* 12, 1 1982.

50. **Post, R. M., Lockfeld, A., Squillace, K. M., and Contel, N. R.,** Drug-environment interaction: context dependency of cocaine-induced behavioral sensitization, *Life Sci.,* 28, 755, 1981.

51. **Kornetsky, C. and Esposito, R. U.,** Reward and detection thresholds for brain stimulation: dissociative effects of cocaine, *Brain Res.,* 209, 496, 1981.

52. **Winger, G. S. and Woods, J. H.,** The reinforcing property of ethanol in the rhesus monkey. I. Initiation, maintenance and termination of intravenous ethanol-reinforced responding, *Ann. N.Y. Acad. Sci.,* 215, 162, 1973.

Chapter 6

COCAINE KINETICS IN HUMANS

John J. Ambre

TABLE OF CONTENTS

I. COCAINE KINETICS IN HUMANS

Despite its widespread use, there have been few attempts to relate the disposition kinetics of cocaine to the responses that this drug elicits. The euphoric and cardiovascular effects have been reported to decline more rapidly than cocaine leaves the plasma after a single dose.[1] Although this phenomenon may or may not indicate tolerance, other observations indicate that cocaine does exhibit acute tolerance development. An intravenous dose of cocaine given after a 96-mg intranasal dose produces a less intense response than the same intravenous dose administered after a placebo dose.[2] Such a phenomenon is of considerable pharmacological interest and is of critical importance in interpreting cocaine plasma concentrations.

Understanding the dose-effect relationship is a major goal of clinical pharmacology. Considerable progress has been made in the area of pharmacokinetics, the study of the time course of drug concentrations in the body using mathematical models.[3] Recent efforts have focused on pharmacodynamics and modeling of the concentration-effect relationship.[4] Conventional pharmacodynamic models involve the assumption that the model parameters are constant or time independent.[4] As discussed above, this does not appear to be true for cocaine. Others have attempted to deal with this analytical difficulty by modeling cocaine dynamics with the distributed-lags method, a mathematical procedure adopted from econometrics.[5] We have attempted instead to modify conventional pharmacokinetic-pharmacodynamic methods by incorporating a tolerance factor.

The phenomenon of decrease effect with prolonged exposure to a drug is called tolerance, and when it occurs within the time course of a single dose, is called acute tolerance.[6] Possible mechanisms of this phenomenon include physiological adjustment by counterregulatory systems or changes in receptor number or membrane location.[6] Further studies of the underlying mechanisms are likely to be facilitated by more rigorous quantitative description of the phenomenon than the usual approach that provides only a quantal index of subject response rather than a full concentration response curve.

In our previous study, the chronotropic effects of cocaine after a short intravenous infusion were analyzed using the linear-effect pharmacodynamic model.[4,7] The intensity of the chronotropic effects of cocaine declined at a faster rate than the decline in plasma concentrations, as discussed above. In the simplest case, biophase and plasma concentrations of cocaine would fall in parallel. Since other studies noted above indicated that tolerance develops to cocaine in the time course of a single dose, we evaluated the possibility that this phenomenon of acute tolerance could be represented by a linear model with progressive attenuation in the intensity of the effect for a given biophase concentration of cocaine. This attenuation process was incorporated into the model as another first-order process influencing the decay of the chronotropic effect (in addition to first order plasma disappearance of cocaine) and was designated a tolerance factor. We propose to demonstrate the validity of this approach by performing steady-state experiments in which the tolerance factor can be calculated directly.

Single-dose, nonsteady-state studies provide information on distribution to biophase. However, cocaine is usually taken in repeated intravenous or intranasal doses at short intervals.[6] Single-dose studies provide no information about the effects of repeated doses since tolerance development is not likely to continue indefinitely. Fischmans studies have shown that a second dose of cocaine produces less response than the first dose of the same size given 1 hr earlier.[2] This is a qualitative description and does not indicate the degree of tolerance development. We are using cocaine infusion studies to determine the degree and persistence of the tolerance phenomenon, the chronotropic effect under steady-state conditions.

In these studies we are also applying our pharmacokinetic-pharmacodynamic approach to the characterization of the concentration-response relationship for the euphoric effect of

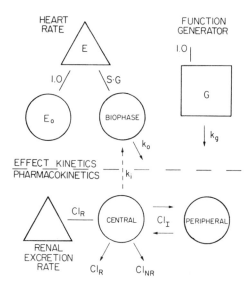

FIGURE 1. Pharmacokinetic-pharmacodynamic model used for analysis of chronotropic response to intravenous dose of cocaine. (From Chow, M. J. et al., *Clin. Pharmacol. Ther.*, 38, 318, 1985. With permission.)

cocaine. We intuitively expect that model parameters for this biophase will differ from those for the chronotropic effect. Steady-state experiments will again define the degree and persistence of tolerance to cocaine-induced euphoria.

Other experiments will deal with the possibility that the tolerance factor exhibits dose dependency by studying higher steady-state levels. We will study the duration or persistence of the tolerance induced acutely and whether the character of the response is altered by readministration of cocaine as early as the following day. Depending to some extent on what we find in these studies we will attempt other studies to discover the mechanism of acute tolerance. We will take advantage of the opportunity to collect blood and urine specimens from subjects, receiving precisely known doses of cocaine to acquire data on the time course of cocaine and metabolite excretion.

Our previous studies of the pharmacokinetics-pharmacodynamics of cocaine have been described in a paper published elsewhere.[7] Five healthy subjects with histories of intravenous cocaine use were given 30 mg of cocaine HCl by a short (2-min), intravenous infusion. Blood samples were drawn at frequent intervals and all urine voided over the next 3 hr was collected. Heart rate was determined directly from a continuously monitored electrocardiogram. Kinetic analyses were made with SAAM 23 digital computer program developed by Berman and Weiss[8] and implemented on a Control Data Corporation Cyber 170/730 computer.

Cocaine distribution and elimination kinetics were modeled with a two-compartment, open system with elimination from the central compartment as shown in Figure 1. Kinetic parameters are shown in Table 2.

The chronotropic effects of cocaine were analyzed using the linear-effect pharmacodynamic model Holford and Sheiner,[4] modified so that there was no net cocaine transfer from the central compartment to the hypothetical biophase. The parameters k^1 and k^0 were used to relate the rise and fall of plasma cocaine concentration to the waxing and waning of cocaine-induced cardioacceleration. The parameter S was used to relate biophase concentrations to the observed intensity of this effect. Biophase and plasma concentrations would be expected to decline in parallel after distribution as shown in Figure 2. The apparent progressive attenuation in the intensity of the effect of a given biophase concentration of

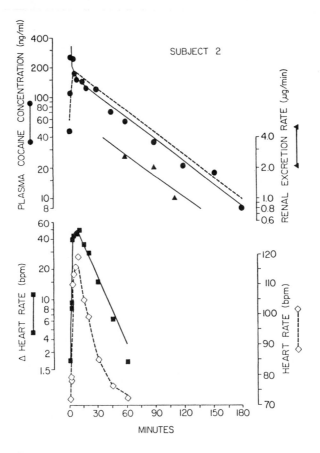

FIGURE 2.   Kinetic analysis in Subject 2 of plasma cocaine concentrations (circles) and renal excretion rate (triangles) is shown in the top panel. In the bottom panel are shown the observed heart rate (open diamonds) and the change in heart rate (Δ heart rate) attributed to the chronotropic effect of cocaine (solid squares). The lines are least-squares fits of the measured values shown by the data points. Hypothetical biophase cocaine concentrations are indicated in the top panel by the broken line. Progressive attenuation of the chronotropic effect of cocaine is evident because Δ heart rate declines faster than biophase cocaine concentrations. (From Chow, M. J. et al., *Clin. Pharmacol. Ther.*, 38, 318, 1985. With permission.)

cocaine was incorporated into the model using a function generator shown in Figure 1 as a square. The contents of the function generator (G) have an initial value of 1, then fall exponentially at a rate described by k_g. The chronotropic effects of cocaine (ΔE) are thus described by the equation:

$$\Delta E = (G)(S)(Cb)$$

where Cb is the biophase concentration of cocaine. The measured heart rate (E) could be analyzed from the relationship:

$$E = EO + [(G)(S)(Cb)]$$

where EO is the baseline heart rate before cocaine administration.

The results of the analysis of cocaine pharmacokinetics in Subject 2 are shown in Figure

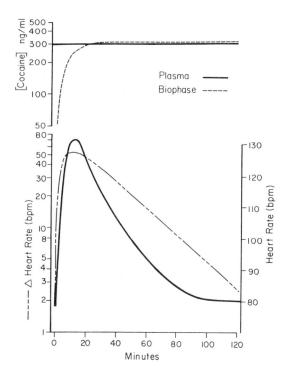

FIGURE 3.   Model-predicted cocaine concentrations and chronotropic response to cocaine in the proposed steady-state experiments.

2. Plasma cocaine concentrations (circles) and renal excretion rate (triangles) are shown in the top panel. The observed heart rate (open diamonds) and change in heart rate (delta heart rate) attributed to the chronotropic effect of cocaine (solid squares) are shown in the bottom panel. The lines are least-squares fits of the measured values. Hypothetical biophase cocaine concentrations are indicated in the top panel by the broken line.

Parameter estimates for the model system relating these effects to plasma cocaine concentrations are shown in Table 3. Estimates of S indicated that biophase concentrations initially accelerate heart rate by 0.3 bpm (beats per minute) on the average, for each 1 ng/mℓ. The constant characterizing the rate of attenuation of the intensity of this effect (k_g) had a mean value of 0.0294 min^{-1}, corresponding to a half-time of 24 min. We are attempting to determine this parameter directly in steady-state experiments. We are making similar observations on the euphoric effect of cocaine.

A steady-state drug plasma concentration can be produced immediately and maintained by using the bolus and exponentially tapering infusion technique described by Ridell. Results from our single-dose studies (mean kinetic parameters) were used to design an infusion regimen (for a target concentration of 300 ng/mℓ) consisting of an initial bolus cocaine dose of 7.8 mg followed by cocaine infusion that begins at a rate of 10.2 mg/min and tapers to a final rate of 0.63 mg/min. The plasma levels, biophase concentrations, and pulse rates expected to result from this dose regimen have been simulated in Figure 3.

Pilot studies have shown that this approach is feasible and have provided useful preliminary information. A young male subject was given cocaine according to the protocol described below with a target cocaine plasma concentration of 300 ng/mℓ. The resulting data are shown in Figure 4. The desired concentration was obtained immediately and then maintained virtually constant at a level of approximately 325 ng/mℓ. As predicted in the above simulation, the heart rate rose abruptly to a peak at 10 to 12 min and then declined in apparent

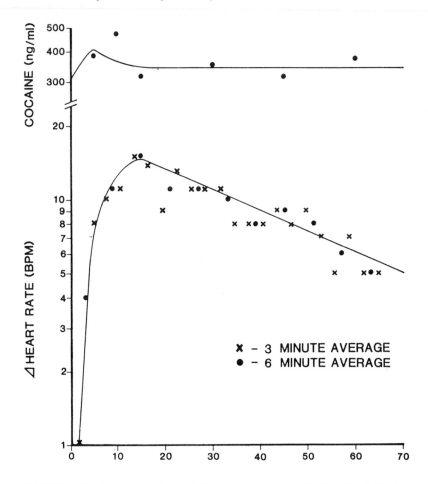

FIGURE 4.   Cocaine concentrations and chronotropic response in the first subject. Cocaine target level was 300 ng/mℓ. Points are actual measured values and the lines are computer fitted values. Heart rate is shown as both 3- and 6-min running averages of continuously recorded electrocardiographic rate data.

logarithmic fashion. The experiment was terminated at 75 min at the request of the subject who was disappointed that he was unable to appreciate any psychological effect. Despite the minimal heart rate response, its decline from peak was clearly exponential with a half-life of 27 min, very close to the mean value of the tolerance factor (24 min) we found in the single-dose studies.[7] This result appears to confirm directly the validity of our tolerance factor.

Because the 300-ng/mℓ level appeared insufficient to produce euphoria in all subjects, the steady-state target level was raised to 500 ng/mℓ. Approval of the Institutional Review Board was obtained for this modification of the protocol. Another young male subject was studied under identical conditions except for the new target level. This regimen consists of an initial bolus cocaine dose of 13 mg, followed by an infusion that beings at a rate of 17 mg/min and tapers to a final rate of 1.05 mg/min. The data obtained are presented in Figure 5. The cocaine plasma level rose within 5 to 10 min to a virtually constant level of approximately 525 ng/mℓ. The heart rate (Figure 6) rose to a peak at 10 min and then declined exponentially toward a plateau at approximately 60% of the peak level. The half-life of its decline was 30 min, again very close to the mean value of the tolerance factor (24 min) we found in the single-dose studies. The finding of the plateau is an interesting result and

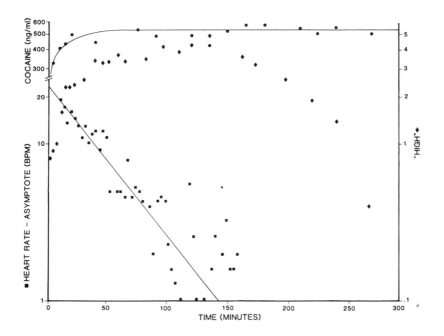

FIGURE 5. Cocaine concentrations, chronotropic response, and self-ratings of ''high'' in the second subject. Cocaine target level was 500 ng/mℓ. Round points are measured cocaine levels and the line is computer-fitted data. Rhomboid points are self-rating ''high''. The square data points are derived from heart rate measurements as the difference between the measured rate at early time points and the eventual plateau (asymptote) rate. The line represents a least-squares regression fit of the derived data points.

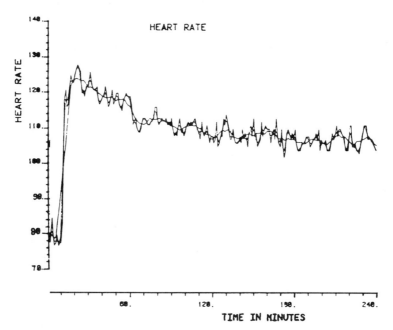

FIGURE 6. Plot of continuously recorded beat-to-beat determination of heart rate in the subject and 3- and 6-min running averages. Illustrates how averaging damps the moment-to-moment variation in rate, but preserves the general contour of the heart rate response to cocaine infusion.

indicates precisely the degree of tolerance that develops acutely. The results also suggest that there is no dose dependency of the tolerance factor with an approximate doubling of the cocaine concentration.

Computer fit of the heart rate data using SAAM program is also shown in the Figure 6. In order to model the incomplete development of tolerance in the heart rate (approach to a plateau or asymptote rather than the baseline), the function generator of the single-dose study model was replaced with a two-compartment closed system with initial input to the first compartment.

The euphoric effect, as measured by the linear analogue scale had a more prolonged rising phase with a relatively stable intensity between 50 and 150 min and subsequent decline almost to baseline at 270 min. Decline approximates exponential process, but the data are not as clearcut. More frequent data points on the declining phase may help to define the line since the euphoric effect, like the heart rate, appears to cycle continuously over a range of constant absolute magnitude. This can be seen during the rising phase, where measurements were taken at about 5-min intervals. These results seem to indicate that the tolerance factor is a useful concept for modeling the euphoric effect of cocaine and that, unlike the cardiovascular effect, total tolerance may develop acutely (effect approaches baseline rather than a plateau). Placebo injection (saline) had no detectable effect on either the heart or psyche in this subject.

II. THE URINARY EXCRETION OF COCAINE AND METABOLITES IN HUMANS: A KINETIC ANALYSIS OF PUBLISHED DATA

There is very little information available on the time course of cocaine or its metabolites in the human body. Since analyses applied to urine samples for the purpose of identifying the cocaine user are aimed at detection of cocaine metabolites,[9,10] knowledge of the time course of metabolite excretion is of more than theoretical interest. Questions frequently arise regarding the interpretation of cocaine and metabolite levels in blood and urine samples. Empirical data from the literature are of little help in answering these questions. Tabular drug concentration data are valid only for the specific experimental conditions under which they were obtained. They allow only qualitative evaluation of concentrations found in isolated samples.

Pharmacokinetic analysis is an attempt to describe experimental data in terms of a kinetic model and its parameters and thereby characterize the dose — drug/metabolite — time relationship. The kinetic parameters can in turn be used to make predictions of a more general and quantitative nature.

We have undertaken a pharmacokinetic analysis of previously published data (including our own) in an attempt to gain further insight into the disposition of cocaine in humans and to present what is known in the most useful format. Literature data form the basis for selection of the kinetic model and the underlying assumptions. Equations appropriate for the kinetic model were used to construct model-predicted excretion and concentration profiles. These were then compared with the experimental data to test the validity of the model. Finally, the possibility of using the model to provide answers to very practical problems is discussed.

A. Literature Data

Kogan et al.[11] reported data from three subjects given 100 mg of cocaine HCl intravenously. Plasma levels of cocaine and benzoylecgonine (BZ) were determined at various times for 24 hr after the dose. Hamilton et al.[12] reported cocaine and BZ urinary excretion data from six subjects given 1.5 mg/kg of cocaine HCl intranasally. Ambre et al.[13] reported cocaine, BZ, and ecgonine methyl ester (EME) urinary excretion data from two subjects given several

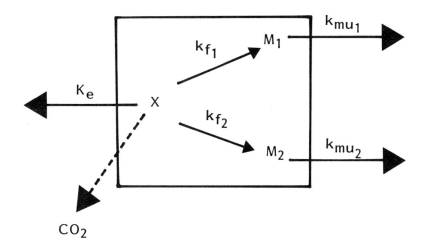

FIGURE 7. A one-compartment open pharmacokinetic model with first-order rate constants characterizing the processes of metabolism and renal excretion. In this scheme, cocaine (x) is converted (k_{f1} and k_{f2}) to two major metabolites (M_1 and M_2) which are excreted into urine without further modification (k_{mu1} and k_{mu2}). Some cocaine is excreted unchanged and some is converted to and excreted as CO_2.

doses (48 and 96 mg intranasally and 48 mg intravenously) of cocaine HCl. Urine was collected for 48 hr after the dose.

The above studies were the only ones found in the literature which provided plasma or urinary concentration data over an extended period after known doses of cocaine.

Studies reported in references[12-15] support the assumption that the majority of a dose of cocaine can be accounted for by measurement of BZ, EME, and unchanged cocaine in the urine. Based on these studies, the following values were assigned to the products of cocaine excretion: BZ 46%, EME 41%, and unchanged cocaine 3%. The remaining 10% consists of demethylated products and ecgonine.

Studies by Wilkinson et al.[16] and Van Dyke et al.[17] presented some data to indicate a linear relationship between cocaine dose, cocaine plasma levels, and peak BZ concentrations in the urine. Only one study[18] challenges the assumption of linearity of cocaine kinetics. In that study, the conclusion that cocaine kinetics exhibited dose dependency above 1.1 mg/kg was based on limited plasma level data in two subjects.

B. Kinetic Analysis

Rigorous analysis of cocaine disposition requires a two-compartment model. However, distribution is essentially complete within 5 min after the dose, and cocaine plasma level decline thereafter exhibits a single phase. Depicting the body as a single, kinetically homogenous unit is a useful approach for the analysis of drugs that distribute rapidly.[21] For the purpose of this study cocaine disposition was represented by a one-compartment open model with first-order rate constants characterizing the elimination processes of metabolism and renal excretion (Figure 7). Absorption of cocaine from the nasal mucosa is very fast, relative to the processes of elimination,[16] so that the absorption step for intranasal cocaine was ignored. The constant K, the overall elimination rate constant, can be determined from the terminal linear portion of a semilog plot of cocaine plasma concentrations against time or the slope of a plot of cocaine excretion rates against time.[21] Rate constants for the overall elimination of the metabolites (k^m) are the sum of the rate constant for renal elmination (k_{mu}) and the rate constant for nonrenal elimination of the metabolite (k_{nr}). Since the metabolites are excreted only in the urine, $k_m = k_{mu}$. Therefore, k_m can be determined from the slope

Table 1
KINETIC PARAMETERS FOR COCAINE AND
METABOLITES

Constant	Value calculated from published data (1/hr)	Mean (1/hr)	$T^{1}/_{2}$ (hr)	Ref.
Cocaine (C)				
K^a	−0.5206			3
	−0.4073	−0.4640	1.5	
	−0.4636			16
Benzoylecgonine (BZ)				
k_m^b	−0.0920			3
	−0.0926	−0.0923	7.5	4
k_f^c	0.2134			5
Ecgonine methyl ester (EME)				
k_m^b	−0.1650		3.6	5
k_f^c	0.1902			5

[a] K = The apparent first-order elimination rate constant for the parent drug, cocaine.
[b] k_m = The elimination rate constant for metabolite.
[c] k_f = The rate constant for metabolite formation.

of the linear portion of a semilog plot of metabolite excretion rates against time.[21] Since K, the elimination rate constant for the parent drug, is greater than k_m, metabolite concentrations in the plasma decline more slowly than the concentration of unchanged drug, and k_m could also be estimated from the terminal slope of a semilog plot of metabolite plasma concentrations against time.[21] The metabolite formation rate constants, k_{f1} and k_{f2}, can be determined from the relationship:

$$kf = K \frac{Mu}{Xo} \tag{1}$$

where Mu is the total amount of metabolite excreted in the urine, Xo is the intravenous dose, and K is the overall elimination rate constant for the parent drug.[21]

According to the above scheme, the equation

$$\frac{dMu}{dt} = \frac{kmu\ (kf)\ Xo}{km - K}\ [e^{-K(t)} - e^{-km(t)}] \tag{2}$$

describes the time course for the appearance of the metabolite in the urine.[21]

Plasma level data for cocaine and BZ reported by Kogan et al.[11] were plotted on a semilog graph against time. Elimination rate constants were calculated by linear regression analysis. Urinary excretion rates for cocaine calculated from urine concentration data for each collection period were reported by Hamilton et al.[12] The resultant values were plotted at the midpoint of the urine collection period on a semilog graph. Elimination rate constants were calculated from the terminal linear portions of these plots by regression analysis. The BZ and EME urinary excretion data of Ambre et al.[13] was plotted in a similar manner. Elimination half-lives were calculated from elimination rate constants by the formula: $T^{1}/_{2} = 0.693/k$.

The theoretical curves illustrating excretion data were calculated from Equation 2 by inserting values for the kinetic constants derived as described above.

The various kinetic rate constants calculated from the literature data are shown in Table 1. These values were used to calculate the theoretical curves.

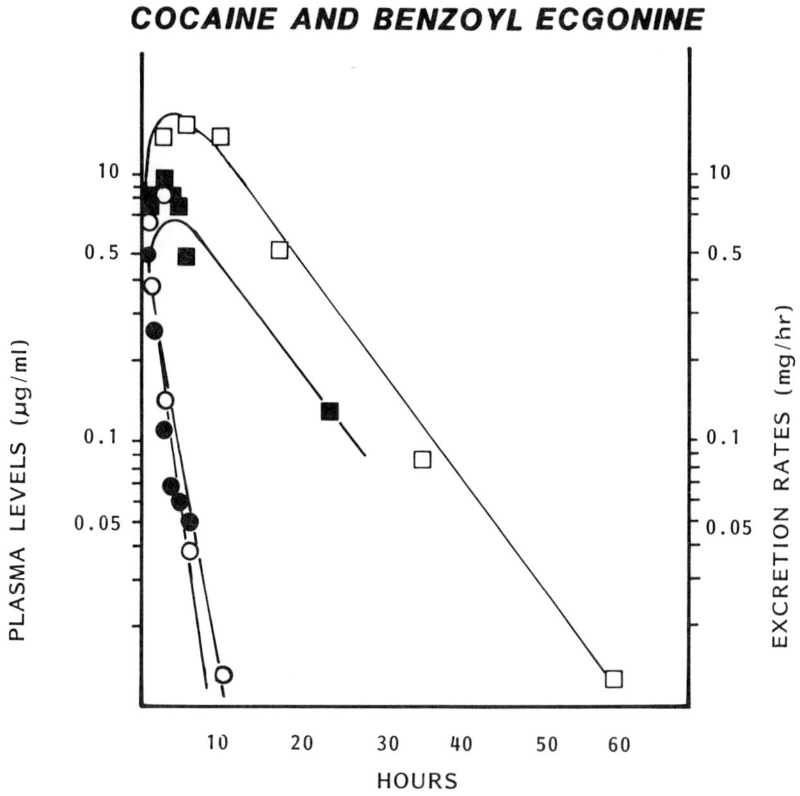

FIGURE 8.   A semilog plot of cocaine and benzoylecgonine plasma levels and urinary excretion rates. Plasma levels (100 mg i.v. cocaine dose): ■, BZ; ●, cocaine. Urine excretion rates (15 mg/kg i.n. cocaine dose): □, BZ; ○, cocaine.

A semilog plot of the plasma level (Kogan et al.) and urinary excretion data (derived from Hamilton et al.) is shown in Figure 8. These are plotted together to show that, as predicted, the decline of the excretion rate plot parallels the plasma level disappearance curve for both cocaine and BZ.

EME excretion rate (Ambre et al.) plot is shown in Figure 9. There is more variation in this data, but, again, the theoretical curves fit the experimental points reasonably well. The similarity of the slopes of these curves provides additional evidence for the linearity of cocaine disposition in this dose range.

Figure 10 is a simulation of the excretion rate curves for cocaine, BZ, and EME after a single 100-mg intravenous cocaine dose. Fischman and Schuster have found that intravenous doses of 16 mg were rated by cocaine users as similar in effect to their usual "street" dose.[22] Such doses, however, are usually taken repeatedly at about 30-min intervals so that much larger total doses are common. The curves in Figure 10 indicate the relative amounts of cocaine, BZ, and EME in urine at any time after a cocaine dose. Since these substances are present in the same volume, the curves also indicate the urine concentration ratio. In Table 2, the predicted concentration ratio of EME to BZ is compared with the experimentally determined ratio calculated from the data of Ambre et al.[13] The average deviation of experimental from predicted values is 30%. Theoretically and experimentally determined ratios of EME to cocaine (Ambre et al.)[13] and BZ to cocaine (Hamilton et al.)[12] concentrations are also compared. The poorer correlation of these ratios may be due to the influence of urine pH on cocaine excretion.[14] Making the assumption that the volume of urine output is 1 mℓ/min,[23] urine concentrations can be estimated for a given dose. Table 3 compares

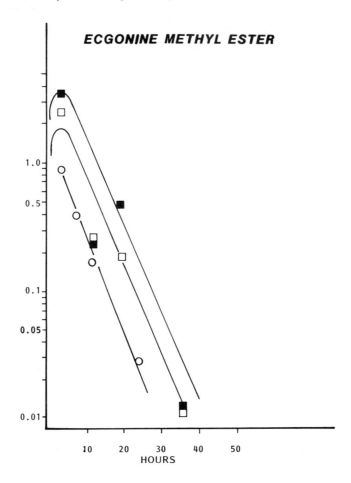

FIGURE 9.   A semilog plot of ecgonine methyl ester urinary excretion rates. Urine excretion rates: ■, 96 mg i.n. cocaine dose; □, 48 mg i.n. cocaine dose; ○, 32 mg i.v. cocaine dose. Units for Y axis expressed in milligrams per hour.

predicted and experimentally determined concentration values. Urine volume is, of course, highly dependent on the state of hydration of the subject and this is a source of potentially large variation. The average deviation of the BZ data, however, is only 25%. The EME and cocaine experimental values match the predicted values reasonably well with average differences of 45 and 42% respectively.

Certain questions arise frequently regarding the detection of the cocaine user. Those responsible for drug treatment programs want to know, for example, the duration of positivity of various screening tests with varying levels of sensitivity aimed at metabolite detection; or the frequency of testing required to detect intermittent cocaine use. The forensic analyst wants an indication of how recently the drug was taken or the time between drug use and death. In the past, attempts to answer these questions have taken the empirical rather than the kinetic approach.

The goal of our kinetic analysis was to define a model of cocaine disposition which would provide a basis for interpretation of cocaine and/or metabolite concentrations in individual or isolated plasma or urine samples. The model might also allow predictions which obviate the need to collect large amounts of empirical data. For example, if the detection limits for the EMIT assay and an RIA assay method for BZ are known to be 1.0 and 0.025 mg/ℓ,

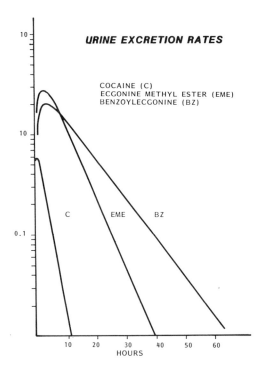

FIGURE 10. A simulation of the excretion rate curves for cocaine ben-zoylecgonine and ecgonine methyl ester after a single 100-mg intravenous cocaine dose. Units for Y axis expressed in milligrams per hour.

respectively, the RIA assay should be positive approximately six BZ half-lives or 48 hr longer than the EMIT assay after a cocaine dose. This is the same conclusion that Hamilton et al.[12] arrived at by the empirical method of testing multiple urine samples from six subjects by both methods over a period of several days.

The illustration in Figure 4 shows that in the first 10 to 12 hr after the last cocaine dose, identification of EME in urine may be an analytically easier method of confirming positive urine screening test results,[10] since the EME concentrations are similar to or higher than BZ concentrations. Almost equal amounts of BZ and EME are produced from cocaine. The reason that BZ can be detected longer by urine testing is due to its slower excretion into urine rather than its greater prominence as a metabolite.

The relative concentrations of cocaine, BZ, and/or EME in a single urine sample may provide an indication of the length of time since the dose of cocaine. Cocaine will generally be detectable only in the first few hours after the last dose. If cocaine (C) is detectable, but the EME/C or the BZ/C ratio is greater than 100, this is also evidence that the dose was more than 10 hr ago. Conversely, EME/C ratio less than 100 would suggest the dose was less than 10 hr ago. An EME/BZ ratio greater than 1.0 ratio would be additional evidence in that regard. If the EME and BZ concentrations are similar (the EME/BZ ratio is greater than 0.5), the dose was likely taken within the last 20 hr. Conversely, an EME/BZ ratio less than 0.5 would indicate more than 20 hr since the dose. EME will usually not be detectable more than 48 hr after the last dose. If EME is detectable, but the EME/BZ ratio is less than 0.1, this is also an indiciation that the dose was more than 48 hr ago. These ratios will not apply if the cocaine dose is repeated over an extended period (several hours), since the extent of accumulation will differ for EME and BZ. In such cases, the ratios must be calculated directly from the model.

Table 2

URINE CONCENTRATION RATIOS FOR COCAINE (C), BENZOYLECGONINE (BZ), AND ECGONINE METHYL ESTER (EME) AT VARIOUS TIMES AFTER DOSE

	Time (hr)								
Concentration ratios	**0.5** (0—1)	**1.5** (1—2)	**3** (2—4)	**4** (0—8)	**6** (4—8)	**10** (8—16)	**12** (8—16)	**20** (16—24)	**36** (24—48)
EME/BZ									
Experimental mean[a]	—	—	—	1.9	—	—	0.51	0.37	0.11
Predicted	—	—	—	1.3	—	—	0.81	0.46	0.14
EME/C									
Experimental mean[a]	—	—	—	9.5	—	—	—	—	—
Predicted	—	—	—	16.8	—	97.9	—	—	—
BZ/C									
Experimental mean[b]	5.9	17.3	12.7	—	109.8	130.5	—	—	—
Predicted	0.9	3.2	8.0	—	27.0	105.0	—	—	—
Experimental mean[a]	—	—	—	10.6	—	—	—	—	—
Predicted	—	—	—	12.5	—	—	—	—	—

[a] Experiment by Ambre et al; n = 2.
[b] Experiment by Hamilton et al; n = 6.

From Ambre, J., *J. Anal. Toxicol.*, 9, 243, 1985. With permission.

Because of the evidence cited earlier that cocaine exhibits first-order kinetics over a wide dose range, Figure 10 provides a base for construction of a nomogram. Figure 11 shows a nomogram for BZ urine concentrations. This might be used to estimate urine metabolite concentrations that would result from various cocaine doses (with additional assumption that urine volume is 1 mℓ/min).

When information is available about the size and timing of intermittent or repeated doses, the model might allow an estimate of the urine levels of cocaine and/or metabolites that would result. Conversely, measured urine levels might allow estimation of dose timing. It is important to note, however, the uncertainty in using the nomogram for doses above 200 mg, since this involves the assumption of linear kinetics. Although this is a reasonable assumption, as pointed out earlier, there is no experimental data to substantiate it.

Finally, this analysis indicates the kind of information needed to improve our understanding of cocaine disposition. Specifically, controlled studies involving precisely known cocaine doses and accurately collected specimens of body fluids will permit refinement of the kinetic model and better definition of the kinetic constants. It will be particularly important to determine whether cocaine exhibits nonlinear kinetcs at higher dose levels.

Table 3
URINE CONCENTRATIONS OF BENZOYLECGONINE, ECGONINE METHYL ESTER, AND COCAINE AT VARIOUS TIMES AFTER A 100-mg COCAINE HCl DOSE[a]

Concentration (mg/ℓ)	Time (hr)												
	0.5 (0—1)	1 (0—2)	1.5 (1—2)	3 (2—4)	4 (0—8)	5 (4—6)	6 (4—8)	10 (8—12)	12 (8—16)	18 (12—24)	20 (16—24)	36 (24—48)	60 (48—72)
Benzoylecgonine													
Experimental mean													
Ambre (n = 2)	—	—	—	—	32.0	—	—	—	20.5	—	18.5	2.1	—
Kogan (n = 2)	—	43.5	—	52.5	—	34.4	—	—	—	—	—	—	—
Hamilton (n = 4)	19.1	—	32.4	—	—	—	39.8	35.2	—	14.8	—	2.2	0.45
Predicted[b]	14.4	25.1	32.9	45.1	47.4	47.1	45.4	34.3	28.8	16.7	13.9	3.2	0.35
Ecgonine methyl ester													
Experimental mean													
Ambre (n = 2)	—	—	—	—	32.4	—	—	—	10.4	—	5.4	0.2	—
Predicted[b]	—	—	—	—	63.1	—	—	—	23.5	—	6.5	0.5	—
Cocaine													
Experimental mean													
Ambre (n = 2)	—	—	—	—	6.6	—	—	—	0.20	—	—	—	—
Kogan (n = 2)	—	9.3	—	4.0	—	2.4	—	—	—	—	—	—	—
Hamilton (n = 4)	9.6	—	3.8	—	—	—	0.7	0.48	—	—	—	—	—
Predicted[b]	15.6	12.7	10.4	5.6	3.8	2.5	1.6	0.33	0.14	—	—	—	—

[a] Cocaine HCl doses in the experimental subjects: Ambre et al., subjects A and B received 96 mg each; Kogan et al., subjects O.L. and A.M. received 100 mg each, and Hamilton et al., subjects C,D,E, and F received 90, 96, 104, and 110 mg, respectively (mean 100 mg).

[b] Predictions based on the assumption that urine output volume is 1 mℓ/min.

From Ambre, J., *J. Anal. Toxicol.*, 9, 243, 1985. With permission.

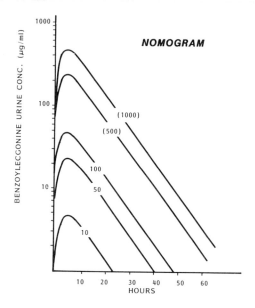

FIGURE 11.   A nomogram for relating benzoylecgonine urine concentrations to the size of and time interval since the cocaine dose. The cocaine
dose may be single or repeated and cumulative. If taken within a relatively
short period (relative to BZ excretion) of a few hours. Extrapolate between
curves for other doses. Doses of 500 mg and above are in parenthesis to
indicate that although kinetics are probably similar above 200 mg, there
are no data available at the present time. (From Ambre, J., *J. Anal.
Toxicol.*, 9, 243, 1985. With permission.)

REFERENCES

1. **Fischman, M. W. and Schuster, C. R.,** Cocaine self-administration in humans, Fed. Proc. *Fed. Am. Soc. Exp. Biol.*, 41, 241, 1982.
2. **Fischman, M. W., Schuster, C. R., Javaid, J., Hatano, Y., and Davis, J.,** Acute tolerance development to the cardiovascular and subjective effects of cocaine, *J. Pharmacol. Exp. Ther.*, 235, 677, 1985.
3. **Gibaldi, M. and Perrier, D.,** *Pharmacokinetics,* 2nd ed., Marcel Dekker, New York, 1982.
4. **Holford, N. H. G. and Sheiner, L. B.,** Understanding the dose-effect relationship: clinical application of pharmacokinetic-pharmacodynamic models, *Clin. Pharmacokinet.*, 6, 429, 1981.
5. **Zahler, R., Wachtel, P., Jatlow, P., and Byck, R.,** Kinetics of drug effect by distributed lags analysis: an application to cocaine, *Clin. Pharmacol. Ther.*, 31, 775, 1982.
6. **Jaffe, J. H.,** Drug addiction and drug abuse, in *The Pharmacological Basis of Therapeutics,* 6th ed., Goodman, L. S., Gilman, A., Eds., Macmillan, New York, 1980.
7. **Chow, M. J., Ambre, J. J., Ruo, T. I., Atkinson, A. J., Jr., Bowsher, D. J., and Fischman, M. W.,** Kinetics of cocaine distribution, elimination, and chronotropic effects, *Clin. Pharmacol. Ther.*, 38, 318, 1985.
8. **Berman, M. and Weiss, M. F.,** SAAM Manual, PHS Publ. No. 1703, Public Health Service, Washington, D.C., 1967.
9. **Wallace, J. E., Hamilton, H. E., Christenson, J. G., Shimek, E. L., Jr., Land, P. L., and Harris, S. C.,** An evaluation of selected methods for determining cocaine and benzoyl-ecgonine in urine, *J. Anal. Toxicol.*, 1, 20, 1977.
10. **Ambre, J. J., Ruo, T.-I., Smith, G. L., Backes, D., and Smith, C. M.,** Ecgonine methyl ester a major metabolite of cocaine, *J. Anal. Toxicol.*, 6, 26, 1982.
11. **Kogan, M. J., Verebey, K. G., DePace, A. C., Resnick, R. B., and Mulé, S. J.,** Quantitative determination of benzoylecgonine and cocaine in human biofluids by gas-liquid chromatography, *Anal. Chem.*, 49, 1965, 1977.

12. **Hamilton, H. E., Wallace, J. E., Shimek, E. L., Jr., Land, P., Harris, S. C., and Christenson, J. G.,** Cocaine and benzoylecgonine excretion in humans, *J. Forensic Sci.,* 22, 697, 1977.
13. **Ambre, J. J., Fischman, M., and Ruo, T.-I.,** Urinary excretion of ecgonine methyl ester, a major metabolite of cocaine in humans, *J. Anal. Toxicol.,* 8, 23, 1984.
14. **Fish, F. and Wilson, W. D.,** Excretion of cocaine and its metabolites in man, *J. Pharm. Pharmacol.,* 21, 135S, 1969.
15. **Inaba, T., Stewart, D. J., and Kalow, W.,** Metabolism of cocaine in man, *Clin. Pharmacol. Ther.,* 23, 547, 1978.
16. **Wilkinson, P., Van Dyke, C., Jatlow, P., Barash, P., and Byck, R.,** Intranasal and oral cocaine kinetics, *Clin. Pharmacol. Ther.,* 27, 386, 1980.
17. **Van Dyke, C., Byck, R., Barash, P., and Jatlow, P.,** Urinary excretion of immunologically reactive metabolites after intranasal administration of cocaine, as followed by enzyme immunoassay, *Clin. Chem.,* 23, 241, 1977.
18. **Barnett, G., Hawks, R., and Resnick, R.,** Cocaine pharmaco-kinetics in humans, *J. Ethnopharmacol.,* 3, 353, 1981.
19. **Stewart, D., Inaba, T., Lucassen, M., and Kalow, W.,** Cocaine metabolism: cocaine and norcocaine hydrolysis by liver and serum esterases, *Clin. Pharmacol. Ther.,* 25, 464, 1979.
20. **Holmstedt, B., Lindgren, J., and Rivier, L.,** Cocaine in blood of cocoa chewers, *J. Ethnopharmacol.,* 1, 29, 1979.
21. **Gibaldi, M. and Perrier, D.,** *Pharmacokinetics,* 2nd ed., Marcel Dekker, New York, 1982, 1.
22. **Fischman, M. W. and Schuster, C. R.,** Cocaine self-administration in humans, *Fed. Proc.* Fed. Am. Soc. Exp. Biol., 41, 241, 1982.
23. **Brenner, B. M. and Hostetter, T. H.,** Mechanisms of renal excretory function with normal and reduced nephron mass, in *Harrison's Principles of Internal Medicine,* 10th ed., Petersdorf, R. et al., Eds., McGraw-Hill, New York, 1983, 1599.
24. **Javaid, J. I., Mahmoud, N. M., Fischman, M., Schuster, C. R., and Davis, J. M.,** Kinetics of cocaine in humans after intravenous and intranasal administration, *Biopharm. Drug Dispos.,* 4, 9, 1983.

Chapter 7

COCAINE PHARMACOLOGY AND TOXICOLOGY

Randall L. Commissaris

TABLE OF CONTENTS

I. INTRODUCTION

A. Cocaine History in Brief

Cocaine has been used for centuries by natives of the Andes Mountains in South America. In Peru and Bolivia cocaine has been chewed for untold generations by natives for its invigorating effects and as a part of religious ceremonies.[1,2]

Cocaine was not used in the western world, however, until the mid 1800s. Sigmund Freud has been indicated as being responsible for much of the problem of cocaine in Europe. This is only partially true because cocaine was introduced to Europe in the 1860s and Freud was born in 1859. As a young child Freud did not influence bringing cocaine to Europe. It is true, however, that Sigmund Freud was important in *promoting* cocaine use in Europe. Freud advocated the use of cocaine in many medical conditions. It was Freud who initially argued that cocaine could be used as a local anesthetic. He advocated the use of cocaine in other conditions as well, including asthma, digestive disorders, and even as an aphrodisiac.[2] Freud also argued that cocaine had no toxic effects at any doses. Unfortunately, in this regard he was quite incorrect. In fact, one patient under Freud's care died following an overdose from cocaine.[55] Freud also advocated the use of cocaine as a "cure" for morphine addiction. A collegue of his, Dr. Ernst von Fleischl-Marxow, was reported to have been the first morphine addict "cured" by cocaine; unfortunately, Dr. von Fleischl-Marxow became perhaps the first cocaine addict in Europe.[1,2] Presently, cocaine has only limited clinical applications as a local anesthetic in primarily oral-related surgery.[3]

B. Cocaine Forms and Routes of Administration

1. Cocaine Hydrochloride

Cocaine hydrochloride is a fine, white powder. This compound can be administered intranasally (i.e., "snorted") in what are called "lines". A line of cocaine is approximately 20 to 30 mg of the substance, usually spread out in a 3- to 5-cm line. In addition to snorting, cocaine hydrochloride can be dissolved in water or saline and administered intravenously.

2. Cocaine Free Base

Another form of cocaine used on the street is cocaine "free base". The process of "freebasing" is undertaken to increase the volatility of the substance (cocaine hydrochloride is much less volatile than is the cocaine free base). Cocaine free base can be obtained through one of two methods. First, cocaine free base can be prepared by the user via an extraction through ether. This process involves heat and extremely volatile substances and can be very dangerous. A second form of cocaine free base is the so-called "crack" or "rock". This is cocaine which has been prepared by the dealer and sold to the user in the "free base" form.

Cocaine free base is administered by inhalation (i.e., smoked). Perhaps one of the reasons that cocaine free base has become so prevalent is based on pharmacokinetics. Intranasal administration ("snorting") of cocaine will result in a peak plasma concentration of roughly 150 to 200 ng/mℓ.[4] In contrast, it has been reported that cocaine administration via inhalation (smoking) can result in plasma concentrations of greater than 900 ng/mℓ.[4]

C. Cocaine-Heroin Drug Combinations — Speedballs

Cocaine is often taken in combination with other drugs. One very frequent combination is the so-called "speedball", which consists of cocaine plus heroin.[5-7] The use of speedballs is common among individuals who start out as heroin-only users or as cocaine-only users. The use of this combination can often result in a dual addiction. One reason for this combination of cocaine and heroin is that the cocaine seems to decrease the "nods" associated with heroin use, while the heroin takes the "edge" off the cocaine effect.[5,6]

The present paper will address the pharmacology and toxicology of cocaine from three perspectives: (1) acute effects, (2) "spree" use, and (3) long-term chronic administration.

II. COCAINE PHARMACOLOGY — ACUTE EFFECTS

A. Specific Pharmacological Actions of Cocaine

1. Blockage of Sodium Channels

Cocaine has two pharmacological actions in the body. The first is to block sodium channels in the membranes of excitable cells (e.g., neurons, muscles) within the body.[8-10] This blockade of sodium channels results in an inability of the cell to propagate action potentials to neighboring cells.[8-10]

2. Blockade of Catecholamine Reuptake

The second action of cocaine is to block the reuptake of the catecholamines dopamine and norepinephrine into presynaptic nerve terminals.[11,12] Since this active reuptake of catecholamines is the primary mechanism by which the effects of these neurotransmitters are terminated, this blockade of catecholamine reuptake results in an increase in norepinephrine and dopamine-mediated effects both in the brain and in the periphery.[11,12]

B. Cocaine Effects and the Mechanism(s) Behind the Effects

To date, all of the effects of cocaine have been attributed to either or both of the pharmacological actions described above. The various effects of cocaine in the body and the mechanisms behind those effects can be divided into effects in the periphery and effects in the central nervous system.

1. Effects in the Periphery

Local anesthetic effects — Cocaine has marked local anesthetic effects.[3,12] These effects are unquestionably the result of the blockade of sodium channels in axons, thus preventing the conduction of action potentials along these axons. This effect of cocaine on sodium channels is shared with lidocaine, procaine, and other local anesthetic agents.[3,10]

Localized ischemia — Cocaine also produces localized ischemia. This is due to localized vasoconstrictor actions resulting from the blockade of norepinephrine reuptake at sympathetic nerve terminals in the periphery.[3,13] Perforated nasal septum due to ischemic injury is a potential problem associated with the chronic intranasal use of cocaine,[14] although the frequency of this problem may be somewhat exaggerated.[15]

Cardiovascular effects — Cocaine also produces marked cardiovascular effects, both in terms of blood pressure and cardiac rhythm. Cocaine can markedly elevate blood pressure;[13,15-18] this effect is related to the norepinephrine reuptake-blocking effects of cocaine at sympathetic terminals in the vasculature in combination with the cardioacceleratory effects associated with increased catecholamines at sympathetic terminals in the heart.[13] Second, cocaine produces alterations in cardiac rhythm. These alterations in cardiac rhythm seem to be related to both the norepinephrine reuptake blockade and the sodium channel blockade. The norepinephrine reuptake blockade produces a Beta-1 sympathomimetic (cardioacceleratory) effect,[3,12] while the sodium channel blockade produces a "local anesthetic"-type effect similar to that seen with Class I anti-arrhythmic agents.[19] These arrhythmogenic effects of cocaine can be very deleterious, as evidenced by the so-called "cocaine cardiac" syndrome.

2. Effects in the Central Nervous System

Cocaine has marked effects in the central nervous system also. The noneuphoric effects appear to relate to the ability of cocaine to block the presynaptic reuptake of dopamine. The precise mechanism for the "euphoric" effects of cocaine is, unfortunately, less well understood.

Noneuphoric effects — Cocaine increases arousal and produces a marked hyperactivity.[5,12,20] These effects seem to be related to dopamine reuptake blockade.[20] Second, cocaine produces anorexia (i.e., decreased appetite); this effect also relates to dopamine reuptake blockade.[12,21] Finally, cocaine decreases plasma prolactin, an effect which is due to an increase in synaptic dopamine in the brain.[22] Thus, the arousal, hyperactivity, anorexia, and hypoprolactinemia all relate to the increased dopamine and/or norepinephrine in the brain.

Cocaine-induced "euphoria" — The last effect of cocaine which is mediated in the brain, perhaps its most important effect, is the *least well understood*. Cocaine produces marked euphoria; however, the mechanism for this euphoric effect is still not completely understood.

C. Cocaine Controversy — Mechanism for the Euphoria

There is still considerable controversy regarding the specific mechanism(s) by which cocaine produces its euphoric effects. This controversy stems primarily from the results of clinical studies examining the contribution of the catecholamine reuptake blockade effects vs. the sodium channel-blocking effects of cocaine. A number of studies have been conducted attempting to determine the mechanism behind the euphoric effects of cocaine. These studies have examined agents which share one, but not both, actions of cocaine. The two agents which have been used in these studies are *d*-amphetamine and lidocaine. *d*-Amphetamine was selected because it has a marked effect on catecholamines in the brain, but has no sodium channel-blocking (i.e., local anesthetic) effects. Lidocaine was selected because it has marked sodium channel-blocking (i.e., local anesthetic) effects, but has no effects on catecholamines. These two compounds have been compared with cocaine in human studies attempting to delineate the mechanism behind cocaine-induced "euphoria".

1. Cocaine High = Catecholamine Increase?

The first studies to be described were conducted by Marian Fischman and co-workers[17] at the University of Chicago and were first published in 1976. The hypothesis of the Fischman group was that the cocaine high was related to an increase in synaptic catecholamines (predominantly dopamine) in the brain. The rationale behind this hypothesis comes from the observation that *d*-amphetamine is a highly abused stimulant agent in its own right.[5,12,23] Moreover, *d*-amphetamine produces a number of noneuphoric effects similar to cocaine: hyperactivity, an increase in arousal, anorexia and peripheral sympathomimetic effects.[11-13]

Fischman and co-workers[4,17,24] conducted a study in which experienced cocaine users were administered either cocaine or *d*-amphetamine by the intravenous route in a double-blind manner. The subjects were asked to rate the "high" produced by these two treatments. These investigators reported that, for a brief period following injection, 16 mg of cocaine and 10 mg of *d*-amphetamine were rated as *identical* by experienced cocaine users.[17,24] Since the half-life of cocaine is much shorter than that of *d*-amphetamine, at later time intervals the subjects could distinguish the cocaine from the *d*-amphetamine.[24] These data support the hypothesis that cocaine-induced highs are related to a pharmacological action shared by both cocaine and *d*-amphetamine (i.e., increases in synaptic catecholamines).

2. Cocaine High = Local Anesthetic Effects?

An alternative to the catecholamine hypothesis is the so-called local anesthetic hypothesis for the euphoric effects of cocaine. This hypothesis has been supported most by the studies of Byck and colleagues[1,15] at Yale University. The rationale behind these studies is as follows: (1) procaine and lidocaine are often found in forensic analyses resulting from police arrests containing substances which were supposed to contain cocaine,[12,25] (2) nonhuman primates will self-administer procaine,[12] which has marked local anesthetic effects and minimal effects on catecholamines (this drug self-administration procedure, described earlier by Brown [see

Chapter 5] has been a very important research tool in predicting the euphoric and/or abuse potential of drugs),[26-28] and (3) lidocaine and/or procaine are frequently used without much objection by experienced cocaine users (cocaine addicts).

Byck and co-workers[1,15] conducted a series of studies comparing the effects of intranasally administered cocaine, lidocaine, and saline. These investigators tested experienced cocaine users in a double-blind procedure and administered either cocaine, lidocaine, or saline intranasally. The subjects were then asked to rate the "highs" associated with the various treatments. As expected, saline administered intranasally was perceived as having no effect. This did not surprise anyone. Consistent with Byck's hypothesis, these experienced cocaine users could not discriminate between the effects of intranasal cocaine or intranasal lidocaine, as both agents were reported to produce marked "highs" in these subjects.[29,30]

To summarize the studies on the so-called cocaine controversy, although there is evidence supporting a catecholamine hypothesis for the euphoric actions of cocaine, there is also evidence suggesting that perhaps some portion of the euphoria or high produced by cocaine is related to its sodium channel-blocking (i.e., local anesthetic) actions. It should be pointed out, however, that these two hypotheses are not mutually exclusive. Indeed, an hypothesis based on a dually mediated "euphoria" for cocaine might actually explain the intensity of the reward associated with cocaine administration.[31] Clearly, the complete answer to the question of how cocaine produces its euphoric effects must await the results of further research.

D. Acute Cocaine Intoxication: Cocaine "Body Packers"

Information regarding cocaine pharmacology and toxicology comes from numerous sources. Much of what is known about the pharmacological and toxicological effects of cocaine has come from animal studies. In addition, clinical reports have contributed greatly to what we know about the pharmacology and toxicology of cocaine. These clinical reports can be classified into two types. First, there are voluntary self-administration situations where either in a clinical laboratory or on the "street" an individual will take cocaine. As discussed above, clinical laboratory studies employing cocaine self-administration in man have been conducted in attempts to delineate the mechanism of action for the "euphoric" effects of cocaine. In addition to these situations of voluntary self-administration, there are recent reports of the phenomenon of cocaine "body packers" who will accidentally self-administer cocaine. Much of what is known about the most severe toxicological consequences of cocaine in man comes from reports relating to these cocaine "body packers".[25,56,57]

Cocaine can be smuggled into the U.S. in very small packages. One recently discovered route of smuggling is that of putting a small amount of cocaine in a sealed vessel (e.g., a balloon or perhaps a condom). Smugglers will often put between 3 to 6 g of fairly pure cocaine in a package. The individual will swallow the package(s) or insert them rectally, get on the airplane, and return to the U.S. Upon getting through the customs checkpoints, the smuggler will go to a rest room and expel the packages.

These cocaine "body packers" do not carry just one of these packages; they will smuggle mutiple containers of cocaine. (The maximum number reported by one author is 175 bags of cocaine.) This cocaine is quite pure, often between 85 to 90%. Based on the street value of cocaine, one can make the following calculations: if an individual takes in 100 bags of cocaine at 5 g per bag, that is close to 500 grams of cocaine at an approximate value of $30,000 per trip. Thus, there is a tremendous financial incentive motivating these "body packers".

Being a cocaine "body packer" is not without its hazards, however. If a package ruptures or if there is significant leakage from one of these smuggled packages, death is often not far behind. The progression from initial signs of acute toxicity to death is usually very rapid. The initial signs and symptoms observed are those normally seen in stimulant overdose:

hyperthermia, hypertension, tachycardia, and mydriasis, first, followed by acute agitation (sometimes considered delirium), followed by grand mal seizures and respiratory arrest. The last two are by far the most dangerous and are normally found to be the major determinants of death.

Treatment of these cocaine ''body packers'' requires multiple drug therapy. First, one must treat the seizures. This is usually done with diazepam or short-acting barbiturates.[56,58] Second, high doses of propranolol have been used to counteract the cardiac sympathomimetic effects of cocaine.[56] Finally, treatment with oxygen and/or sodium bicarbonate is employed to correct for metabolic and respiratory acidosis.[57,58]

III. COCAINE PHARMACOLOGY — SUBCHRONIC ADMINISTRATION (''SPREE'' USE)

Cocaine and other stimulants (e.g., *d*-amphetamine, methylphenidate) are often administered in what are called ''sprees'' or ''runs''.[5,12,32] This is a situation where an individual will administer a fairly high dose for a brief period of time. Often associated with this spree use of the drug is a phenomena called the ''stimulant-induced psychosis''. Another problem associated with the spree use of stimulants is that of convulsions and death from accidental overdose. A third potential problem associated with spree use of cocaine is the permanent loss of midbrain dopamine neurons. Finally, spree use of cocaine has been reported to be associated with the so-called ''cocaine crash''. The present section will address these four aspects of the subchronic administration of cocaine.

A. Stimulant-Induced Psychosis

The stimulant-induced psychosis is a syndrome which was initially linked to the spree use of *d*-amphetamine, with perhaps the most impressive reports from cross-country truck drivers and other individuals using stimulant agents to remain awake for prolonged periods of time. This syndrome consists of five principle components: (1) marked hyperactivity and stereotyped behavior patterns, (2) ''delusions of parasitosis'', (3) visual hallucinations, (4) a desire to tinker, and (5) aggressive and/or assaultive behaviors. It should be noted that this ''stimulant-induced psychosis'' is a problem associated only with the stimulant agents, specifically amphetamine, cocaine, and methampetamine. High doses of marijuana, hallucinogens, opiates, ethanol, or other sedative hypnotics do not produce this syndrome.

Sterotyped behaviors and hyperactivity — Stereotyped behavior patterns are associated with increases in dopamine neurotransmission in the nigrostriatal dopamine tract in the brain.[11,33] These stereotyped behaviors are repetitive motor activites like pacing and/or head bobbing. Although cocaine-induced stereotyped behaviors are of no real harm to the patient, they can serve to signal the onset of other more potentially harmful effects. Hyperactivity is also observed following the spree use of cocaine; this effect probably is the result of the dopamine reuptake-blocking actions of cocaine in the mesolimbic dopamine tracts.[34-36]

Delusions of parasitosis — Delusions of parasitosis are another very prominent aspect of the stimulant-induced psychosis associated with cocaine spree use. Individuals experiencing this aspect of the stimulant-induced psychosis will report the presence of ''bugs under my skin''.[5,12,32] In its most intense form, these individuals are so convinced of the existence of these ''cocaine bugs'' under their skin that they will use a knife and inflict wounds upon their body in attempt to dig out these bugs.[12] The precise mechanism behind the ''delusions of parasitosis'' has yet to be ascertained.

Visual hallucinations — Visual hallucinations are also a prominent part of the stimulant-induced psychosis. This has been referred to as the ''snow lights'' or the ''snow blindness'' when the stimulant agent is cocaine;[32] but these visual hallucinations also occur following the ''spree'' administration of amphetamine or methamphetamine.[12]

Desire to Tinker — Another hallmark of stimulant-induced psychosis associated with cocaine spree use is the "desire to tinker" or the fascination that a cocaine user will have with mechanical devices.[12] These individuals will often spend hours taking apart a mechanical device like a toaster or some other household appliance. (Of course, these individuals fully *intend* that they will put the appliance back together.)

Aggressive/assaultive behaviors — Perhaps one of the most severe problems associated with the stimulant-induced psychosis is the emergence of aggressive and/or assaultive behaviors associated with paranoid delusions and excitement.[12,37,38] These individuals can become very belligerent and can be dangerous either to themselves or the public. Angrist et al.[38] have reported that dopamine antagonists such as haloperidol can attenuate this aspect of the stimulant-induced psychosis, suggesting that a dopaminergic mechanism is involved.

B. Convulsions

In addition to the so-called stimulant-induced psychosis, cocaine spree use (or a high single dose for that matter) can be associated with the phenomena of stimulant-induced convulsions. As mentioned above in the section on cocaine "body packers", convulsions can occur following large doses of cocaine. These convulsions can lead to postictal respiratory depression and death if not treated. As indicated above, management of these convulsions usually is accomplished by the administration of benzodiazepines or barbiturates.

C. Permanent Loss of Midbrain Dopamine

In addition to the convulsant effects of high doses of cocaine, it has been shown in laboratory animals that high doses of cocaine or other stimulants can result in a permanent loss of midbrain dopamine.[39,40] This loss of midbrain dopamine can result in neuroendocrine dysfunction, such as hyperprolactinemia. This loss of midbrain dopamine has been proposed as being responsible for the phenomena of "cocaine cravings", which are discussed in the section on cocaine addiction (see Section IV.B).

D. "Cocaine "Crashes"

Cocaine crashes represent yet another problem associated with the spree use of cocaine. These cocaine crashes often occur between runs or sprees of cocaine and are characterized by irritability, a ravenous appetite, tiredness, excessive sleep, and an emotionally depressed state, possibly including suicidal ideation.[11,12] In a "typical" cocaine spree use pattern, an individual will have a run of cocaine, go into a crash, come back to normal, and then repeat this run-crash-normal cycle. There is anecdotal evidence that during a "crash" additional cocaine will not produce a euphoric effect. That is, once the crash phase has begun the cocaine addict cannot experience the euphoria, even if additional drug is administered. Good clinical studies investigating this observation are lacking, however.

A number of investigators have suggested these "cocaine crashes" are actually minor withdrawals associated with repeated cocaine use.[41-43] Other investigators, who define drug withdrawal as that behavioral and physiological state associated with the abrupt discontinuation following the *long term* administration of drug,[5] argue that the term withdrawal is not appropriate, since these cocaine crashes can be observed after less than 1 week of continuous cocaine.[12] Regardless of whether one views them as a form of cocaine withdrawal or not, there is little known regarding the neuropharmacological basis of these cocaine crashes. Again, this area is in need of additional clinical and animal research.

IV. COCAINE PHARMACOLOGY — TRUE CHRONIC ADMINISTRATION

A. Tolerance and Sensitization

Both tolerance and sensitization have been reported to occur following chronic cocaine administration. Tolerance is that process whereby the magnitude of the drug effect diminishes as a function of chronic administration, while sensitization is the process whereby the effect of the drug *increases* as a function of chronic administration.[5,12] Whether tolerance, sensitization, or no change in the response to cocaine occurs following its chronic administration depends upon the drug effect being measured as well as situational and experiential considerations.[12,44]

Tolerance has been reported to occur to the local anesthetic effects of cocaine.[45] There is also significant tolerance to the hypertensive effects of cocaine in chronic cocaine users.[12] There is less evidence for tolerance to the arrhythmogenic effects of cocaine. There is considerable tolerance to the anorexic effects of cocaine or any CNS stimulant agent used for appetite suppression.[12,46-49]

In contrast, chronic cocaine administration results in *sensitization* to the stimulant effects of the drug.[44,50-52] There are few definitive studies regarding possible tolerance to the effects of cocaine on generalized arousal and plasma prolactin concentrations. Lastly, there is evidence for at least moderate tolerance to the "euphoric" effects of cocaine.[5]

B. Cocaine Addiction

Addiction can be defined in terms of an overwhelming involvement with the procurement and use of a drug.[5] One term often considered to be synonomous with drug addiction is drug craving. Based upon this definition, cocaine is a powerfully addicting substance. The specific answer to the question, "Why is cocaine addicting?" is presently unknown. However, Gold and co-workers[41-43] at the Fair Oaks Clinic have postulated that the craving for cocaine and perhaps cocaine addiction itself is related to the loss of midbrain dopamine.

Neuroendocrine changes during cocaine cravings — As stated above, acute administration of cocaine often results in hypoprolactinemia due to increases in synaptic dopamine in the brain. Consistent with his hypothesis that dopamine depletion is a potential cause of cocaine cravings, Gold and collegues have reported that cocaine addicts exhibit elevated plasma prolactin during their cocaine cravings.[43]

Pharmacological manipulation of cocaine cravings — Gold has also reported that dopaminergic drugs can effect cocaine cravings. First, the dopamine agonist bromocriptine will reduce cocaine cravings.[41-43] Second, the dopamine receptor-blocking drug thioridazine will increase cocaine cravings.[43] These data are also consistent with the fact that cravings are related to an insufficiency in brain dopaminergic activity. Clearly, these interesting findings warrant additional research in both man and animals.

C. Cocaine Dependence and Withdrawal

Finally, we should consider the phenomena of cocaine dependence and withdrawal. Clearly, this is a very serious problem. However, it also quite true that there are only limited studies characterizing true cocaine dependence and withdrawal in man or in animals.[2,39,53,54] Again, there is a need for considerable additional research in this area.

V. SUMMARY AND CONCLUSIONS — UNANSWERED QUESTIONS

The present paper can be summarized most effectively in terms of the unanswered questions it has posed regarding cocaine. First, the mechanism behind the "euphoric" actions of cocaine is still not specifically identified or delineated. Once the mechanism behind the euphoric effects of cocaine can be identified, perhaps selective antagonists can be developed and applied and we might be able to pharmacologically manipulate cocaine problems. A second question that remains unanswered is, Why is cocaine so addictive? Of course, this question is much broader than just cocaine. If we knew why any drug was addicting we'd probably have the answer for cocaine and many other drugs. There is hope for an answer soon, however, as indicated in Brown's chapter regarding the possible role of dopamine in the general process of addiction (Chapter 5). The third question which needs to be answered concerns the specific nature and consequences of cocaine withdrawal. Very few studies in man or animals have specifically identified the nature and/or consequences of the long-term chronic administration of cocaine.

REFERENCES

1. **Byck, R., Ed.,** *Cocaine Papers: Sigmund Freud,* Stonehill Publishing, New York, 1974.
2. **Petersen, R. and Stilman, R.,** Cocaine: An overview, in Cocaine: 1977, Petersen, R. and Stillman, R., Eds., DHEW Publ. No. (ADM) 77-471, National Institute on Drug Abuse. Department of Health, Education and Welfare, Washington, D.C., 1977.
3. **Ritchie, J. M. and Greene, N. M.,** Local anesthetics, in *The Pharmacological Basis of Therapeutics,* Goodman, A. G., Goodman, L. S., Rall, T. W., and Murad, F., Eds., Macmillan, New York, 1985.
4. **Fischman, M.,** The behavioral pharmacology of cocaine in humans, in Cocaine: Pharmacology, Effects and Treatment of Abuse, Grabowski, J., Ed., National Institute on Drug Abuse Research Monogr. Ser., DHHS Publ. No. (ADM) 84-1326, Department of Health and Human Services, Washington, D.C., 1984.
5. **Cox, T., Jacobs, M., LeBlanc, A., and Marshman, J., Eds.,** Drugs and Drug Abuse: A Reference Text, *Addiction Research Foundation Press,* Toronto, 1983.
6. **Smith, D. and Wesson, D.,** Cocaine, *J. Psychedelic Drugs,* 10, 351, 1978.
7. **Nakamura, G. and Noguchi, T.,** Fatalities from cocaine overdose in Los Angeles County, *Clin. Toxicol.,* 18, 895, 1981.
8. **Hille, B.,** Common mode of action of three agents that decrease the transient change in sodium permeability in nerves, *Nature (London),* 210, 1220, 1966.
9. **Hille, B.,** Local anesthetics: hydrophilic and hydrophobic pathways for the drug-receptor reaction, *J. Gen. Physiol.,* 69, 497, 1977.
10. **Matthews, J. and Collins, A.,** Interactions of cocaine and cocaine congeners with sodium channels, *Biochem. Pharmacol.,* 32, 455, 1983.
11. **Cooper, J., Bloom, F., and Roth, R.,** *The Biochemical Basis of Neuropharmacology,* Oxford University Press, New York, 1975.
12. **Jaffe, J.,** Drug addiction and drug abuse, in *The Pharmacological Basis of Therapeutics,* Goodman, A. G., Goodman, L. S., Rall, T. W., and Murad, F., Eds., Macmillan, New York, 1985.
13. **Weiner, N.,** Norepinephrine, epinephrine and the sympathomimetic amines, in *The Pharmacological Basis of Therapeutics,* Goodman, A. G., Goodman, L. S., Rall, T. W., and Murad, F., Eds., Macmillan, New York, 1985.
14. **Messinger, E.,** Narcotic septal perforations due to drug addiction, *JAMA,* 179, 964, 1962.
15. **Byck R. and VanDyke, C.,** What are the effects of cocaine in man?, in cocaine: 1977, Petersen, R. and Stillman, R., Eds., DHEW Publ. No. (ADM) 77-471, National Institute on Drug Abuse, Department of Health, Education and Welfare, Washington, D.C., 1977.
16. **Post, R., Kotin, J. and Goodwin, F.,** The effects of cocaine on depressed patients, *Am. J. Psychiatry,* 131(5), 511, 1974.
17. **Fischman, M., Schuster, C., Resenekov, L., Shick, J., Krasnegor, N., Fennel, W., and Freedman, D.,** Cardiovascular and subjective effects of intravenous cocaine in humans, *Arch. Gen. Psychiatry,* 33, 983, 1976.
18. **Resnick, J., Kestenbaum, R., and Schwartz, L.,** Acute systemic effects of cocaine in man: a controlled study by intranasal and intravenous routes, *Science,* 195, 696, 1977.
19. **Bigger, J. T. and Hoffman, B. F.,** Antiarrhythmic drugs, in *The Pharmacological Basis of Therapeutics,* Goodman, A. G., Goodman, L. S., Rall, T. W., and Murad, F., Eds., Macmillan, New York, 1985.
20. **Scheel-Kruger, J., Braestrup, C., Nielson, M., Golembiowska, K., and Mogilnicka, E.,** Cocaine: discussion on the role of dopamine in the biochemical mechanism of action, in *Cocaine and Other Stimulants,* Ellinwood, E. and Kilbey, M., Eds., Plenum Press, New York, 1976.
21. **Zigmund, M., Heffner, T., and Stricker, E.,** The effect of altered dopaminergic activity on food intake in the rat: evidence for an optimal level of dopaminergic activity for behavior, *Prog. Neuropsychopharmacol.,* 4, 351, 1980.

22. **Murad, F. and Haynes, R.,** Hormones and hormone antagonists, in *The Pharmacological Basis of Therapeutics,* Goodman, A. G., Goodman, L. S., Rall, T. W., and Murad, F., Eds., Macmillan, New York, 1985.

23. **Ellinwood, E. and Kilbey, M., Eds.,** *Cocaine and Other Stimulants,* Plenum Press, New York, 1976.

24. **Fischman, M. and Schuster, C.,** Cocaine self-administration in humans, *Fed. Proc. Fed. Am. Soc. Exp. Biol.,* 41, 241, 1982.

25. **Wetli, C. and Fishbain, D.,** Cocaine-induced psychosis and sudden death in recreational cocaine users, *J. Forensic Sci.,* 30, 873, 1985.

26. **Deneau, G., Yanagita, T., and Seevers, M.,** Self-administration of psychoactive substances by the monkey — a measure of psychological dependence, *Psychopharmacologia,* 16, 30, 1969.

27. **Schuster, C. and Thompson, T.,** Self-administration of and behavioral dependence on drugs, *Annu. Rev. Pharmacol.,* 9, 483, 1969.

28. **Griffiths, R., Brady, J., and Bradford, L.,** Predicting the abuse liability of drugs with animal drug self-administration procedures: psychomotor stimulants and hallucinogens, in, *Advances in Behavioral Pharmacology,* Thompson, T. and Dews, P., Eds., Academic Press, New York, 1978.

29. **Van Dyke, C., Jatlow, P., Ungerer, J., Barash, P., and Byck, R.,** Cocaine and lidocaine have similar psychological effects after intranasal application, *Life Sci.,* 24, 271, 1979.

30. **Van Dyke, C., Ungerer, J., Jatlow, P., Barash, P., and Byck, R.,** Intranasal cocaine: dose relationships of psychological effects and plasma levels, *Int. J. Psychiatr. Med.,* 12, 1, 1982.

31. **Ainger, T. and Balster, R.,** Choice behavior in Rhesus monkeys: Cocaine versus food, *Science,* 201, 534, 1978.

32. **Siegel, R.,** Cocaine hallucinations, *Am. J. Psychiatry,* 135, 309, 1978.

33. **Ernst, A. and Smilek, P.,** Site of action of dopamine and apomorphine on compulsive gnawing behavior, *Experientia,* 22, 837, 1966.

34. **Pijnenburg, A., Honig, W., Van der Heyden, J., and VanRossum, J.,** Inhibition of d-amphetamine-induced locomotor activity by injection of haloperidol into the nucleus accumbens of the rat, *Psychopharmacologia,* 41, 87, 1975.

35. **Pijnenburg, A., Honig, W., Van der Heyden, J., and Van Rossum, J.,** Effects of chemical stimulation of the mesolimbic dopamine system upon locomotor activity, *Eur. J. Pharmacol.,* 35, 45, 1976.

36. **Kelly, P. and Iversen, S.,** Selective 6-OHDA-induced destruction of mesolimbic dopamine neurons: abolition of psychostimulant-induced locomotor activity in rats, *Eur. J. Pharmacol.,* 40, 45, 1976.

37. **Post, R.,** Cocaine psychoses: a continuum model, *Am. J. Psychiatry,* 132, 225, 1975.

38. **Angrist, B., Sathananthan, G., Wilk, S., and Gershon, S.,** Amphetamine psychosis: behavioral and biochemical aspects, *J. Psychiatr. Res.,* 8, 13, 1974.

39. **Ellinwood, E.,** Amphetamines/anorectics, in Handbook on Drug Abuse, Dupont, R., Goldstein, A., and O'Donnell, J., Eds., National Institute on Drug Abuse, U.S. Government Printing Office, Washington, D.C., 1979.

40. **Seiden, L. and Vosmer, G.,** Formation of 6-hydroxydopamine in caudate nucleus of the rat brain after a single large dose of methylamphetamine, *Pharmacol. Biochem. Behav.,* 21, 29, 1984.

41. **Gold, M. and Dackis, C.,** Bromocriptine as a treatment of cocaine abuse, *Lancet,* May 18, 1985.

42. **Gold, M. and Dackis, C.,** Dopamine deficiency with chronic cocaine abuse: bromocriptine reverses cocaine withdrawal, *Neurosci. Abstr.,* 11(7), 6, 1985.

43. **Gold, M. and Dackis, C.,** Bromocriptine treatment for cocaine abuse: the dopamine depletion hypothesis, *Int. J. Psychiatry Intern. Med.,* 15(2), 125, 1985.

44. **Kilbey, M. and Ellinwood, E.,** Chronic administration of stimulants: Response modification, in *Cocaine and Other Stimulants,* Ellinwood, E. and Kilbey, M., Eds., Plenum Press, New York, 1976.

45. **Castellani, S., Ellinwood, E., and Kilbey, M.,** Behavioral analysis of chronic cocaine intoxication in the cat, *Biol. Psychiatry,* 13, 203, 1978.

46. **Wolgin, D.,** Tolerance to amphetamine anorexia: role of learning versus body weight settling point, *Behav. Neurosci.,* 97, 549, 1983.

47. **Panskepp, J. and Booth, D.,** Tolerance in the depression of food intake when amphetamine is added to the rat's food, *Psychopharmacologia,* 29, 45, 1973.

48. **Poulos, C., Wilkinson, D., and Cappell, H.,** Homeostatic regulation and Pavlovian conditioning in tolerance to amphetamine-induced anorexia, *J. Comp. Physiol. Psychol.,* 95, 735, 1981.

49. **Woolverton, W., Kandel, D., and Schuster, R.,** Tolerance and cross-tolerance to cocaine and d-amphetamine, *J. Pharmacol. Exp. Ther.,* 205, 525, 1978.

50. **Tatum, A. and Seevers, M.,** Experimental cocaine addiction, *J. Pharmacol. Exp. Ther.,* 36, 401, 1929.

51. **Downs, A. and Eddy, N.,** The effect of repeated doses of cocaine in the rat, *J. Pharmacol. Exp. Ther.,* 46, 199, 1932.

52. **Stripling, J. and Ellinwood, E.,** Cocaine: physiological and behavioral effects of acute and chronic administration, in *Cocaine: Chemical, Biological, Clinical, Social, and Treatment Aspects,* Mule, S., Ed., CRC Press, Boca Raton, Fla., 1976.

53. **Kleber, H. and Gawan, F.,** Cocaine abuse: a review of current and experimental treatments, in *Cocaine: Pharmacology, Effects and Treatment of Abuse,* Grabowski, J., Ed., National Institute on Drug Abuse Mongr. Ser., DHHS Publ. No. (ADM) 84-1326, Department of Health and Human Services, Washington, D.C., 1984.

54. **Tomasello, T.,** Cocaine dependence and treatment: the pharmacological aspects, *Pharmalert,* 15, 1, 1984.

55. **Woods, J. H. and Downs, D. A.,** The psychopharmacology of cocaine, in Drug Use in America: Problem in Perspective, U.S. Government Printing Office Washington, D.C., 1973, 116.

56. **Fishbain, D. E. and Wetli, C. V.,** Cocaine intoxication, delerium and death in a body packer, *Ann. Emergency Med.,* 10(10), 531, 1981.

57. **McCarron, M. M. and Wood, J. D.,** The cocaine ''body packer'' syndrome, *JAMA,* 250(11), 1417, 1983.

58. **Jonsson, S., O'Meara, M., and Young, J. B.,** Acute cocaine poisoning, *Am. J. Med.,* 75(12), 1061, 1983.

Chapter 8

COCAINE USE IN MAN: SUBJECTIVE EFFECTS, PHYSIOLOGIC RESPONSES, AND TOXICITY

Karen M. Kumor, Michael A. Sherer, and Nicola G. Cascella

TABLE OF CONTENTS

I. PATTERNS OF COCAINE USE

In the U.S., the principle methods of self-administration of cocaine are smoking, intranasal snorting, and intravenous injection. Resnick and Schuyten-Resnick have described five patterns of cocaine using behavior: experimental (short-termed and without pattern), recreational (use in social settings with friends), circumstantial (use for a special purpose), intensified (daily use), and compulsive (high frequency and intensity).[1] These patterns of use can be found among users adhering to each route of cocaine administration, intranasal, smoking, and injection. Thus, serious dependence can be supported by intranasal as well as intravenous and smoking use.

The customs of drug self-administration are related to the pattern of cocaine use. Experimental, recreational, and circumstantial users tend to buy small amounts of cocaine, use it, and then stop or seek more drug. Intensified and compulsive users generally buy a cache of drug and use it by self-administering the drug at short intervals estimated to range between 2 and 60 min until the drug is gone. The interval appears to be determined by the route of administration. Smokers and intravenous users dose themselves at shorter intervals than intranasal users. These bouts or binging episodes may last from a few minutes to days and the amount of drug used may amount to several grams. Bingers report that they stop only when they run out of money or drug, become paranoid, experience fearful dysphoric feelings, or become exhausted. During binges, alcohol, marijuana, and other drugs are frequently used to self-treat the excessive stimulation induced by cocaine.[2]

The longitudinal patterns of use have been studied by Seigel who followed a group of social-recreational intranasal cocaine users (1 g/month) for 9 years.[3] In the study, 50% (25/50) of the subjects still enrolled in the study at 9 years remained social-recreational users, but 32% (16/50) became circumstantial-stituational users, 8% (4/50) became intensified users, and 10% (5/50) became compulsive users. The subjects who became compulsive users had all become free base smokers. These statistics give credence to the view that cocaine is a highly addictive substance and that smoking free base is particularly addicting. Furthermore, the compulsive free base smokers developed a paranoid profile with features of depression, impulsiveness, easy frustration, poor social adjustment, and sleep disturbances. Siegel also reported that all forms of chronic cocaine use were associated with increasingly negative (dysphoric) drug effects. Although many subjects were lost to follow-up, these findings suggest that long-term compulsive use is associated with decrements in mental well being. As is the case with other drugs of abuse, it is not certain if the association is one of cause and effect.

II. SUBJECTIVE EXPERIENCE

A. Euphoria

The use of cocaine is associated with sensations that are experienced as pleasurable or euphoric. All drugs of abuse have this characteristic that can be measured with self-report techniques in at least some segment of the general population. The psychopharmacologic effects of cocaine that reward drug-seeking behavior are necessary elements in the development of addictive behavior.

There are some differences in the subjective experience depending on the route of administration. Generally, cocaine users state that they take cocaine to get "high". This pleasurable state of altered sensation is evident in the moments after cocaine use, and persists for a periods up to several hours. In addition, users report a euphoric but distinct sensation often termed "rush", an intensely pleasurable sensation that is sometimes likened to a sexual orgasm. Unlike the cocaine "high", however, cocaine "rush" dissipates rapidly.[4-6] Addicts who have experienced cocaine by snorting, smoking, and injecting, report that snorting produces little or no sensation of rush, although they do experience the "high" feelings. Injecting or smoking free base generates a "rush" which these users describe as the most desirable effect of cocaine. This probably explains the fact that the more serious patterns of drug abuse are associated with smoking free base and intravenous injection. At the current time, it is unclear whether cocaine high and rush represent different intensities generated from the same electrochemical brain events, or separate feeling states emanating from different root occurrences.

A problem arising from the study of self-reported feelings and drug culture language is a lack of specificity. Thus, although rush appears to have a generally accepted meaning among cocaine users, this same word is used to express the initial pleasurable sensation experienced after injecting heroin.[6] However, users who have experience with both heroin and cocaine insist that the rush of the two drugs is entirely different. Some even express that they are opposite sensations. A cocaine-induced rush is described as exciting and "up"; the heroin-induced rush is described as down, mellow, and relaxing.

1. Tolerance

Pharmacologic tolerance seems to be an important determinant of the subjective response to cocaine. Early studies of the acute subjective and physiologic responses after a slow intravenous injection of cocaine reported that the drug high or euphoria and heart rate fell faster than the serum concentration of cocaine.[7-9] This was interpreted as evidence of acute tolerance or homeostatic mechanisms. In another study, responses to slow intravenous injections of cocaine were diminished after a pharmacologically active intranasal dose of cocaine as compared to a small subthreshold dose of intranasal cocaine.[10] The hypothesis of acute tolerance to the subjective and physiologic responses of cocaine was studied by Kumor et al.,[11] in a double-blind randomized study of 7 subjects which employed bolus loading doses of cocaine, 40, 60, and 80 mg, followed by steady-state infusions of cocaine or placebo. During the period of cocaine plasma concentration plateau between 12 and 240 min of active cocaine infusions, most subjective and physiologic measures demonstrated robust increases from baseline that were sustained without decline. Conditions in which bolus doses of cocaine were followed by placebo infusions did not demonstrate sustained responses. Instead, the responses declined to baseline over several hours. Thus, this study failed to demonstrate clinically important tolerance to most subjective and physiologic responses to cocaine including heart rate and blood pressure and self-rated good, energetic, and anxious feelings. "Rush" was an exception to this pattern. The magnitude, time course, and duration of "rush" was completely unaltered by a continuous infusion of cocaine following the injection of drug as compared with a placebo infusion following the injection. Thus, "rush" alone demonstrated an apparent refractory period or acute tolerance.

We have studied the apparent tolerance to "rush" in a study of paired injections of 30-mg doses of cocaine. When the interval between two doses was 70 min, we found that rush was greatly diminished following the second dose. This was not true for ratings of cocaine "high" (as measured with self-reports of good and energetic feelings), and cardiovascular responses, which were not different from the first injection. However, when the interval between doses was increased to 3 hr, the effects following the second injection were similar to those which followed the first injection. Thus, like the infusion experiments, the repeated dosing experiments demonstrated tolerance to "rush", but not to other sensations associated with cocaine.

2. Sensitization

Sensitization, or reverse tolerance, is the process of augmented or enhanced response with repeated or continued exposure to a drug. A number of the effects of central stimulants have shown such a pattern of response, including locomotor activity and stereotypy (for review, see Post[12]).

The principle behavioral toxicity of cocaine and other central stimulants is the clinical syndrome resembling paranoid schizophrenia with or without a clear sensorium which is observed after prolonged or repeated use.[12,13] During our 4-hr infusions of cocaine, but not following single doses of cocaine, variable degrees of suspiciousness were noted, occasionally to the point of paranoia.[14] Preceding the development of paranoia, most subjects reported dysphoric and anhedonic sensations; sensory disturbances were common, and a number of subjects experienced both visual and auditory illusions. In a number of cases, there may have been hallucinations. Two of the eight subjects experienced disturbances in reality testing during the latter phases of the infusion, with one subject developing both persecutory and nonpersecutory paranoid delusions.

We were particularly interested in examining factors antecedent to the development of suspiciousness. There was no close correlation between the plasma cocaine concentrations during the cocaine infusions and the amount of suspiciousness noted by nurse observers. Similarly, we did not note an association between subjects reported drug or psychiatric history and propensity to experience paranoid behavior during the infusions. However, the amount of cocaine that subjects had received during the study on our ward prior to receiving the 40-mg injection with subsequent cocaine infusion was significantly related to the severity of the reaction that day. Additionally, once suspiciousness had been noted, reactions on subsequent cocaine infusion exposures were invariably scored as increased in suspiciousness. Clinical observations of similar phenomena have lead several authors to suggest that the suspiciousness which develops during the course of stimulant abuse may represent a form of behavioral sensitization to the effects of the drug.[12,15]

Possible biologic mechanisms underlying the induction of sensitization to the effects of cocaine remain poorly understood. The main biochemical effect of cocaine is on receptor-mediated transmitter reuptake in noradrenergic and dopaminergic neurons. Chronic, or even brief, exposure of receptors to cocaine can result in changes in both the number of available receptors, as well as the binding characteristics of these receptors. Cocaine has been shown to induce a number of changes in receptor sensitivity. Banergee et al.[16,17] reported in animal studies that cocaine, but not amphetamine, can induce alterations in beta adrenergic sensitivity following acute and chronic exposure to the drug. Under certain circumstances, the induced changes may persist for a period of weeks.[18] In recent years particular attention has been paid to presynaptic inhibitory receptors in the adrenergic and dopaminergic systems. These receptors are part of inhibitory feedback systems, and desensitization of these receptors results in enhanced transmitter release and enhanced responses. Although uptake inhibitors such as cocaine do not effect these receptors directly, a number of studies have shown that treatment with uptake blockers does alter subsequent responses of drugs which do act at these sites.[19,20] Finally, it is known that biochemical effects vary among brain areas, with sensitization developing in some but not other dopaminergic pathways. It is possible that changes in the functional balance between these various receptors could account for changes in the effects of cocaine over time, including behavioral sensitization. Although the specific mechanisms underlying sensitization are not well understood, a variety of biological mechanisms have now been demonstrated which could account for sensitization.[12]

B. Craving

Free base smokers and intravenous users of cocaine consistently report that following a dose of cocaine subsequent to the "rush", they experience a craving for more drug. Binging episodes of repeatedly administering the drug may be intimately related to these sensations. Although the concept of drug craving is frequently discussed, there has been very little experimental validation of this concept. Some 10 years ago, Ludwig and Wikler reviewed this subject and discussed the concepts of "irresistable desire", "overpowering urge", "needs", "appetite", and "psychological dependence".[21]

In general terms, factors contributing to continued drug-seeking behavior can include both environmental (exteroceptive) variables, and internal (enteroceptive) drives, some of which may be induced by the abused drug. Examples of environmental stimuli which have been demonstrated to increase drug-seeking behavior have included the setting in which previous abuse has occurred,[22-24] drug paraphernalia, and preparatory activities associated with prior drug use.[25-33] Enteroceptive cues that have been related to drug-seeking behavior have included various mood states[33] and the stimulus properties of the abused drug.[34-36]

In addition, clinical reports and laboratory experimentation indicate that the desire to continue using cocaine is greatest in the moments following cocaine use and several weeks after discontinuation.[37] These findings raise the possibility that craving may be induced either by the drug itself or as part of the withdrawal phenomenon.

Recently, we have studied the role of direct (enteroceptive) stimulation in the genesis of craving for cocaine. We studied nine subjects, aged 21 to 35, who received intravenously 40 mg of cocaine or placebo under double-blind conditions.[38] Subjects were asked about both their *desire* for the drug and their *need* for the drug. As surmised from clinical reports, administration of cocaine not only failed to satiate drug craving, but served to increase the amount of craving reported.

The evidence of earlier studies and our own studies taken together support the idea that subjective responses are complex and probably determined by strong conditioned and pharmacological components. They may offer an explanation of how binging behavior associated with smoking or injecting drug is molded. The feelings of craving become intense after the ''rush'' wanes. The user hungrily attempts to repeat that first ''rush'' sensation by dosing again, but is disappointed because the intensity of ''rush'' declines with repeated injection. Yet, the desire for drug rush is sustained, and more injections follow.

The neurochemistry of drug-induced craving, specifically the role of dopaminergic transmission, is the subject of much active inquiry. Dackis and Gold have recently proposed treatment of addiction with noneuphorigenic dopaminergic agonists.[39] The same authors have suggested the effectiveness of bromocriptine in the treatment of craving, while others have reported success in reducing craving with amantadine.[40] We gave cocaine users oral pretreatment with bromocriptine or placebo 2 hr prior to the administration of cocaine or placebo. Bromocriptine did not reduce basal cocaine craving in a laboratory setting. Bromocriptine did, however, significantly attenuate cocaine-induced increases in desire and need for cocaine. Since we administered cocaine under double-blind conditions, we believe we were able to isolate the contributions to cocaine ''wanting'' and ''craving'' which originated from internal or drug-induced cues. The increases in ratings of cocaine craving appear related to the actions or stimulus properties of the administered cocaine. This finding is consistent with a large body of literature in animals demonstrating that once an animal is familiar with cocaine, further drug administration can play a major role in reinstituting drug-seeking behavior which has been previously extinguished. In a prototypic study, deWit and Stewart demonstrated that once cocaine administration had reinforced particular behavioral repertoires, subsequent administration of cocaine — even in low doses, in noncontingent circumstances, and following extinction trials, led to rapid and sustained increases in the index behaviors.[41] This phenomenon is not limited, however, to cocaine. Similar processes have been demonstrated following administration of other abused drugs.[42,43]

Our findings do partially support the hypothesis of a dopaminergic component to cocaine craving. Dackis and Gold, and Gold and Dackis have articulated most fully the possible roles of dopamine in the pathogenesis of cocaine-induced craving.[44,45] In their speculation, they have noted that chronic abuse of cocaine leads to a functional depletion of dopamine; decreased levels of brain dopamine have indeed been noted in animals following repeated administration of cocaine.[46] Increases in dopaminergic receptor binding have also been reported following administration of cocaine.[47-49] There is frequently a reciprocal relationship between basal level of a neurotransmitter and the corresponding receptor binding. Thus, these increases can be seen as partial evidence for alterations in basal dopaminergic levels. The observations by Dackis and Gold[50] of pseudo-Parkinsonism in regular cocaine users, and our own observation of an increased frequency of dystonia following haloperidol among cocaine users,[51] provide indirect evidence for alterations in basal dopaminergic function during the course of chronic cocaine abuse. Conceivably, a functional hypodopaminergic state among chronic users could predispose to the occurrence of such dystonic reactions.

However, the attenuation of cocaine-induced craving by acute doses of bromocriptine does not necessitate a specific dopaminergic mechanism. It is possible that the experience of bromocriptine pretreatment and cocaine is sufficiently different from cocaine alone as to disrupt conditioned cocaine "cueing", without this process having any pharmacological specificity. Although it is possible that side effects of bromocriptine, including nausea, vomiting, headache, and general malaise, may have caused reduced desire for cocaine, subjects did not report dysphoric sensations on questionnaires. In general terms, our findings are consistent with previous clinical reports on the effect of bromocriptine on chronic and environmentally evoked craving for cocaine.

III. PATHOPHYSIOLOGY OF COCAINE POISONING

A. Cardiovascular

In recent years, the incidence of serious cocaine poisoning has been increasing.[52] This is related to the increase in cocaine use and probably the increase in intravenous and free base use. There have been numerous reports of self-administered cocaine poisoning. Principally, there appear to be two common syndromes of serious cocaine toxicity: cardiovascular and central nervous system. The cardiovascular toxicity appears to involve myocardial ischemia, and there are several reports of myocardial infarctions in young persons who used cocaine close to the time of infarction.[53-62] Some of these individuals were demonstrated to have normal coronary vasculature by coronary arteriography.[54,59,62] This suggests that the pathophysiology of the infarction is related to coronary spasm. This theory is supported by the autopsy report of a 21-year-old cocaine user who had experienced nausea and chest pain within a minute of his second cocaine injection.[57] Within an hour he was *in extremis* and died before reaching the hospital. At autopsy, he was found to have severe chronic intimal proliferation of the coronary arteries and multiple acute platelet thrombi. Additionally, subendocardial fibrosis, granulation tissue, and myocyte contraction bands (which are indicative of acute myocardial ischemia) were present. The authors propose that cocaine-induced coronary artery spasm caused focal endothelial injury and favored platelet adherence and aggregation which resulted in death. Chronic platelet thrombosis causes intimal proliferation which in turn is implicated as increasing the risk of further platelet thrombosis.[63] The importance of the chronicity of the process implies that the risk to the cocaine user of myocardial ischemic heart disease increases with the duration of the cocaine abuse and the experienced abuser may be at greater risk than the novice.

Arrhythmias are often reported in cases of cocaine toxicity. It appears they are most often secondary to myocardial infarction or the ischemia and acidosis caused by seizure activity and hypoventilation. There exist few reports of arrhythmia without associated seizures, coma, or myocardial ischemia.[64,65] From our own practice we have seen one case of a man who had bigeminy on a routine electrocardiogram obtained for admission to our research ward. He gave a history of having injected cocaine just prior to appearing for his admission appointment. He was in no distress and there were no ischemic changes on his electrocardiogram. The bigeminy resolved after several hours and he was released after a normal electrocardiogram was obtained. We have also observed a case of a 25-year-old man who developed a high frequency of premature junctional beats (>20/min), sometimes occurring in pairs or triplets, after a 20-mg injection of cocaine administered as part of a research protocol. The dysarrhythmia lasted for several hours before resolving. It is unclear how these arrhythmias relate to serious cocaine toxicity, but they are consistent with the widely held opinion that cocaine can cause primary arrhythmias.

B. Central Nervous System

The CNS toxicity of cocaine has both psychiatric and neurologic manifestations. Many, perhaps most, fatal cocaine poisonings reported involve central nervous system dysfunction. Patients may experience paranoia including auditory, visual, or olfactory hallucinations. Generally, cocaine-induced hallucinations occur in the presence of a clear sensorium in contradistinction to the confusion and disorientation that accompanies a toxic psychosis. The paranoia may cause violent or dangerous behavior and may be a prodrome to seizures and coma. Sander reported several cases of paranoid behavior, followed by a quiet period of behavior, and then convulsions which quickly resulted in death.[66]

The convulsions can appear between 30 min to several hours after the last dose of cocaine, and cases of cocaine-induced neurotoxicity can involve intravenous and intranasal routes of administration. It is puzzling that the fatal consequences of cocaine administration can be delayed after peak plasma concentrations have been achieved.[67] This may be due to toxic metabolites, but none have been identified. Other possibilities exist, such as neurological sensitization or the accumulation of cocaine into a critical anatomical area during the elimination phase.[68]

The seizures induced by cocaine can cause acidosis, which is important in the pathophysiology of cardiac dysfunction. Catravas and Waters in an interesting set of experiments in conscious dogs found that hyperthermia and acidosis were related causally with a fatal outcome for cocaine poisoning in the animals.[69] Chlorpromazine and diazepam were found to counteract the hyperthermia in the dogs probably as a result of the sedative and anticonvulsant properties of these drugs at the doses used. In the same experiments, propranolol was determined to be without benefit despite counteracting the increases in heart rate and blood pressure induced by cocaine. Although some authors have suggested propranolol treatment for cocaine toxicity,[70] there is a report of propranolol-induced hypertension in a case of cocaine overdose.[71] This case has engendered controversy about the role of beta blockers for cocaine intoxication.[72] There is evidence that calcium channel blockers are beneficial in a rat model of cocaine toxicity.[73]

Other kinds of cocaine-related medical complications have been reported. These include cerebral vascular accidents both in adults and infants of cocaine-using mothers, aortic rupture, infection, abruption placentae, and intestinal ischemia.[74] Free base smoking has been associated with pneumomediastinum, pneumopericardium, decreased exchange capacity, and pulmonary edema.[74]

Altogether there is a paucity of knowledge about the pathophysiology of cocaine toxicity and optimal methods of treatment of cocaine overdose. Published information is based on case reports and the clinical experience of physicians committed to the care of drug abusers. Based on the evidence available, it is probable that prevention and treatment of acidosis is of great importance in cocaine poisoning. Hyperthermia, while important in dogs, does not seem to be a frequent feature of human cocaine posioning, although its presence requires immediate attention and treatment.[75] Since cocaine psychosis may precede the fatal consequences of the drug, psychosis should be treated as a sign of grave toxicity. It seems justified based on medical case reports and animal studies that such patients be treated with chlorpromazine and/or diazepam both as treatment for psychosis and agitation as well as for prevention of seizures. There is a consensus that diazepam is the drug of choice for cocaine-induced seizure activity. Furthermore, at the present time the available evidence supports the use of calcium channel blockers in the treatment of myocardial spasm and arrhythmias caused by cocaine.

C. Toxicity and Plasma Concentrations

The range of cocaine blood concentrations associated with fatal cocaine poisoning is difficult to establish for several reasons. First, cocaine may be incidental in many cases of accidental death or deaths where multiple drugs were involved and the causative role the drug held in the death was difficult to judge. Even the exclusion of these cases does not much improve estimates of the fatal concentrations because cocaine is metabolized in blood vessels by serum esterases as well as by the liver. Thus, it can be metabolized in the blood even when the circulation has stopped. The time the sample is taken after death is rarely reported,[57] and the time between the last dose of cocaine prior to death is usually unknown. These unknown time-related factors tend to underestimate, probably grossly, the peak plasma concentration which was associated with fatality. Lastly, there is some concern among investigators that there exist unaccountable differences in assay results between laboratories and even within the same laboratory.[76,77] These kinds of technical problems have been a continuing focus of investigation in laboratory medicine for drugs of abuse, and cocaine is no exception.[78]

It is possible that cocaine toxicity is related both to plasma concentration and the duration of the acute exposure. Increasing susceptibility to convulsions and progressively stereotypic behavior have been observed in animals chronically treated with once-daily injections of cocaine.[79,80] Although the once-daily injection research design is unlike human binging behavior, it raises the possibility that duration of acute exposure may be an important element in toxicity.

Another element contributing to toxicity of cocaine is the nonlinearity of cocaine kinetics. Barnett et al. first reported this in their study of intravenous injections of cocaine.[81] In our studies of cocaine continuous infusions, we observed that the cocaine clearance decreased in six of seven subjects at the higher dose. For drugs with linear kinetics, the drug half-life is a constant. Drugs with nonlinear kinetics have a half-life that varies as a nonlinear function of the drug concentration. In this case, the more drug that is accumulated, the longer the half-life, which in turn causes further accumulation on repeated dosing. This process can easily result in very large plasma concentrations of drug and toxicity.

In summary, several features appear to have importance in the development of cocaine toxicity. First, the behavioral pattern of repeated dosing is very probably a consequence of attempts to achieve euphoric sensations, especially rush. In addition, craving for cocaine increases dramatically, shortly after cocaine dosing, further compelling the user to continue dosing. Despite the tolerance to rush, heart rate and blood pressure do not demonstrate an important degree of tolerance to cocaine during, at least, the first several hours, indicating a continuing responsiveness of the cardiovascular system to cocaine concentration. At the same time there may be sensitization of the nervous system to the effects of cocaine. Finally, the cocaine concentrations can accumulate in a precipitous way during binging because of the nonlinearity of cocaine metabolism. The interaction between these complex behavioral and physiological events set the stage for serious cocaine intoxication.

IV. DRUG INTERVENTION AND TREATMENT

The treatment of cocaine dependence is of considerable clinical importance. While pharmacologic interventions may become useful, the mainstay of treatment must still rest on support or deconditioning therapy to reduce drug craving and drug-seeking behavior. Studies of animal behavior,[82] as well as clinical work with humans,[83] highlight the importance of environment in conditioning and drug-taking behavior. It is often necessary to enforce a period of abstinence before long-term reduction in drug craving can occur. The patient attempting to give up cocaine must make the drug "psychologically" unavailable since it is difficult to make it physically unavailable. Hospitalization is important for some patients because it forms a buffer period during which the patient is freed from drug craving stimuli and life stress and may be better able to confront his drug problem. Hospitalization has been recommended for certain high-risk cocaine-using populations:[50]

1. Chronic free base or intravenous users
2. Concurrent dependence on alcohol or other drugs
3. Psychiatric or medical problems of a serious nature
4. Psychosocial impairment of a severe nature
5. Lack of motivation
6. Lack of family or social supports
7. Repeated outpatient failures

The proper use of pharmacologic intervention is within a planned therapeutic strategy as part of a program of treatment. Tricyclic antidepressants, bromocriptine, and amantadine have been reported to be useful as anticraving agents in patients seeking treatment. In some patients, those with attention deficit disorders, dysthymic, and cyclothymic disorders, methylphenidate and lithium may diminish cocaine self-medication.

Tennant and Rawson reported that desipramine facilitated abstinence in 14 cocaine abusers.[84] However, in their study, 11 of the 14 subjects received desipramine for less than 7 days. Such short-term treatment would not be expected to have a major effect on receptor binding, but suggests the mechanism of catecholamine reuptake blockade is involved.

Gawin and Kleber reported prolonged desipramine treatment in six subjects, all of whom demonstrated prolonged abstinence and decreased craving.[85] The onset of action for the desipramine was consistent with an effect on neuroreceptor binding. Rosecan studied 25 subjects treated with imipramine and obtained an average period of abstinence and decreased craving in 80% of the sample studied.[86] However, these studies were carried out as open pilot trials and thus, the conclusions can only be tentative until completion of larger scale, double-blind placebo control trials.

Several studies have investigated craving for drug in an experimental laboratory setting. Dackis and Gold have postulated a hypodopaminergic state underpinning the craving for cocaine during abstinence.[50] Based on this hypothesis, they showed a decrease in craving for cocaine after a single administration of 0.625 mg of bromocriptine in a single-blind, uncontrolled experiment involving two patients.[39] Tennant and Sagerian, in a double-blind study of amantadine (100 mg) and bromocriptine (2.5 mg) twice-daily, subjects reported a decrease in craving, but the study had no placebo control.[88] In a double-blind controlled laboratory study we found that cocaine wanting and craving, induced by an intravenous injection of cocaine, was decreased after pretreatment with 2.5 mg of bromocriptine.[38]

In addition to drugs which may block feelings of drug craving, drugs which interfere with the euphorigenic properties of cocaine may become useful drug treatments. Lithium treatment blocks behavioral,[89] electrophysiologic,[90] and neurochemical[93] effects of acute cocaine or amphetamine in animal experiments. Some early clinical trials of lithium blockade of cocaine- or amphetamine-induced euphoria reported partial efficacy.[87,91,92] However, a subsequent trial failed to demonstrate an effect.[94] Despite this disappointment, lithium may have a place in the treatment of those cocaine-dependent patients with cyclothymic or dysthymic disorders.[85]

Based on the hypothesis that cocaine euphoria is mediated by dopaminergic neurotransmission, Gawin and Kleber proposed that neuroleptics might block effectively cocaine euphoria.[37] In animal studies, Woolverton and Balster found that chlorpromazine and haloperidol at doses therapeutically active in man did not effect drug-seeking behaviour in baboons.[95] Gawin treated as outpatients four cocaine addicts troubled with episodes of paranoia related to cocaine use; two with haloperidol, 5 to 20 mg orally, and two with chlorpromazine, 100 to 500 mg orally.[96] These patients reported that the neuroleptic drug blocked their feelings of paranoia and lessened the feelings of uncomfortable stimulation, but they detected no effect upon cocaine euphoria. In our double-blind randomized laboratory study of five cocaine users, we found no effect of haloperidol (8 mg) on drug "rush", but haloperidol did significantly decrease other pleasant sensations (good feelings).[97] These findings are similar to those of Nurnberger et al. who found that haloperidol attenuated the "high" feelings after intravenous amphetamine.[98] Although these interactions are scientifically interesting, they are of doubtful clinical utility because "rush", a major component of cocaine euphoria, is not blocked, and the blockade of other euphoric sensations is only partial. Despite this, such work promises an increased understanding of the neuropharmacologic mechanisms involved in drug-seeking feelings and behavior.

Other interesting drugs which interact with the dopaminergic system and may prove useful include pyridoxine, a coenzyme in dopamine synthesis; agonist and antagonist analogues of CCK, a brain peptide that modulates dopaminergic function; arginine vasopressin analogues which may be active in modulating brain reward systems; and atypical stimulants such as pemoline.[5]

For the present, these treatments remain experimental as none has been clearly demonstrated effective. One novel aspect of recent cocaine treatment research has been the focus on pharmacological interactions with feelings of drug craving. This approach has not been directly addressed previously for cocaine or other drugs of abuse. Nevertheless, drug abuse treatment, like other areas of clinical medicine, requires double-blind treatment trials that follow patients for long periods of time. There is a dearth of such studies because of their great expense and effort. For ordinary drugs, this kind of work is supported by the pharmaceutical industry which carries out such trials in cooperation with the FDA. This process facilitates the acquisition of new treatments, and, together with government funding, provides an optimal system of new treatment research. It is hoped that more resources will be invested into well-designed treatment trials in order that more effective therapies can be provided to persons with drug dependence.

REFERENCES

1. **Resnick, R. B. and Schuyten-Resnick, E.,** Clinical aspects of cocaine: assessment of cocaine abuse behavior in man, in *Cocaine: Chemical, Biological, Clinical, Social, and Treatment Aspects,* Mule, S. J., Eds., CRC Press, Boca Raton, Fla., 1976.
2. **Fischman, M. W.,** Personal communication, 1987.
3. **Siegel, R. K.,** Changing patterns of cocaine use: longitudinal observations, consequences, and treatment, in Cocaine: Pharmacology, Effects, and Treatment of Abuse, Grabowski, J., Ed., NIDA Res. Monogr. No. 50, DHHS Publ. No. (ADM) 84-1326, Department of Health and Human Services, Washington, D.C., 1984, 92.
4. **Spotts, J. V. and Shontz, F. C.,** The Life Styles of Nine American Cocaine Users: Trips to the Land of Cockaigne, DHEW Publ. No. (ADM) 76-392, Department of Health, Education and Welfare, Washington, D.C., 1976.
5. **Angrist, B.,** Clinical effects of central nervous system stimulants: a selective update, in *Brain Reward Systems and Abuse,* Engel, J., Oreland, L., Ingvar, D. H., Pernow, B., Rossner, S., and Pellborn, L. A., Eds., Raven Press, New York, 1987, 109.
6. **Seecof, R. and Tennant, F. S.,** Subjective perceptions to the intravenous "rush" of heroin and cocaine in opioid addicts, *Am. J. Alcohol Drug Abuse,* 12 (1 & 2), 79, 1986.
7. **Javaid, J. I., Fischman, M. W., Schuster, C. R., Dekirmenjian, H., and Davis, J. M.,** Cocaine plasma concentration: relation to physiological and subjective effects in humans, *Science,* 202, 227, 1978.
8. **Fischman, M. W., Schuster, C. R., and Hatano, Y.,** A comparison of the effects of cocaine and lidocaine in humans, *Pharmacol. Biochem. Behav.,* 18, 123, 1983.

9. **Chow, M. J., Ambre, J. J., Tsuen, I. R., Atkinson, A. J., Bowsher, D. J., and Fischman, M. W.,** Kinetics of cocaine distribution, elimination, and chronotropic effects, *Clin. Pharmacol. Ther.,* 38, 318, 1985.

10. **Fischman, M. R., Schuster, C. R., Javaid, J., Hatano, Y., and Davis, J.,** Acute tolerance development to the cardiovascular and subjective effects of cocaine, *J. Pharmacol. Exp. Ther.,* 235, 677, 1985.

11. **Kumor, K. M., Sherer, M. A., Gomez, J., Cone, E., and Jaffe, J. H.,** Continuous infusion of cocaine. I. Subjective effects, 1987, submitted.

12. **Post, R. M.,** Central stimulants: clinical and experimental evidence on tolerance and sensitization, in *Research Advances in Alcohol and Drug Problems,* Vol. 6, Israel, Y., Ed., Plenum Press, New York, 1981, 1.

13. **Jaffe, J. H.,** Drug addiction and drug abuse, in *The Pharmacologic Basis of Therapeutics,* 7th ed., Gilman, A. G., and Goodman, L. S., Eds., Macmillan, New York, 1985, 532.

14. **Sherer, M. A., Kumor, K. M., Cone, E. J., and Jaffe, J. H.,** Continuous intravenous infusion of cocaine. II. Cocaine induced suspiciousness, *Arch. Gen. Psychiatry,* 45, 673, 1988.

15. **Kramer, J. C.,** Introduction to amphetamine abuse, in *Current Concepts on Amphetamine Abuse,* Ellinwood, E. H. and Cohen, S., Eds., DHEW Publ. No. (HSM) 72-9085, Department of Health, Education and Welfare, Washington, D. C., 1972.

16. **Banerjee, S. P., Sharma, V. K., Kung-Cheung, L. S., Chanda, S. K., and Riggi, S. J.,** Cocaine and *d*-amphetamine induce changes in central beta-adrenoceptor sensitivity: effects of acute and chronic drug treatment, *Brain Res.,* 175, 119, 1979.

17. **Banerjee, S. P., Sharma, V. K., and Kung-Cheung, L. S.,** Amphetamine induces adrenergic receptor supersensitivity, *Nature (London),* 271, 380, 1976.

18. **Antelman, S. M. and Chiodo, L. A.,** Dopamine autoreceptor subsensitivity — a mechanism common to the treatment of depression and the induction of amphetamine psychosis?, *Biol. Psychiatry,* 16, 717, 1981.

19. **Martres, M. P., Costentin, J., Baudry, M., Marcais, H., Protais, P., and Schwartz, J. C.,** Longterm changes in the sensitivity of pre- and postsynaptic dopamine receptors in mouse striatum evidenced by behavioral and biochemical studies, *Brain Res.,* 136, 319, 1977.

20. **Nahorski, S. R.,** Altered responsiveness of cerebral beta-adrenoreceptors assessed by adenosine cyclic $3'5'$ monophosphate formation and [3H] propranolol binding, *Mol. Pharmacol.,* 13, 679, 1977.

21. **Ludwig, A. M. and Wikler, A.,** Craving and relapse to drink, *Q. J. Stud. Alcohol,* 35, 108, 1974.

22. **McAuliffe, W. E. and Ch'ien, J. M. N .,** Recovery training and self help: a relapse-prevention program for treated opiate addicts, *J. Subst. Abuse Treat.,* 3, 9, 1986.

23. **O'Brien, C. P., Testa, T., O'Brien, T. J., Brady, J. P., and Wells, B.,** Conditioned narcotic withdrawal in humans, *Science,* 195, 1000, 1977.

24. **Ludwig, A. M. and Start, L. H.,** Subjective and situational aspects, *Q. J. Stud. Alcohol,* 35, 899, 1974.

25. **Teasdale, J.,** Conditioned abstinence in narcotic addicts, *Int. J. Addict.,* 8, 273, 1973.

26. **O'Brien, C. P.,** Experimental analysis of conditioning factors in human narcotic addiction, *Pharmacol. Rev.,* 27, 533, 1975.

27. **O'Brien, C. P., Greenstein, R., Ternes, J., McLellan, A. T., and Grabowski, J.,** Unreinforced selfinjections: effects on rituals and outcome in heroin addicts, in Committee on Problems of Drug Dependence, Harris, L. S., Ed., NIDA Monogr. No. 27, DHEW Publ. No. (ADM) 80:901, Department of Health, Education and Welfare, Washington, D. C., 1980, 275.

28. **Sideroff, S. and Jarvik, M. E.,** Conditioned responses to a videotape showing heroin-related stimuli, *Int. J. Addict.,* 15(4), 529, 1980.

29. **Baker, T. B. and Cannon, D. S.,** Taste aversion therapy with alcoholics: techniques and evidence of a conditioned response, *Behav. Res. Ther.,* 17, 229, 1979.

30. **Cannon, D. S. and Baker, T. B.,** Emetic and electric shock alcohol aversion therapy: assessment of conditioning, *J. Consult. Clin. Psychol.,* 49, 20, 1981.

31. **Ternes, J. W., O'Brien, C. P., Grabowski, J., Wellerstein, H., and Jordan-Hayes, J.,** Conditioned drug responses to naturalistic stimuli, in Committee on Problems of Drug Dependence, Harris, L. S., Ed., NIDA Monogr. No. 27, Department of Health, Education and Welfare, Washington, D. C., 1980, 282.

32. **McCaul, M. E., Turkkan, J. S., and Stitzer, M. L.,** Psychophysiologic effects of alcohol-related stimuli, in Committee on Problems of Drug Dependence, Harris, L. S., Eds., NIDA Monogr. No. 27, DHHS Publ. No. (ADM) 87—1508, Department of Health, Education and Welfare, Washington, D.C., 1987, 131.

33. **Childress, A. R., McLellan, A. T., and O'Brien, C. P.,** Assessment and extinction of conditioned opiate responses in an integrated treatment for opiate dependence, in Committee on Problems of Drug Dependence, NIDA Res. Monogr. No. 55, Department of Health, Education and Welfare, Washington, D.C., 1984, 202.

34. **McLellan, A. T., Childress, A. R., Ehrman, R., and O'Brien, C. P.,** Extinguishing conditioned responses during opiate dependence treatment turning laboratory findings into clinical procedures, *J. Subst. Abuse Treat.,* 3, 27, 1986.

35. **Kaplan, R. F., Cooney, N. L., Baker, L. H., Gillespie, R. A., Meyer, R. A., and Pomerleau, O. F.**, Reactivity to alcohol-related cues: Physiological and subjective responses in alcoholics and non-problem drinkers, *J. Stud. Alcohol,* 46, 267, 1985.

36. **Ludwig, A. M. and Wikler, A.**, The first drink. Psychobiological aspects of craving, *Arch. Gen. Psychiatry,* 30, 539, 1974.

37. **Kleber, H. and Gawin, F.**, Psychopharmacological trials in cocaine abuse treatment, *Am. J. Drug alcohol Abuse,* 12, 235, 1986.

38. **Jaffe, J. H., Cascella, N. G., Kumor, K. M., and Sherer, M. A.**, Bromocriptine reduces cocaine-induced craving, *Biol. Psychiatry,* 1987, in press.

39. **Dackis, C. A., Gold, M. S., Davies, R. K., and Sweeney, D. R.**, Bromocriptine: treatment for cocaine abuse: the dopamine depletion hypothesis, *Int. J. Psychiatry Med.,* 15(2), 125, 1985.

40. **Tennant, F. S. and Sagherian, A. A.**, Double-blind comparison of amantadine and bromocriptine for ambulatory withdrawal from cocaine dependence, *Arch. Intern. Med.,* 147, 109, 1987.

41. **deWit, H. and Stewart, J.**, Drug reinstatement of heroin reinforced responding in the rat, *Psychopharmacology,* 75, 134, 1981.

42. **Gerber, G. J. and Stretch, R.**, Drug-induced reinstatement of extinguished self-administration behaviour in monkeys, *Pharmacol. Biochem. Behav.,* 3, 1055, 1975.

43. **Davis, W. M. and Smith, S. G.**, Role of conditioned reinforcers in the initiation, maintenance, and extinction of drug-seeking behavior, *Pavlovian J. Biol. Sci.,* 11, 222, 1976.

44. **Dackis, C. A. and Gold, M. S.**, Pharmacological approaches to cocaine addiction, *J. Subst. Abuse Treat.,* 2, 139, 1985.

45. **Gold, M. S. and Dackis, C. A.**, New insights and treatments: opiate withdrawal and cocaine addiction, *Clin. Ther.,* 7, 6, 1984.

46. **Taylor, D. and Ho, B. T.**, Neurochemical effects of cocaine following acute and repeated injection, *J. Neurosci. Res.,* 3, 95, 1977.

47. **Memo, M., Pradhan, S., and Hanbauer, I.**, Cocaine induced supersensitivity of striatal dopamine receptors: role of endogenous calmodulin, *Neuropharmacology,* 20, 1145, 1981.

48. **Borison, R. L., Hitri, A., Klawans, H. L., and Diamond, B. I.**, A new animal model for schizophrenia: behavioral and receptor binding studies, in *Catecholamines, Basis and Clinical Frontiers,* Usdin, E., Kopin, I. J., and Barchas, J. Eds., Pergamon Press, New York 1979, 719.

49. **Taylor, D. B., Ho, T., and Fagen, J. D.**, Increased dopamine receptor binding in rat brain by repeated cocaine injections, *Commun. Psychopharmacol.,* 3, 137, 1979.

50. **Dackis, C. A. and Gold, M. S.**, New concepts in cocaine addiction: the dopamine depletion hypothesis, *Neurosci. Biobehav. Rev.,* 9, 469, 1985.

51. **Kumor, K. M., Sherer, M. A., and Jaffe, J. H.**, Haloperidol-induced dystonia in cocaine addicts, *Lancet,* II, 1341, 1986.

52. **Adams, E. H. and Durell, J.**, Cocaine: a growing public health problem, in Cocaine: Pharmacology, Effects, and Treatment of Abuse, Grabowski, J., Ed., NIDA Res. Monogr. No. 50, DHHS Publ. No. (ADM)84—1326, Department of Health and Human Services, Washington, D.C., 1984, 9.

53. **Pasternack, P. R., Colvin, C. B., and Bauman, F. G.**, Cocaine induced angina pectoris and acute myocardial infarction in patients younger than 40 years, *Am. J. Cardiol.,* 55, 847, 1985.

54. **Cregler, L. L. and Mark, H.**, Cardiovascular dangers of cocaine abuse, *Am. J. Cardiol.,* 57, 1185, 1986.

55. **Gould, L., Chitra, G., Chandrakant, P., and Betzu, R.**, Cocaine-induced myocardial infarction, *N.Y. State J. Med.,* 99, 660, 1985.

56. **Boag, F. and Havard, C. W. H.**, Cardiac arrhythmia and myocardial ischemia related to cocaine and alcohol consumption, *Postgrad. Med. J.,* 61, 997, 1985.

57. **Simpson, R. W. and Edwards, W. D.**, Pathogenesis of cocaine-induced ischemia heart disease, *Arch. Pathol. Lab. Med.,* 110, 479, 1986.

58. **Nanji, A. A. and Filipenko, J. D.**, Asystole and ventricular fibrillation associated with cocaine intoxification, *Chest,* 85, 132, 1984.

59. **Howard, R. E., Hueter, D. C., and Davis, G. J.**, Acute myocardial infarction following cocaine abuse in a young woman with normal coronary arteries, *JAMA,* 254, 95, 1985.

60. **Coleman, D. L., Ross, T. F., and Naughton, J. L.**, Myocardial ischemia and infarction related to recreational cocaine use, *West. J. Med.,* 136, 444, 1982.

61. **Kossowsky, W. A. and Lyon, A. F.**, Cocaine and acute myocardial infarction. A probable connection, *Chest,* 86, 729, 1984.

62. **Schachne, J. S., Roberts, B. H., and Thompson, P. D.**, Coronary-artery spams and myocardial infarction associated with cocaine use, *N. Engl. J. Med.,* 310, 1665, 1984.

63. **Schwartz, S. M. and Ross, R.**, Cellular proliferation in artherosclerosis and hypertension, *Prog. Cardiovasc. Dis.,* 26, 355, 1984.

64. **Benchimol, A., Bartall, H., and Desser, K. B.**, Accelerated ventricular rhythm and cocaine abuse, *Ann. Intern. Med.,* 88, 519, 1978.

65. **Isner, J. M., Estes, M., Thompson, P. D., Costanzo-Nordin, M. R., Subramanian, R., Miller, G., Katsas, G., Sweeney, K., and Sturner, W. Q.,** Acute cardiac events temporally related to cocaine abuse, *N. Engl. J. Med.,* 315, 1438, 1986.

66. **Sander, R., Ryser, M. A., Lamoreaux, T. C., and Raleigh, K.,** An epidemic of cocaine associated deaths in Utah, *J. Forensic Sci.,* 30(2), 478, 1985.

67. **Wetli, C. V. and Wright, R. K.,** Death caused by recreational cocaine use, *JAMA,* 241, 2519, 1979.

68. **Noe, D. A. and Kumor, K. M.,** Drug kinetics in low-flux (small) anatomic compartments, *J. Pharm. Sci.,* 72, 718, 1983.

69. **Catravas, J. D. and Waters, I. W.,** Acute cocaine intoxification in the conscious dog: studies on the mechanism of lethality, *J. Pharmacol. Exp. Ther.,* 217, 350, 1981.

70. **Gay, G. R.,** Clinical management of acute and chronic cocaine poisoning, *Ann. Emergency Med.,* 11, 562, 1982.

71. **Ramoska, E. and Sacchetti, A. D.,** Propranolol-induced hypertension in treatment of cocaine intoxification, *Ann. Emergency Med.,* 14, 1112, 1985.

72. **Correspondence:** Management of the cocaine-intoxicated patient, *Ann. Emergency Med.,* 16, 234, 1987.

73. **Nahas, G., Trouve, R., Demus, J. F., and von Sitbon, M.,** A calcium channel blocker as antidote to the cardiac effects of cocaine intoxification, *N. Engl. J. Med.,* 313, 519, 1985.

74. **Cregler, L. L. and Mark, H.,** Medical complications of cocaine abuse, *N. Engl. J. Med.,* 315, 1495, 1986.

75. **Roberts, J. R., Quattrocchi, E., and Howland, M.,** Severe hyperthemia secondary to intravenous drug abuse, *Am. J. Emergency Med.,* 2, 373, 1984.

76. **Barnett, G.,** Personal communication, 1987.

77. **Jones, R. T.,** Cocaine and other drug interactions: strategy considerations, in Strategies for Research on the Interactions of Drugs of Abuse, Braude, M. C. and Ginzburg, H. M., Eds., NIDA Res. Monogr. Ser. No. 68, DHHS Publ. No. (ADM) 86-1423, Department of Health and Human Services, Washington, D. C., 1986, 142.

78. **Hansen, H. J., Caudill, S. P., and Boone, J.,** Crisis in drug testing, *JAMA,* 253, 2382, 1985.

79. **Post, R. M.,** Progressive changes in behaviour and seizures following chronic cocaine administration: relationship to kindling and psychosis, in *Cocaine and Other Stimulants,* Ellinwood, E. H. and Kilbey, M. M., Eds., Plenum Press, New York, 1977, 353.

80. **Stripling, J. S., and Ellinwood, E. H.,** Sensitization to cocaine following chronic administration in the rat, in *Cocaine and Other Stimulants,* Ellinwood, E. H. and Kilbey, M. M., Eds., Plenum Press, New York, 1977, 327.

81. **Barnett, M. J., Hawks, R., and Resnick, R.,** Cocaine pharmacokinetics in humans, *J. Ethnopharmacol.,* 3, 353, 1981.

82. **Goldberg, S. R., Spealman, R. D., and Kelleher, R. T.,** Enhancement of drug seeking behavior by environmental stimuli associated with cocaine or morphine injections, *Neuropharmacology,* 18, 1015, 1979.

83. **Wikler, A.,** Dynamics of drug dependence: implications of a conditioning theory for research and treatment, *Arch. Gen. Psychiatry,* 28, 611, 1973.

84. **Tennant, F. S., Jr. and Rawson, R. A.,** Cocaine and amphetamine dependence treated with desipramine, problems of drug dependence, *NIDA Res. Monogr. Ser.,* 43, 351, 1983.

85. **Gawin, F. H. and Klebler, H. D.,** Cocaine abuse treatment: an open pilot trial with lithium and desipramine, *Arch. Gen. Psychiatry,* 41, 903, 1984.

86. **Rosecan, J. S. and Nunes, E. V.,** Pharmacological management of cocaine abuse, in *Cocaine Abuse. New Directions in Treatment and Research,* Spitz, H. I. and Rosecan, J. S., Eds., Brunner/Mazel, New York, 1987, 255.

87. **Cronson, A. J. and Flemenbaum, A.,** Antagonism of cocaine highs by lithium, *Am. J. Psychiatry,* 135, 856, 1978.

88. **Tennant, F. S., Jr. and Sagherian, A. A.,** Double blind comparison of amantadine and bromocriptine for ambulatory withdrawal from cocaine dependence, *Arch, Intern. Med.,* 147, 109, 1987.

89. **Berggren, U., Tallstedt, G., and Ahlenius, S.,** The effect of lithium on amphetamine induced locomotor stimulation, *Psychopharmacology,* 59, 41, 1978.

90. **Cassems, G. P. and Mills, A. W.,** Lithium and amphetamines: opposite effects on threshold of intracranial reinforcements, *Psychopharmacologia,* 30, 283, 1973.

91. **Angrist, B. and Gershon, S.,** Variable attenuation of amphetamine effects by lithium, *Am. J. Psychiatry,* 136, 806, 1979.

92. **Gold, M. S. and Byck, R.,** Lithium, naloxone, endorphins and opiate receptors: possible relevance to pathological and drug induced manic-euphoric states in man, the international challenge on drug abuse, *NIDA Res. Monogr. Ser.,* 19, 192, 1978.

93. **Mandell, A. J., and Knapp, S.,** Neurobiological antagonism of cocaine by lithium, in *Cocaine and Other Stimulants,* Ellinwood, E. H., Jr. Kilbey, M. M., Eds., Plenum Press, New York, 1976, 187.

94. **Resnick, R. B., Washton, A. M., La Placa, R. W., and Ston Washton, N.,** Lithium-carbonate as a potential treatment for compulsive cocaine use: a preliminary report, presented to the 32nd Annu. Convent. and Scientific Meet. Biological Psychiatry, Toronto, 1977.
95. **Woolverton, W. L. and Balster, R. L.,** Effects of antipsychotic compounds in Rhesus Monkeys given a choice between cocaine and food, *Drug Alcohol Depend.,* 8, 69, 1981.
96. **Gawin, F. H.,** Neuroleptic reduction of cocaine-induced paranoia but not euphoria?, *Psychopharmacology,* 90, 142, 1986.
97. **Kumor, K. M., Sherer, M. A., and Jaffe, J. H.,** Haloperidol pretreatment for intravenous cocaine, Soc. Biological Psychiatry Annu. Meet., Chicago, 1987.
98. **Nurnberger, J. I., Simmons-Alling, S., Kessler, L., Jimerson, S., Schreiber, J., Hollander, E., Tamminga, C. A., Nadi, N. S., Goldstein, D., and Gershon, E.,** Separate mechanisms for behavioral, cardiovascular, and hormonal responses to dextroamphetamine in man, *Psychopharmacology,* 84, 200, 1984.

Chapter 9

TREATMENT OF COCAINE ABUSE: MEDICAL AND PSYCHIATRIC CONSEQUENCES

Maria-Elena Rodriguez

TABLE OF CONTENTS

I. INTRODUCTION

Cocaine is no longer viewed as a safe drug. Examples of this fact proliferate daily life with increases in telephone help lines, admissions to emergency rooms and drug treatment centers, as well as cocaine-related deaths. These facts demonstrate the very real danger that cocaine represents to an individual's physical, mental, and social well-being.

It is only in recent years that it has become apparent that cocaine is one of the most addictive of drugs. Animal studies have shown that when there is unlimited access to cocaine, the effect on animals is extreme compulsive use, leading to death if left unchecked. Cocaine appears to be the most rewarding of drugs.

Cocaine users have repeatedly reported that the pleasurable effects from cocaine use are in a class of their own as compared to other illicit drug effects. In fact, the development of a cocaine dependency occurs quite rapidly, sometimes over a period of months rather than years. There appears to be a rapid appearance of tolerance as well. Cocaine becomes the focus of the user's daily life with cycles that alternate between periods of "cocaine use", "cocaine craving", and "cocaine-seeking behavior", often with short periods of recuperation between intervals. Medical or psychiatric complications often follow in a short period of time with detrimental changes in lifestyle and behavior. This profile is in striking contrast, for example, to that of the alcoholic whose chronic and progressive addiction may take decades to develop.

Addiction itself is a complex disorder that involves neurochemical disruptions and alterations that explain both objective and subjective effects of a drug on the organism. Psychological and social factors are also implicated. Cocaine is no exception; therefore, biological, psychological, and social processes, as determinants of cocaine addiction, ought to be taken into consideration when planning a treatment program for the cocaine addict. Indeed, a variety of strategies and treatment alternatives exist ranging from self-help groups and psychological techniques to experimental pharmacologies. Generally speaking, treatment programs include several of these strategies alternating within different stages of the treatment process. Unfortunately, in the area of cocaine abuse treatment, there is no existing research which can give practical guidelines to the clinician about which treatment approach might be more or less effective.

II. MEDICAL AND PSYCHIATRIC CONSEQUENCES OF COCAINE ABUSE

Although the use of cocaine seems to have stabilized among certain groups in recent years, the consequences of its use and abuse are multiplying. Reasons for the increase of some cocaine-related pathologies and deaths are, as yet, not clearly known. These consequences are seen in cocaine users of all ages independent of duration, frequency, or amount of cocaine use. For example, an individual may use cocaine for several years without apparent problems and then succumb to the addiction. Route of administration does not always determine the degree of severity, as problems from cocaine use may occur regardless of the route of administration. Three years ago, when freebasing was not as prevalent, it was believed that intravenous use, smoking coca paste, and freebasing all had the same potential to elicit dependence. Further, it was believed that those who snorted cocaine were not as likely to become heavily addicted in a short span of time. Currently, the view is that freebasing cocaine promotes the development of addiction more quickly than snorting or intravenous use. Clinical experience shows that most cocaine addicts have been using the drug for 2 to 4 years before their situation forces them to enter some type of treatment. Nevertheless, that point in time may have no relation to the type and severity of the consequences, although, generally speaking, freebasers and intravenous users exhibit medical pathologies and levels of psychological distress greater than snorters.

A. Medical Consequences

1. Acute Medical Complications

Sudden death is the most dramatic acute consequence of cocaine use and can occur after administration of cocaine by all routes. It can be preceded by convulsions or mental confusion in some cases, and it may occur with doses approaching 1 g. Persons with inborn deficiency of the enzyme pseudocholinesterase in plasma are especially at risk when they use cocaine because that enzyme is essential for metabolizing the drug. These patients may die even if they have 10 or 20 mg of cocaine administered in connection with a local anesthesia, because the drug is never destroyed. The acute toxic reactions can occur after cocaine use by all routes. It is similar to that caused by amphetamines and consists in nervousness, dizziness, tremor, and blurred vision. In cases of fatal cocaine toxicity, the patient may present an initial agitation, tachycardia, hypertension, hyperthermia, diaphoresis, and acidosis. Sometimes cocaine is just the trigger of some complications of previously existing pathologies. The acute medical consequences of cocaine use are summarized in six categories as follows:

1. Sudden death after
   - Fatal pulmonary edema and respiratory paralysis
   - Convulsive crisis
   - Cardiac dysrhythmias (direct effect of cocaine on the myocardium)
2. Acute intoxication causing
   - Convulsions
   - Cardiac arrhythmias
   - Respiratory arrest
3. Complications of previously existing pathologies such as
   - Focus epilepticus
   - Valvulopathies alternating the cardiac rhythm
   - Abnormalities in the coronary arteries
   - Aneurysms causing hemorrhages
   - Abnormalities in the liver
4. Complications due to the agents used to adulterate cocaine (such as the local anesthetics)
5. "Tanking up" (or administration of an excessive dose of cocaine after a period of abstinence); this is often the way the patient will say "Bye" to the drug before entering a treatment program
6. Other complications:
   - Hypertension
   - Severe hyperpyrexia
   - Status epilepticus (repeated convulsions)
   - Excessive agressiveness (to others and self)
   - Automobile or work-related accidents (sometimes due to paranoid miscalculations or superhuman delusions)

2. Cardiac Complications of Cocaine

The most common complications of cocaine use are acute myocardial infarction (AMI), cardiac arrhythmias, and rupture of the ascending aorta and sudden cardiac death. There is increasing evidence that these complications may occur in young adult users with or without preexisting coronary artery disease, and these complications are not limited to intravenous users. Serious cardiac clinical events (including death) may occur after intranasal use and after freebasing.

The sympathomimetic effects of the drug may induce vasoconstriction and subsequently tachycardia, hypertension, or coronary artery spasm. The latter would explain the complications mentioned above, but the specific cause of each one of them is not clear for some experts and remains under discussion.

The mechanism of how cocaine causes AMI (or coronary occlusion) remains uncertain. Current information suggests that cocaine may induce either coronary spasm or coronary thrombosis (coronary artery embolization). This second possibility is very uncommon in the absence of other sources of emboly in the system. In general, when a young patient with no history of coronary risk factors presents an AMI, we assume that cocaine use has precipitated a coronary spasm and subsequently the AMI. Any individual with underlying fixed coronary artery disease should look at cocaine as a very potential danger due to its effects of increasing the heart rate, systolic blood pressure, and myocardial oxygen demand.

Cardiac arrhythmias are a direct consequence of cocaine use due to the arrhythmogenic property of the drug. The mechanism that more likely explains this effect is the increase in beta stimulation of the cardiac muscle due to cocaine blockage of the reuptake of norepinephrine in presynaptic nerve endings. Arrhythmias may also occur after cocaine-induced myocardial infarction and also as a consequence of hyperpyrexia naturally induced by the drug.

The acute rupture of the ascending aorta as a consequence of cocaine use is not very common and is unlikely to happen in the absence of an important hypertension. It is supposed to occur after a large increase in the systemic arterial pressure because of high levels of cocaine in blood.

Less common complications have been described in case report studies. Lymphocyte myocarditis has been found in a long-term cocaine user who died of myocardial ischemic lesions.[1] Pneumopericardium has been described in a cocaine freebaser in which freebasing air may have leaked either from a ruptured alveolus or along fascial planes of the neck to the mediastimum and pericardial space.[2] These two case report studies concluded that long-term cocaine use may cause dilated cardiomyopathy and recurrent myocardial infarction, even in the absence of atherosclerotic coronary artery disease. The long-term recurrent stimulation of the myocardium by the cocaine-related chatecholamine excess may possibly lead to inflammation of the myocardium and dilated cardiomyopathy.[3] It is thought that substances commonly used as cocaine adulterants may also be responsible for cardiac pathogenesis of the drug.

3. Central Nervous System Complications

The two main complications of cocaine use in the central nervous system are cerebrovascular accidents and seizures.[4-6] Cerebrovascular accidents seem to be related to adrenergic stimulation and may occur as a consequence of the sudden increase in blood pressure due to administration of cocaine. Of course, anyone with arteriovenous malformation or an aneurysm of a cerebral vessel is at risk of developing this kind of pathology.

Seizures can appear after a single dose of cocaine. In most of these cases it seems that cocaine either lowers the threshold for convulsions, or the seizures are secondary to central nervous system-related events. Other complications are not very frequent. An example is the cerebral infarction after using cocaine intravenously and freebasing.[7] Sympathomimetic actions of cocaine are responsible for the vasoconstriction in the cerebral arteries which may cause the infarction. In all the cases where this complication has been described, no other irregularity or previous pathology was noticed.

4. Digestive System Complications

Digestive system complications occur mainly with oral ingestion of cocaine. The most common is the intestinal ischemia.[8] This is a result of the vasoconstriction and reduced blood flow in the mesenteric vasculature following ingestion of a large amount of cocaine.

It is not known whether cocaine has any effect on the enteric nervous system. Norepinephrine and epinephrine are probably involved in the nervous transmission of that area and thus, may be affected by cocaine. By this mechanism, involving catecholamines, cocaine may induce gastrointestinal mucosal ischemia, which may be the cause of pathologies such as pseudomembranous colitis in cocaine addicts.[9]

Some effects on gingiva have been described after the use of cocaine powder on the gingiva.[10] The intensive vasoconstriction action of the drug may cause inflammation of the tissues surrounding the gingiva, gingival bleeding, and desquamation of portions of the epithelium in the mouth.

5. Sexual Dysfunctions

Sexual dysfunctions seem to be related to alterations in dopamine neurotransmission. These complications may include difficulties in maintaining erection, complete sexual disinterest, aberrant sexual behavior such as compulsive masturbation, and multiple sexual marathons. Such behavior usually follows prolonged periods of cocaine use.

6. Obstetrical Complications

Cocaine affects the menstrual cycle, pregnancy and its outcome, the labor process, and the infants of abuser women.

Chronic cocaine abuse is associated with irregularities in the menstrual cycle. The mechanism that would explain this complication is either body fat loss, which is clearly related to cocaine abuse, or general debilitation caused by drug abuse.[11]

Acute onset of labor with abruptio placenta has been studied in women who had used cocaine intravenously. This complication was a result of decrease in the flow of blood to the fetus and an increase in uterine contractions, both of which were due to the action of cocaine as a potent peripheral vasoconstrictor (causing a subsequent abrupt increase in the blood pressure).

Other studies have examined the incidence of miscarriage among pregnant cocaine abusers. Miscarriages were found in 38% of the women subjects.[12] Obstetrical complications are specially important because of the consequences for the baby. This is an area where more research is needed to assess long-term effects of cocaine on infants. What we know now is that the rate of spontaneous abortion among pregnant cocaine abusers is higher than in nonusers (as expected), and is higher than in heroin users.

Some serious studies demonstrate that babies exposed to cocaine during pregnancy are at risk for congenital malformations, perinatal mortality, and neurobehavioral impairments.[13] Newborn babies of cocaine-abusing women have also been found to be less reactive to environmental stimuli and to exhibit depressed interactive behavior. Long-term neurobehavioral deficits have not yet been determined. It is unknown if these effects occur in the fetus or in the neonate. The dosage of cocaine used, the frequency of use, and effects of adulterants may influence the outcome of the pregnancy.

It has been observed that cocaine babies present a higher-than-normal rate of respiratory and kidney troubles, a high incidence of strokes, and it is suspected that there is an increase risk of sudden infant death syndrome.

A case study reported an acute focal cerebral infarction in a neonate 24 hr old.[14] His mother had a large ingestion of cocaine and the infarction could have been caused either by intrauterine and postnatal hypertension and subsequent cerebral hemorrhage, or by peripartum hypotension and bradycardia with subsequent cerebral hypoperfusion.

Cocaine is particularly dangerous for babies because of the continued persistence of benzoylecgonine (a primary metabolite of cocaine) for 4 days in their system. This suggests that babies cannot metabolize the drug as well as adults because of a lack of the necessary enzymes (such as cholinesterases).

There is one study that does not corroborate the findings described above.[15] Out of eight babies whose mothers gave a history of cocaine abuse and whose urines were positive for cocaine, none of them showed evident symptomatology or signs of teratogenicity. Only one of the babies manifested any association with neonatal withdrawal.

7. Pulmonary Complications

Spontaneous mediastinum, also known as mediastinal emphysema (occurrence of air in the mediastinum) and pneumothorax, have been described in cocaine freebasers.[17-19] The spontaneous occurrence of pneumomediastinum is rare. Cocaine freebasers are a group particularly at risk because of the deep, prolonged, and forced inhalations they perform while attempting to enhance the desired effects of the drug. The cause of pneumothorax and pneumomediastinum in cocaine addicts is presumed to be an increase in the airway pressure leading to a rupture of alveolar blebs. Then free air goes to the peribronchial paths into the mediastinum and the pleural cavities.

Another pulmonary pathology that is a result of cocaine use is acute pulmonary edema and acute respiratory failure,[16] conditions that have occurred in intravenous users.

The finding of a significant reduction in lung diffusing capacity suggests that inhalation of free base cocaine may directly damage the pulmonary gas exchange surface. Definitive reductions have been observed in single-breath carbon monoxide diffusing capacity (DLCO, a nonspecific test that screens the gas exchanging capabilities of the patient).[20] Specifically, one study of 19 freebasers showed that more than half of them had respiratory symptoms and dyspnea.[21]

The hypothesis that explains the mechanism of these alterations in the pulmonary gas exchange is based on the pharmacologic properties of cocaine. The intense vasoconstrictor effect of the drug may produce lung damage by a direct effect on the pulmonary vasculature, thus producing a decrease in pulmonary blood flow which then causes the gas exchange abnormality. The absence of any abnormality in the airflow of pulmonary function tests of the subjects studied and reported corroborate this hypothesis.

The author is currently conducting a study that includes looking at forced expiratory volume in one second (FEV1), functional residual capacity (FRC), and total lung capacity (TLC). Free base cocaine use produces abnormalities in the pulmonary gas exchange that in many cases occur after brief periods of abuse. These conditions seem to persist after cessation of free base cocaine, although it is not yet known for how long. With more prolonged use, the damage in the lungs may be proportionally greater. One aspect where attention is being focused is on the role of tobacco abuse in the development of these conditions (most of the cocaine patients studied are heavy tobacco smokers). Agents used to adulterate cocaine should also be taken into account as possible damaging substances.

Pulmonary granulomatosis occurs when drugs intended for oral use are used intravenously. Particles added to the drug, such as talc, are often the most damaging agent. This condition has been found not only in patients who use cocaine intravenously, but also in a case of sniffing cocaine.[22]

Cocaine produces death most of the times from respiratory collapse with all routes of drug administration. Frequently, autopsies reveal pulmonary congestion.

8. Other Complications

System	Pathology	Route	Mechanism
Renal	Heroin-like associated nephropathy	i.v.	Unknown (adulterants probably implicated)
	Renal infarction	i.v.	Increased adrenergic stimulation (existing arterial thrombus)
Liver	Elevated serum transaminase levels	All	Loss of reducing hepatic equivalents/direct effect in the liver; research needed
Endocrine	Several studies looking at prolactin and growth hormone; results are too different to draw any conclusion		

System	Pathology	Route	Mechanism
Skin	Connective tissue disease	i.n., F.B.	Acral vasospasm
	Cocaine-related bullous disease	i.v.	
	Abscess	i.v.	
Nasal	Perforation of the nasal septum (with nose deformity and osteolytic sinusitis in some cases)	i.n.	Vasoconstriction in nasal mucosa
	Persistent nasal congestion and allergies;		
	Complication of routine nasal problems		

9. Infections

Addicts frequently have a variety of uncommon infectious diseases. Individuals using drugs intravenously are specially at risk for contagious diseases. This is because the sharing of needles plays a major role in the transmission of hepatitis B virus, HTLV III virus and other viruses, bacterias, and microorganisms.

In general, all kinds of infections are not uncommon because of the impairment in the inmune system due to poor diet, disruptions of sleep patterns, and other consequences of the changes of lifestyle that impact on individual's health. This explains the fact that users of routes other than intravenous are also at risk for infections. Some of the infections can be very severe and potentially life threatening.

Staphylococcal sepsis resulting from cocaine sniffing has been described in the literature.[23] This is an example of a bacteria that normally would not cause any infection because it colonizes in the mucosa of the nose naturally. It has been suggested that drug users are at a higher risk for infection partially because they carry more bacteria than nonusers due to the administration of the drug itself or to the paraphernalia. In the case of cocaine, the explanation is related to the properties of the drug itself. Cocaine is an intense vasoconstrictor when applied to the mucosa membranes. Thus, long-term cocaine use may cause inflammatory changes with nasal septal perforation. The cocaine-induced mucosal damage in the natural setting of the staphylococcus aureus colonization may easily result in bacteriemia and sepsis.

B. Psychiatric Consequences

The results of psychiatric studies of cocaine addicts are unclear concerning the relationship between cocaine addiction and psychopathology. Except for a few cases, it is not possible to know the sequence of events, i.e., if there was a preexisting psychopathology that facilitated the addictive behavior, or if cocaine abuse was the cause of the disorder. Data from two independent studies using structured interviews and DSMIII criteria are available. They show that at the time of the study, when the cocaine addicts were going through the postcocaine "crash", 30% of them were diagnosed with a depressive disorder (either major depression, atypical depression, or dysthymic disorder), and 20% suffered from a bipolar disorder, including cyclothymic disorder. Even though in some cases researchers obtained extensive historical and corroborating family history data, and repeated observations during periods when cocaine users were neither consuming the drug nor suffering of postcocaine depression, the information did not reveal whether pathology was primary or secondary to the cocaine abuse. In a nonpsychiatric facility, another well-known expert found evidence that 90% of his patients did not show psychiatric diagnoses. In about 90% of the cases, cocaine abuse was not a symptom of underlying psychopathology, but a primary disease. Nevertheless, all experts agree on the need to collect basic information on psychiatric history and psychiatric diagnoses routinely, since it may be very valuable when planning treatment for the patient.

Following are the major results of the main studies concerning psychopathology in cocaine abusers (psychiatric diagnosis).

- Cocaine has been known to precipitate and/or exacerbate depression, mania, and acute psychosis.
- Panic disorder during recreational use of cocaine continues autonomously even after drug use stops.
- Panic attacks occur in as many as 64% of chronic cocaine users, depending on the route of administration and bioavailability of the drug.
- Cocaine use in a normal adolescent sample generated no significant increase or decrease in eight measures of emotional distress.
- Evaluation of 30 chronic cocaine abusers in an outpatient treatment program showed that half of the sample had a DSMIII axis I diagnosis in addition to the cocaine abuse (33% depression, 17% cyclothymia, and 1 subject ADD).
- DSMIII data for 30 inpatient cocaine abusers showed that 50% of them had affective disorders (30% depression, 20% cyclothymia, and 6% ADD).
- Evaluation (other than DSMIII) of a sample of heavy cocaine users showed that 18% of the sample presented depression and anhedonia.
- Out of a sample of 259 cocaine abuser, 22% met DSMIII criteria for bulimia, 7% for bulimia and anorexia nervosa (ANN), and 2% for ANN alone.

III. TREATMENT

Effective drug treatment should have as its foundation a working model of addiction. Over the years, four different models have evolved that offer an etiology or hypothesis of addiction. They have come to be identified as the moral model, the disease model, the behavioral model, and the self-medication model.

The moral model assumes that drug abuse, i.e., cocaine, is due to moral weakness. Thus, for those individuals who become cocaine addicts, the only explanation is one of willfulness. Advocates of this model would most likely say that it is weakness that made him/her use drugs in the first place and lack of willpower that keeps the person using it. In addition to the historical prominence of this model, there has recently been a resurgence of adherents to this view. Under this model, treatment usually consists of punishment, i.e., jail or moral education.

The disease model holds that chemical dependency is a primary illness based on a bio-genetic predisposition. The disease is assumed to be chronic, that is, always present. Like diabetes or schizophrenia, the patient is not considered to be responsible for developing the illness (the addiction) or for maintaining it. Therefore, the treatment goal consists of total abstinence, since the illness is always present. Cocaine addiction, under this model, is no exception. The model is generally endorsed by Cocaine Anonymous and the medical profession.

The behavioral model has been brought to prominence in recent years by psychologist Alan Marlatt. Addiction is viewed as a pattern of maladaptive, learned habits which can be modified by cognitive behavioral techniques. Although these techniques can be used in the service of complete abstinence, the model more popularly embraces the concept of controlled use of substances.

Lastly, there is the self-medication hypothesis which encourages clinicians to look for another primary psychiatric illness, such as affective disorder, attention deficit disorder, schizophrenia, or posttraumatic stress syndrome, for which the patient may be treating himself/herself. This model vs. the disease model would view cocaine addiction as secondary to another disorder.

Independently of the model the clinician embraces, it is important to do a detailed psychiatric assessment of the cocaine abuser. This is often difficult at the beginning of the treatment because some psychiatric symptoms may be a consequence of cocaine itself (for example, the acute depressive reaction that often follows heavy episodes of cocaine use). Patients who are diagnosed with a psychiatric condition, in repeated longitudinal assessments isolated from postcocaine symptomatology, can benefit from appropriate psychotherapy. The medication depends on the psychopathology and the patient's response to the pharmacotherapy. The tendency of the addicts to generally abuse whatever drug is made available to them, is the reason to restrict psychotherapy to those cases who really need it.

A. Treatment Goals

Treatment goals are predicated on the treatment model. Thus, one of the major issues in the treatment of cocaine addiction is whether the goal ought to be total abstinence or controlled use. Here, one confronts the debate between medical and behavioral models. Most clinicians involved in cocaine treatment advocate complete abstinence. This is especially true since cocaine is an illegal drug. Users themselves, however, may enter treatment with different goals and even if they are willing to give up cocaine, may not be willing to give up other substances. This issue presents researchers with an interesting question that has just begun to be addressed. Should the treatment goal include abstinence from all substances and not just cocaine? There has been evidence that the factor most commonly preceding relapse to cocaine use is the use of alcohol and/or marijuana. Because these other drugs have usually been associated with cocaine many times, their use may trigger severe cravings for cocaine. The sequence of events that occur prior to relapse parallel the development of first-time cocaine use, i.e., usually preceded by the use of "gateway" drugs such as cigarettes, alcohol, and marijuana.

Personal clinical experience shows that during periods of cocaine abstinence, patients use other drugs (mostly alcohol) for several reasons (not exclusively to substitute cocaine "highs"). It is interesting to observe that this occurs as well for patients who had never used or abused other drugs previously in their lives. It is important to talk to the patients about this topic at the beginning of the treatment process, and to warn them about the unrealistic notion of controlled use of drugs. The risks associated with occasional use of drugs must also be addressed. One of the most common reasons for relapsing is the patient's attempt to test his control over cocaine. Without any doubt, based on clinical experience, achieving complete abstinence from all drugs is a basic condition for successful treatment.

Other treatment goals are often predicated on the individual needs of the cocaine users, clinical resources, therapeutic ambitions, and may include improvements in employment, interpersonal relationships, and decreases in criminal behaviors. These are psychosocial problems often hard hit by cocaine addiction. The most ambitious of treatments attempt to affect changes in patients' character structures. For groups such as Cocaine Anonymous, spiritual healing is an integral part of the program as well as a treatment goal in itself.

B. The Treatment Setting

It has long been known that "set and setting" are pivotal to addiction, in general, and to its treatment. Treatment settings can be categorized along several dimensions including residential vs. nonresidential, medical vs. nonmedical, and private vs. public vs. self-supported. To date there has been little in the way of research to indicate that inpatient treatment is anymore effective than outpatient treatment, if effective means less of a likelihood of relapse. For cocaine addicts, there is a difference of opinion about which settings are most beneficial for which patients. Once again, however, there has been practically no research on this issue.

One group of researchers, although asserting that most cocaine addicts can be treated as outpatients, have suggested the following guidelines for inpatient treatment.

1.   Chronic free base or intravenous use
2.   Concurrent physical dependency on other addictive drugs or alcohol requiring phar-
      macological detoxification
3.   Serious medical or psychiatric problems
4.   Severe impairment of psychosocial functioning
5.   Intermittent but destructive health-threatening cocaine use
6.   Insufficient motivation for outpatient treatment
7.   Lack of family and social supports
8.   Failure in outpatient treatment

In contrast, other researchers have asserted that only severe depression or psychotic symptoms persisting 1 to 3 days after cocaine cessation necessitate hospitalization.

The advantages of outpatient treatment are lower cost, less stigmatization, less disruption to the life of the patient and family (especially for female addicts), and the need to learn abstinence in the home environment. Inpatient treatment can offer the patient a supportive, therapeutic environment which might otherwise be absent. Further, there is intensive, round-the-clock care for monitoring and treating rapidly changing symptoms as well as a controlled environment to insure against a return to cocaine use.

One of the additional concerns in the question of treatment setting surrounds the issue of whether or not to mix cocaine users with other substance abusers or psychiatric patients. Many substance abuse programs have assimilated cocaine users into their existing program structure by adding a few cocaine groups and lectures on the topic of cocaine. There are some reasons to agree with such an approach: most cocaine abusers are using other substances as well, cocaine abuse is a specific instance of addictive disease in general, and the lack of scientifically proven, specific treatments for cocaine abuse.

Many specialized cocaine abuse treatment programs have been established in response to the demand for such service.These specialized treatment settings provide an alternative to those cocaine addicts who are willing to be in a setting specifically devoted to their problem.

C. Phases in Treatment

Timing in the treatment of cocaine addiction appears to be worthy of careful attention, since the cocaine addict can go through several phases of withdrawal. Some abusers first come to the attention of the health care system because of medical or psychiatric emergencies resulting from acute intoxication. When the acute phase subsides, this is often a good time for intervention to direct the person to more definitive treatment. Most of the patients first seek treatment because their life is no longer manageable. They feel dependent on cocaine to the point that the drug has taken over all other interests in their lives. This life crisis is more or less severe depending on the case. Ideally, the patient should be admitted into treatment right at the moment he asks for help. Often treatment programs have waiting lists of 2 weeks or more. Some professionals in the field believe that this is even advantageous for the patients because it gives them the opportunity to decide if they truly want to attend the program. For other groups of experts, waiting periods are not recommendable. We believe that the moment the addict seeks treatment is a good time to admit him into the program. The goal is to get the person into treatment as soon as possible.

Most experts do recognize a cocaine withdrawal syndrome. From the clinical point of view, having direct contact with patients, there is no doubt about the existence of such a syndrome. Different patients present different symptoms of withdrawal and the intensity varies enormously. The withdrawal period may start several hours after use and continue for several days or up to 1 or 2 weeks thereafter. The patient may experience anxiety, depression, irritability, marked craving, hypersomnia, increased appetite, fatigue, and head-aches. During this time, patients may be more concerned with securing their own personal comfort and may be too easily distracted to participate in treatment activities such as groups, lectures, and readings. If such a program is immediately forced on them, they may drop from treatment. Medication may be useful to treat the symptoms. The goal of this phase is to keep the patient in treatment.

A next phase is the treatment of cocaine abuse per se. At this point, it is important to arrange a time course for the various goals of treatment. For example, providing a support system and learning techniques to maintain abstinence may be followed later by affecting character change and spiritual healing.

There are different opinions about the frequency and duration of various treatment components and timing of treatment settings, for example, the frequency of group and individual therapy in inpatient and outpatient settings, or the duration of an after-care program, or the sequence of different modalities of treatment (some believe that addicts should try outpatient programs first and then be admitted to inpatient units only if outpatient treatment fails, while others believe that in all cases an initial period of inpatient stabilization should precede the after-care program). Unfortunately, there is no information available on this issue that could help the clinician to decide the best alternative for each patient.

It is important to specify the expected length of treatment (12 or 18 months). Although the real length may be longer than the expected, it seems to benefit the patient if he counts on the treatment having some kind of a deadline. Some studies have concluded that there is a proportional relationship between the length of treatment and the chance of remaining abstinent. Some of our patients have relapsed several times and still continued to visit periodically. After resetting the deadlines of the treatment process, and keeping contact with them, they may reach that point where their determination and state of mind to stay abstinent are good enough to abstain from cocaine for long periods of time.

D. Specific Therapeutic Interventions

This is an area for which, once again, a scant amount of research has been conducted. Treatment of cocaine abuse can be grossly divided into somatic therapies and psychotherapies. In addition to these two categories, a third category for adjunctive techniques such as urine monitoring will often be used. Somatic therapies for cocaine abuse include pharmacotherapies, acupuncture, and psychosurgery. However, only pharmacotherapy has even begun to be tested and still remains in an experimental stage. Cocaine exerts its effects neurochemically and, therefore, the treatment of cocaine abusers requires more than psychological interventions. One of the main targets for medication is craving.

Pharmacotherapies include use of antidepressants, lithium, methylphenidate, bromocriptine, amino acids, and vitamins. Some suggested treatments, that have not yet been tested include L-dopa, bupropion, apomorphine, pergolide, lisuride, and lergotrile, Thyroxine has also been proposed.

Antidepressants are probably the best studied of pharmacological treatments to date. There are three articles which describe a total of five case reports using either desipramine or trasodone, three reports of open pilot trials using either imipramine or desipramine, and one published account of a double-blind, placebo-controlled study of desipramine with a small group of 22 cocaine abusers. Interestingly, the case reports and open pilot trials all reported generally positive results, whereas the double-blind, placebo-controlled study concluded that desipramine was no more effective than placebo. The latter study, however, may have used too low of a dose (150 mg) to discern an effect and did not monitor blood levels to ensure that their outpatients were compliant with the medication.

Various neurochemical theories have been advanced to provide a rationale for studying the antidepressants. One early rationale was that cocaine blocks the reuptake of catecholamines, especially norepinephrine, which eventually leads to depletion of norepinephrine. Because antidepressants also block reuptake without causing depletion, it was felt that antidepressants could restore the neurotransmitter depletion. This mechanism of action was supported by evidence that desipramine quickly reversed cocaine withdrawal symptoms corresponding to the rapid action of desipramine as a reuptake blocker of catecholamines. It has been hypothesized that prolonged cocaine use induces catecholamine receptor supersensitivity in the brain and that these receptor changes mediate postcocaine dysphoria and craving. Antidepressants, which are believed to reverse these receptor changes after several weeks of administration, might therefore be useful to cocaine abusers.

One researcher combined these two theories and hypothesized that the neurotransmitter depletion leads to the compensatory receptor supersensitivity. Antidepressants, then, become useful in the short term by blocking reuptake without depletion and in the long-term by reversing receptor supersensitivity. None of these theories, however, explain why trazodone, which impacts on serotonergic (not catecholaminergic) systems, should be effective.

The use of bromocriptine is also based on a theory of neurotransmitter depletion. In this model, the catecholamine dopamine is postulated to mediate cocaine-induced euphoria acutely and then through its eventual depletion, postcocaine dysphoria and withdrawal. Besides animal data, there is evidence of hyperprolactinemia in human cocaine abusers which lends support to the dopamine depletion theory. These findings, however, are at odds with those from other researchers. Under this model, continued, compulsive cocaine use may be considered an attempt to recapture the lost dopamine; the neurochemical parallel of recapturing the lost psychological "high". Accordingly, chemicals which enhance dopaminergic activity without depleting dopamine are postulated to be useful in breaking the cycle of compulsive cocaine use. In addition to bromocriptine, which is a dopamine agonist, this model predicts the utility of apomorphine, L-dopa, bupropion, pergolide, lisuride, lergotrile, and tyrosine. Similarly, it predicts that dopamine blockers, such as the neuroleptics, will exacerbate cocaine craving and dysphoria leading to increased use. Indeed, neuroleptics have been shown to increase self-administration of cocaine in animals. This last point has current clinical significance because many authors recommend the use of neuroleptics to treat cocaine-induced psychosis. Therefore, unless such treatment is undertaken in a controlled treatment setting, another episode of cocaine consumption may be iatrogenically induced by neuroleptics which have a relatively long half-life.

In a preliminary trial of bromocriptine, two female, hospitalized cocaine abusers underwent six single-dose trials, during which they were blindly given either 0.625 mg of bromocriptine or placebo. Cocaine craving markedly decreased following bromocriptine, but not after placebo. Using the same method, cocaine craving increased following two trials with a 50-mg dose of the neuroleptic thioridazine. The authors reported anecdotally that seven cocaine abusers were treated with maintenance doses of bromocriptine (7.5 to 12.5 mg daily) for an unspecified period of time. Follow-up at 3 to 9 months indicated continued cocaine abstinence and decreased craving in six of the patients. The first open-design study of the use of bromocriptine in cocaine withdrawal was conducted in 1986 with 24 patients. Based on the findings, it could be postulated that bromocriptine is effective in reducing cocaine craving and dysphoria during the initial abstinence period (42 days in that study). Nevertheless, clinical experience shows that the dysphoria decreases naturally with abstinence, and craving often appears after several months of abstinence. Therefore, further research is necessary to conclude that bromocriptine is effective in the treatment of cocaine withdrawal.

The use of methylphenidate is based on a diagnostic rationale for which it is hypothesized that some cocaine users may be self-medicating the stimulant-responsive syndrome of attention deficit disorder (ADD). In three cases reported to date, when methylphenidate (the drug of choice for treating ADD) was administered, cocaine craving, cocaine abuse, and ADD pathology diminished. Similarly, it has been reported that polydrug abuse in general and cocaine abuse in particular were the best predictors of improvement with methylphenidate in a group of adults with ADD. Although this approach is of interest, it is unknown what percentage of cocaine abusers also suffer from ADD: the retrospective diagnosis of childhood ADD in adulthood is not an easy one to make; methylphenidate is not always helpful in adults with ADD, and methylphenidate abuse could occur.

Lithium has been reported to block cocaine-induced euphoria as well as to attenuate cocaine abuse in patients with concurrent affective disorders. It has also been proposed for the treatment of cocaine-induced psychosis. The preliminary evidence suggests that patients with concurrent bipolar or cyclothymic disorder are more likely than other cocaine abusers to improve with lithium. Unfortunately, double-blind, placebo-controlled studies have not yet been published.

The use of vitamins and amino acids is also based on restoring chemical depletions. It has been reported that nearly 3/4 of cocaine abusers had at least one vitamin deficiency. The most common deficiencies were in thiamine (B1), pyridoxine (B6), vitamin C, and tyrosine. Whether these deficiencies were due to a lack of nutrition or specific cocaine effects was unclear. Two studies have looked at tyrosine, a precursor in the synthesis of catecholamines, in the treatment of cocaine abusers. In an open trial of six addicts with doses of 100 mg/kg/day, there were consistent antiwithdrawal effects. In another study, using an open trial with 1 g of tyrosine in combination with L-tryptophan and imipramine, the differential effects of the three agents could not be determined. Because of the relatively benign nature of using vitamins and neurotransmitter precursors, it seems necessary that further studies should be undertaken to assess their usefulness.

Although pharmacotherapy can be useful, there are still behavioral and emotional needs that must be addressed by some form of psychotherapy. Psychotherapy can be conducted with individuals, groups, or families. Ideally, the treatment plan should be discussed with the patient's spouse or significant others. Often the recovery process is more successful for patients whose spouses understand the problem of addiction and know of the treatment plan and participate in it to some extent. Unfortunately, the reality is that most of the times, due to the history of the patient's addiction, the relatives refuse to be involved or to collaborate in anything that requires them to have contact with the patient until he "proves" that he is recovered.

Psychotherapy can be conducted from behavioral, supportive, or dynamic orientations. There is to date only one experimental study of psychotherapy in cocaine abusers utilizing the behavioral method of contingency contracting. In this method, patients agree with the therapist upon adverse consequence such as sending a letter to the police, an employer, a licensing board, etc. if the patient admits a relapse or if urine tests are positive for cocaine. The mentioned study showed that 81% of the contracted patients remained in treatment and abstinent for at least 3 months compared to none of the patients without contract. The problem in using this technique is the ethical dilemma of using potentially harmful negative contingencies when approaches utilizing positive reinforcement might have proven to be just as effective. Other psychotherapies have been described for cocaine abusers, but have not been experimentally tested.

Because of the differences in treatment populations, it is not possible to accurately compare treatments across different centers. Nevertheless, there are several reports that show similar percentages of abstinent patients who were following pharmacotherapeutical approaches and patients who were in psychotherapy alone. On the other hand, ongoing studies are very promising about pharmacological approaches resulting in increases in patients' retention in treatment.

The issue of psychotherapy for cocaine addicts leads to a variety of questions. The role physicians, psychologists, nurses, social workers, and recovered substance abusers can play in the process of treatment is still not well defined and systematized. Questions such as the cost-effectiveness for someone to see a psychiatrist individually or a drug counselor who could provide equivalent treatment remain unanswered. It seems that successful treatment for most patients would include both individual and group therapy. The latter has to be conducted by professionals with expertise and specific training in the area of cocaine abuse. Self-help groups led by recovered addicts are very effective for some patients, while others do not seem to benefit from that kind of group approach.

Cocaine abuse appears to be a heterogeneous disorder with different degrees of severity and is acquired by different pathways. Thus, not all cocaine addicts are alike, and different people may be helped by different treatment strategies. The challenge is how to match patients with the different treatments available. This is the crucial question for research on treatment outcome to answer.

The techniques and approaches described here are used in the U.S. to treat cocaine addicts. In some European countries the epidemic of cocaine addiction and its consequences are just starting to appear. Some of the techniques mentioned are expensive and may not be affordable in European countries, where drug addiction is not a high priority in the government budgets. An important priority in treatment research is to develop approaches for cocaine addiction treatment that are inexpensive and effective.

REFERENCES

1. **Simpson, W. R. and Edwards, W. D.,** Pathogenesis of cocaine-induced ischemic heart disease, *Arch. Pathol. Lab. Med.,* 110, 479, 1986.
2. **Adrouny, A. and Magnusson, P.,** Pneumopericardium from cocaine inhalation, *N. Engl. J. Med.,* 313(1), 48, 1985.
3. **Wiener, R. S., Lockhart, J. T., and Schwartz, R. G.,** Dilated cardiomyopathy and cocaine abuse, *Am. J. Med.,* 81, 699, 1986.
4. **Sawicka, E. H. and Trosser, A.,** Cerebrospinal fluid rhinorrhoea after cocaine sniffing, *Br. Med. J.,* 286, 1983.
5. **Lichtenfeld, P. J., Rubin, D. B., and Feldman, R. S.,** Subarachnoid hemmorrhage precipitated by cocaine snorting, *Arch. Neurol.,* 41, 223, 1984.
6. **Myers, J. A. and Earnest, M. P.,** Generalized seizures and cocaine abuse, *Neurology,* 34(5), 675, 1984.
7. **Golbe, L. I. and Merkin, M. D.,** Cerebral infarction in a user of freebase cocaine, *Neurology,* 36, 1602, 1986.
8. **Nalbandian, H., Sheth, N., Dietrich, R., and Georgiou J.,** Intestinal ischemia caused by cocaine ingestion, *Surgery,* 97(3), 374, 1985.
9. **Dello Russo, N. M. and Temple, H. V.,** Cocaine effects on gingiva, *JADA,* 104, 13, 1982.
10. **Fishel, R. et al.,** Cocaine colitis, disease of the colon and rectum, 28(4), 264, 1985.
11. **Rosecan, J. S. and Gross, B. F.,** Newborn victims of cocaine abuse, *Med. Aspects Hum. Sexual.,* November, 1986.
12. **Moser, C.,** Effects of cocaine on the menstrual cycle, *Med. Aspects Hum. Sexual.,* 19(4), 9, 1985.
13. **Chasnoff, I. J. et al.,** Cocaine use in pregnancy, *N. Engl. J. Med.,* 313(11), 666, 1985.
14. **Chasnoff, I. J. et al.,** Perinatal cerebral infarction and maternal cocaine use, *J. Pediat.,* 108(3), 456, 1986.
15. **Madden, J. D., Payne, T. F., and Miller, S.,** Maternal cocaine abuse and effect on the newborn, *Pediatrics,* 77(2), 209, 1986.
16. **Allred, R. J. and Ewer, S.,** Fatal pulmonary edema following intravenous "freebase" cocaine use, *Ann. Emergency Med.,* 10(8), 441, 1981.
17. **Shesser, R., Davis, C., and Edelstein, S.,** Pneumomediastinum and pneumothorax after inhaling alkaloidal cocaine, *Ann. Emergency Med.,* 10(4), 213, 1981.
18. **Bush, M. et al.,** Spontaneous pneumomediastinum as a consequence of cocaine use, *N.Y. State J. Med.,* 84(12), 618, 1984.
19. **Hunter, J. G. et al.,** Spontaneous pneumomediastinum following inhalation of alkaloidal cocaine and emesis, *M. Sinai J. Med.,* 53(6), 491, 1986.
20. **Weiss, R. D. et al.,** Pulmonary dysfunction in cocaine smokers, *Am. J. Psychiatry,* 138(8), 1110, 1981.
21. **Itkonen, J., Schnoll, S., and Glassroth, J.,** Pulmonary dysfunction in "freebase" cocaine users, *Arch. Intern. Med.,* 144, 2195, 1987.

22. **Copper, C. B., Bai T. R., and Heyderman, E.,** Cellulose granulomas in the lungs of a cocaine sniffer, *Br. Med. J.,* 286, 2022, 1983.
23. **Silverman, H. S. and Smith, A. L.,** Staphylococcal sepsis precipitated by cocaine sniffing, *N. Engl. J. Med.,* 312(26), 1706, 1985.

Chapter 10

MARIJUANA PHARMACOKINETICS AND PHARMACODYNAMICS

C. Nora Chiang and Gene Barnett

TABLE OF CONTENTS

I. INTRODUCTION

Marijuana is perhaps the most widely used illicit drug in our society, in large part because it produces a psychological "high" effect which reinforces recreational use. Marijuana is a crude drug made from the herbaceous annual plant *Cannabis sativa* and is most commonly consumed as the cigarette. Other preparations of cannabis, such as hashish, a resinous form of extract from the plant, are not as common as marijuana cigarettes in the U.S. Marijuana contains more than 420 chemical compounds including at least 61 cannabinoids, a class of chemicals unique to the cannabis plant.[1] Among cannabinoids, delta-9-tetrahydrocannabinol (THC) is the major psychoactive component ingested. The THC content is quite variable among varieties of the cannabis plant. The average THC content of sinsemilla, the most potent form of marijuana, has increased to about 6%, with some samples as high as 14% compared to an average of 2% in 1976.[2] Because of the complexity of the chemistry of marijuana, research on the pharmacology, pharmacokinetics, and pharmacodynamics of cannabis has been carried out primarily based on the THC content of cannabis or with the pure synthetic THC molecule. This chapter provides a critical summary of current findings on the pharmacokinetics and pharmacodynamics of cannabis in humans.

II. PHARMACOKINETICS

A. Physicochemical Properties

Delta-9-tetrahydrocannabinol (THC; see Figure 1) is the major psychoactive component of marijuana. It is a resinous oil with a pKa of 10.6 that is extremely lipophilic and extensively protein-bound (ca. 99%) in plasma.[3] THC is poorly distributed into red blood cells as in vitro experiments suggest that only approximately 10% of THC is bound to the cells.[3,4] A comparison of hemolyzed blood and plasma concentrations from split specimens show the average blood/plasma ratio of THC concentrations is approximately 0.5.[5,6] As the hematocrite is approximately 0.5, this ratio confirms that THC is preferentially in plasma and the concentrations in hemolyzed blood are essentially a dilution with the volume of red blood cells.

B. Disposition Kinetics

Following a single intravenous dose, THC is rapidly distributed into tissues and also rapidly metabolized, as plasma THC levels decline very rapidly over the first few minutes and then at a much slower rate. A multiexponential equation and a four-compartment model was proposed by Hunt and Jones[7] for the description of THC plasma levels, indicating at least four different composites of tissues into which THC is distributed with different rates of permeation and tissue-binding strengths. The rapid initial decline of plasma THC levels results from the rapid distribution into other tissues as well as the rapid metabolism of THC. After psuedoequilibrium is reached between plasma and tissues, THC is eliminated from the body at a slow rate with a terminal plasma half-life of about 19 hr.[7] This slow elimination process is primarily due to the slow return of THC from sequestered tissues to blood.

The terminal half-life of THC in plasma was first reported to be 28 hr for chronic marijuana users and 57 hr for naive smokers by Lemberger et al.[8,9] In their pioneering studies, the analytical methods used were nonspecific, which likely accounts for the lack of agreement. In recent studies using specific methods, the half-life of THC is approximately 1 day with no differences between moderate users and users who have been exposed to THC doses for 2 weeks.[7] Studies by Ohlsson et al.[10,11] found a similiar half-life, estimated as greater than 20 hr, and Wall et al.[12] suggested a terminal half-life of 25 to 36 hr.

The steady-state volume of distribution of THC is estimated to be 10 ℓ/kg, and the average plasma clearance is about 800 to 900 mℓ/min.[7,10,12] Since THC is preferentially distributed

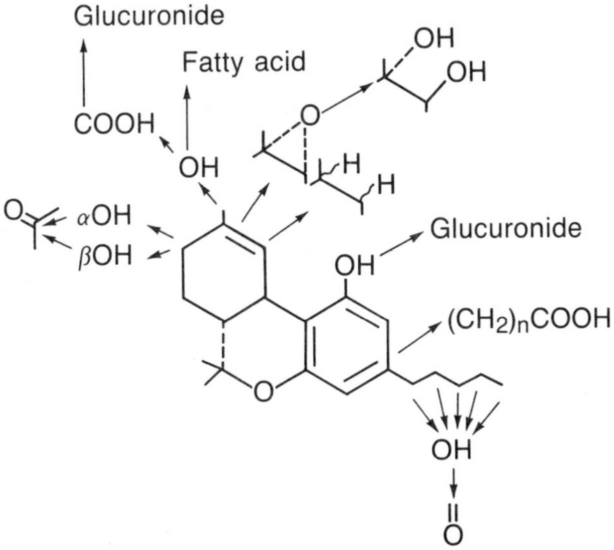

FIGURE 1. The molecular structure of delta-9-tetrahydrocannibinol (THC) is presented along with the sites on the molecule where metabolic changes have been found to occur. (From Harvey, D. J., in *Marijuana in Science and Medicine*, Nahas, G. G. et al., Eds., Raven Press, New York, 1984, 38. With permission.)

in plasma, the estimated blood clearance is 1.5 to 1.6 ℓ/min, close to the hepatic blood flow. This indicates that THC is rapidly metabolized. The rate of metabolism of THC is clearly dependent on hepatic blood flow to the liver, and enzyme induction/inhibition appears to have little effect on metabolic clearance.[7,10,12]

C. Metabolism and Excretion

THC is completely metabolized and excreted as metabolites in feces and urine. Figure 1 shows the metabolic sites of the THC molecule.[13] Approximately 65% of the dose was excreted in feces and 20% in urine during the first 5 days following an intravenous dose.[7,12,14]

More than 60 metabolites have been identified for THC in animals and in vitro liver preparations.[13,15] The metabolic pathways shown in Figure 1 include allylic and aliphatic hydroxylations, epoxidation of the double bonds, reduction of double bonds, and conjugation with glucuronic acid or fatty acids. The hydroxylation products may undergo further oxidation to aldehyde and carboxylic acids. Several monohydroxy metabolites have been found to be psychoactive.[16]

More than 24 metabolites of THC have been identified in human urine and feces, and there is still a significant portion of the dose in both specimen that has not been identified.[12,14,17-19] The pattern of metabolites in urine is different from that in feces. All urine metabolites identified are acidic in nature, including 18 carboxylated products and 2 glucuronic acid conjugates.[17,18] There are neutral, acidic, and acid polar compounds in feces, including one carboxylated metabolite and various hydroxylated metabolites.[12,14] The major metabolite in both urine and feces is 11-nor-9-carboxy-delta-9-THC (9-carboxy-THC). Except for this 9-carboxy-THC, all carboxylated metabolites identified in the urine involve oxidation in the side chain. In feces, 11-hydroxy-THC and 9-carboxy-THC are the major metabolites, while 8-beta and 8-alpha-hydroxy and 8,11-dihydroxy metabolites of THC have also been identified.

While 9-carboxy-THC is the major known metabolite, it is not psychoactive. The monohydroxy metabolites, 11-hydroxy-THC and 8-beta-hydroxy-THC, were found to be psychoactive.[16,20,21] The 11-hydroxy-THC is equipotent to THC, while 8-beta-hydroxy-THC is much less potent.

III. ABSORPTION

A. Oral

Absorption of THC by the oral route is slow and erratic. Peak THC concentrations occur at 1 to 6 hr after ingestion of THC in chocolate cookies,[11,22] and a mean peak concentration at about 2 hr after ingestion of THC in sesame oil.[12] The bioavailability of THC is in the range of 10 to 20% when administrated in sesame oil solution.[12] The low bioavailability of THC may result in part from degradation of THC in the GI tract, but it is more likely due to the "first-pass effect"[23] (see Figure 2). THC is a drug with high hepatic clearance, close to that of hepatic blood flow. The absorbed oral dose, which must first pass through the liver, is extensively metabolized before it reaches the systemic circulation.

The patterns of metabolites in the plasma for an oral dose is different than that for an intravenous dose because of this first-pass effect. After an intravenous dose, the 11-hydroxy-THC metabolite is detectable at levels less than 15% of THC,[7,12] while after an oral dose 11-hydroxy-THC levels are about 50% of THC for the first 6 hr.[12] The ratio of 9-carboxy-THC to THC after an oral dose is also considerably higher (about four times) than that after an intravenous dose. As 11-hydroxy-THC is about equipotent to THC, this metabolite probably does not contribute significantly to the psychoactive effects of THC after an intravenous or smoking dose, but it certainly contributes to the effect after an oral dose.

It has also been shown that THC is absorbed via the ophthalmic route of administration in rabbit studies, although it is slow and quite variable, with a bioavailability of 6 to 40%.[24]

B. Smoking

For the smoking route, THC is inhaled and absorbed from the lungs or respiratory tract into the circulation very rapidly (see Figure 2). Peak plasma concentrations are reached even while the subject is still smoking, and the plasma profile (see Figure 3) is very similar to that of an intravenous dose.[11,25,26]

The amount of THC absorbed is affected by the burning characteristics of the cigarette, depth of inhalation, puff duration, and probably other factors, and can therefore be quite variable. During the smoking process, part of the dose is lost by pyrolysis and in side stream smoke. In vitro smoking studies showed about 69% of THC was recovered when the whole cigarette is consumed as a simulated single puff. This indicates that about 30% of THC is degraded during smoking and the bioavailability will not exceed 70% of the THC content of the cigarette. For puff volume and puff duration simulated to that of a typical marijuana smoker, about 16 to 19% of the THC was recovered in the smoke condensate.[27]

The THC bioavailability from actual smoking of a 1 to 2% marijuana cigarette is variable, depending on the experience of the smokers. Experienced smokers seem to inhale marijuana more efficiently than nonexperienced ones, as the average bioavailability is 27% (range 16 to 40%) for heavy users and 14% (range 13 to 14%) for light users.[10,11]

1. "Dose"-Potency Relationships for Marijuana

The dose of drug absorbed by smoking cannot be readily specified and there is considerable variability in both blood levels and pharmacologic response.[22,25,26,28] In a study of six subjects who smoked three marijuana cigarettes containing 1.3, 2.0, and 2.5% THC by weight in their usual fashion, the amount of THC consumed was estimated by measuring the amount in the portion of the remaining cigarette after the subject stopped smoking. This showed considerable variability as it ranged over 7 to 12, 7 to 16, and 11 to 19 mg for 1.3, 2.0,

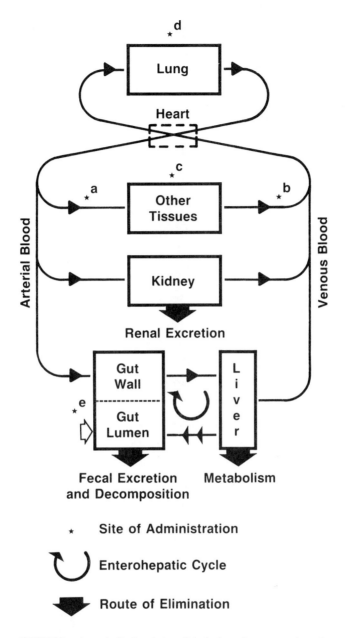

FIGURE 2.   A symbolic description of the body to demonstrate the pathways for drug entry into the body by various routes of administration. (From Rowland, M. and Tozer, T. N., *Clinical Pharmacokinetics Concepts and Applications,* Lea & Febiger, Philadelphia, 1980. With permission.)

and 2.5% cigarettes, respectively.[26] Area under the plasma time curve until 6 hr after smoking (AUC), which is proportional to the dose absorbed, showed a two- to threefold range across subjects for each potency and generally increased with potency for individuals (see Figure 4). When AUC is normalized for potency (AUC/potency), it shows a decrease with increasing potency, suggesting that the fraction of THC inhaled from higher potency cigarettes is relatively less, although the absolute amount absorbed may still be greater. This is further confirmed by a study (four subjects) using marijuana cigarettes of 1 and 3.8% THC content, where the ratio of mean plasma AUC was found to be only 1:1.8, which suggests that the total amount of THC inhaled was about half of the expected value.[16]

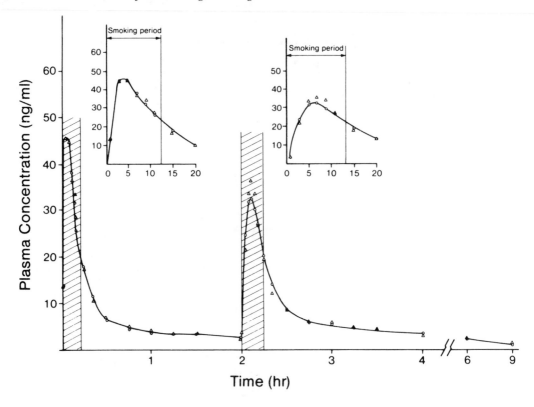

FIGURE 3. Concentration vs. time curve are shown for delta-9-tetrahydrocannabinol in plasma, for one subject, as the result of smoking one marijuana cigarette at time t = 0 and a second at t = 2 hr. The shaded areas are the time intervals when the subject was actively smoking. (From Barnett, G., Chiang, C. N., Perez-Reyes, M., and Owens, S. M., *J. Pharmacokinet. Biopharm.*, 10, 495, 1982. With permission.)

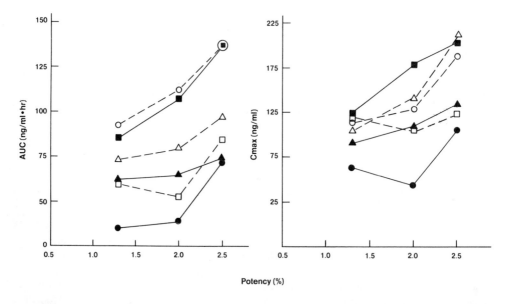

FIGURE 4. The relationship for individual subjects between AUC (left panel) and C_{max} (right panel) vs. potency for three males (dark symbols) and three females (light symbols). Each subject smoked one marijuana cigarette on three different occasions of THC potencies 1.3, 2.0, and 2.5% in a double-blind crossover study design, as described in the text.

Table 1
HEART RATE RESPONSE TO SMOKING ONE MARIJUANA CIGARETTE

Subject	Potency (% THC)	Baseline (bpm) (range)	HR_{max} (bpm)	t^{hr}_{max} (min)	t^{hr}_{end} (min)	AUC_{hr} (bpm × min)
F1	1.3	81 (76—92)	136	21	120	3150
	2.0	91 (86—97)	128	24	54	999
	2.5	73 (68—82)	146	24	120	4190
F2	1.3	83 (78—92)	118	23	45	865
	2.0	96 (90—104)	140	9	50	1270
	2.5	88 (82—92)	148	13	71	1755
F3	1.3	84 (80—88)	123	15	51	1062
	2.0	81 (76—88)	110	26	40	993
	2.5	88 (83—93)	125	20	51	1053
M1	1.3	74 (67—81)	111	18	51	837
	2.0	77 (74—80)	110	15	39	717
	2.5	70 (66—74)	140	19	85	2383
M2	1.3	81 (78—94)	148	10	55	1823
	2.0	87 (82—91)	135	11	57	1431
	2.5	84 (78—88)	139	28	106	2522
M3	1.3	70 (62—82)	122	20	52	1403
	2.0	81 (72—86)	138	15	45	1298
	2.5	68 (64—78)	130	20	87	2343

IV. PHARMACODYNAMICS

It is well established that marijuana produces a broad range of psychological and biological effects. The pharmacological responses vary over time and result in complex pharmacodynamic profiles. Since the dose of drug absorbed by smoking cannot be specified, it is not surprising that there is considerable variability in both blood levels and response. In general, pharmacodynamic analysis of drug response is less well developed as a quantitative research tool than pharmacokinetic analysis. This problem is exacerbated in the case of studying effects due to smoking a marijuana cigarette, and data are usually presented as mean values. We discuss the pharmacodynamic analysis of heart rate response to smoking marijuana, based on objective observational data, and the psychological "high" response which is based on subjective self-reported data. Pharmacodynamics of behavioral response for measures related to safety in operating complex machinery is also discussed. There is also interest in determining the relationships that exist between the pharmacokinetics and the pharmacodynamics, as it offers hope of gaining further understanding of mechanisms of actions.

To illustrate the variability and "dose"-potency relationships from smoking, the experimental data from a three-potency, double-blind crossover study are discussed in considerable detail,[26] along with other previously reported studies. Six subjects smoked three marijuana cigarettes containing 1.3, 2.0, and 2.5% THC by weight and were instructed to smoke as much of the cigarette as they wished in their usual fashion. Heart rate and psychological "high" effects were measured and blood samples were collected, all over a considerable time span. After the start of smoking, heart rate accelerates very rapidly to maximum values in 9 to 28 min and returns to baseline values in 39 to 120 min. Psychological high has a slower onset and a more extended duration than effect on heart rate, as time to maximum effect is 10 to 45 min and duration of effect is up to 6 hr. Correlations are seen between pharmacologic measure and THC plasma levels even with individual subject data.

A. Heart Rate Acceleration

The pharmacodynamics of heart rate, HR, acceleration due to smoking a marijuana cigarette are presented in Table 1 for the three female and three male volunteers. Since baseline rates, in beats per minute (bpm), have considerable fluctuations, especially with individual data as opposed to mean values, the 10-min average and range is reported. The HR accelerates very rapidly after the start of smoking to maximum values of 110 to 148 bpm, for HR_{max} where the increase is 30 to 50% over baseline. The time of the observed maximum effect t_{max}^{hr} is 9 to 28 min and is generally less than a twofold range within subjects. The time required for HR to return to within the baseline range t_{end}^{hr} is 39 to 120 min. Within subjects, t_{end}^{hr} is much greater for the 2.5% than the 1.3% cigarette and the range is less than twofold. Some subjects may have been accelerated during baseline measurements due to clinical preparations for the study, thus t_{end}^{hr} is probably an underestimate of the duration of tachycardia. The area under the heart rate vs. time curve, AUC_{hr}, is usually largest for the 2.5% cigarette and may be thought of as the added heart burden over the period t = 0 until t_{end}^{hr} due to smoking marijuana. The ratio AUC_{hr}/t_{end}^{hr} is then an average heart rate increase above baseline during the duration of pharmacologic effect and has the range 16 to 34 bpm across subjects, usually increasing with increasing THC potency of the cigarette.

The relationship between HR and THC plasma concentration for the individual subjects is presented in Figure 5 for the time points t = 30, 60, 90, and 120 min. After an initial upswing of the phase plot (see, e.g., Reference 29), there is a strong linear correlation from the highest THC concentrations with a range of 19 to 71 ng/mℓ at 30 min through 2 hr where the concentration range is 4 to 12 ng/mℓ. Least-squares analysis of the data gives the correlation coefficients (range 0.76 to 0.91) and slopes (range 0.6 to 2.5) shown in the figure. In all cases there is a single valued relationship between effect and THC levels within individual subjects, but not among subjects.

B. Psychological "High"

Psychological "high" (PH), also known as the subjective self-reported level of intoxication, has a slower onset and a more extended duration of effect than heart rate, as seen in Table 2. The maximum self-reported psychological "high", PH_{max}, ranges from 35 to 105% of each subject's "best ever" previous experience. Four subjects reported an almost equal response across potencies, although this varied greatly between subjects, with ranges from 35 to 40% for subject F1 to 90 to 105% for M2. The time to reach maximum effect, t_{max}^{ph}, has a range of 0.17 to 0.75 hr, but the within-subject ranges are much less. In all cases the "high" effect lasts for several hours, usually up to 6 hr. Area under the "high" vs. time curve from t = 0 until t_{end}^{ph}, AUC_{ph}, is always greatest for the most potent cigarette. The ratio AUC_{ph}/potency decreases for two subjects, suggesting that they self-limit drug effect.

Figure 6 shows a plot of the relationship between PH and THC plasma levels for the time points t = 0.5, 1.0, 1.5, 2.0, and 4.0 hr. For THC levels of 20 ng/mℓ and less there is a rapid decrease in PH with THC levels, but at higher plasma concentrations the PH tends to plateau. Attempts to fit the data by least-squares analysis gave poor results for a log-linear fit, but description of the data with a Michaelis-Menton type of function, $PH = k_1 * C/(k_2 + C)$, gives good results for subjects F1, F2, and M3, a weak fit for F3 and M2, and no fit for M1. In the latter two cases, the subjects had plasma levels below 25 ng/mℓ and only a suggestion of a plateau.

In a pharmacokinetic and pharmacodynamic compartmental model analysis,[29] the "high" effect was satisfactorily correlated with the entire plasma THC curve, where the pattern of the PH showed a slower rise and a slower decline than the THC plasma levels. This delay of the effect suggests that the site of action of THC is not easily accessible to the plasma. When this is taken into consideration in the compartmental model analysis, the effects correlate well with plasma THC levels. Estimation of the degree of intoxication from a single THC plasma level is of questionable value due to time dependence in both effects and plasma levels.

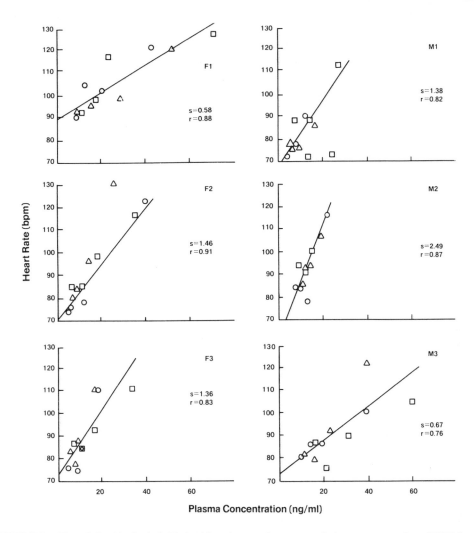

FIGURE 5. The relationship for individual subjects between heart rate and plasma concentration of THC from smoking as described in Figure 4. The symbols represent measurements with cigarettes of potencies 1.3% (circles), 2.0% (triangles), and 2.5% (squares) for females (left side) and males (right side). The slope (s) and correlation coefficient (r) is reported for each subject on each graph as determined by linear least-squares analysis.

C. Performance Decrement

Marijuana use has been associated with decrements in behavior and cognitive performance. Information about the effects of marijuana on performance impairment has been collected from epidemiology studies as well as clinical laboratory studies in an effort to determine if marijuana use is detrimental to safe operation of a motor vehicle. Epidemiological studies done on blood specimens obtained from drivers involved in fatal automobile crashes were analyzed for detectable levels of THC in fatally injured drivers, but it was not possible to establish marijuana as a cause from such studies because of the general high incidence of alcohol intoxication shown in the victims.[30-32]

Laboratory investigations have reported that THC may affect complex performance skills for up to 24 hr after drug ingestion. One study reports a "hangover" effect on the morning following a dose of marijuana, 9 hr after smoking a marijuana cigarette of 3% THC,[33] while mean data on performance of pilots in a flight simulator showed a trend toward impairment at 24 hr after smoking a cigarette of 2% THC.[34]

Table 2
PSYCHOLOGICAL HIGH RESPONSE TO SMOKING ONE MARIJUANA CIGARRETTE

Subject	Potency (% THC)	PH_{max} (%)	t^{ph}_{max} (hr)	t^{ph}_{end} (hr)	AUC_{ph} (% high × hr)
F1	1.3	35	.50	6	97
	2.0	40	.75	6	87
	2.5	37	.33	6	98
F2	1.3	40	.33	4	44
	2.0	60	.25	6	97
	2.5	50	.17	6	189
F3	1.3	80	.17	6	172
	2.0	95	.25	6	129
	2.5	105	.50	6	251
M1	1.3	20	.25	4	25
	2.0	40	.25	2	40
	2.5	70	.33	6	140
M2	1.3	90	.33	6	194
	2.0	100	.50	6	172
	2.5	105	50	6	234
M3	1.3	55	.75	6	122
	2.0	60	.25	6	110
	2.5	50	.50	6	160

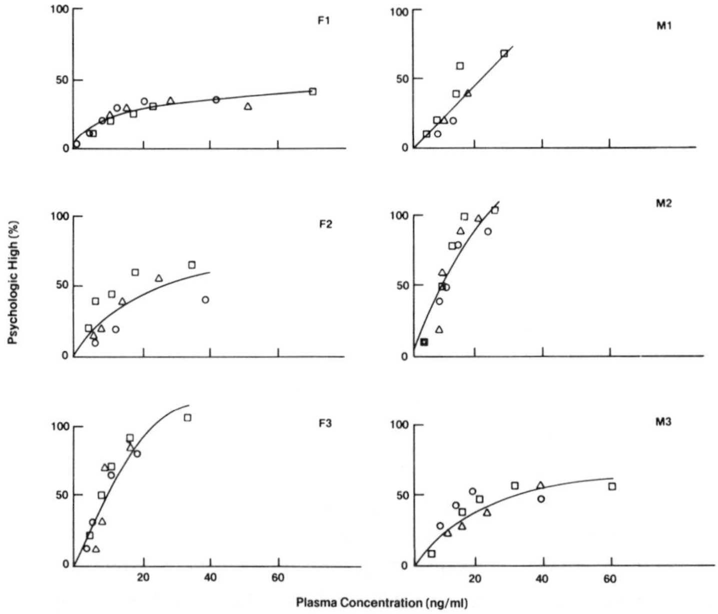

FIGURE 6.   The relationship for individual subjects between psychological high and plasma concentration of THC from smoking as described in Figure 4. The symbols represent measurements with cigarettes of potencies 1.3% (circles), 2.0% (triangles), and 2.5% (squares) for females (left side) and males (right side).

Another laboratory study demonstrated a quantitative correlation between impaired performance and THC plasma concentrations, shown in Figure 7, from smoking one marijuana cigarette.[35] The results for a three-way crossover study design show a correlation of THC plasma levels immediately after smoking one marijuana cigarette with impaired performance which continues for approximately 7 hr. Over this time interval, the THC plasma levels fall

CRITICAL TRACKING
Break Point (rad/sec)

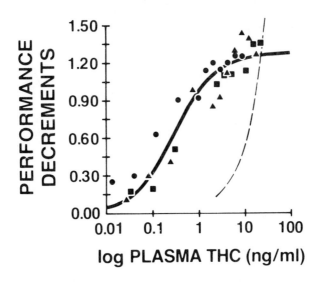

FIGURE 7. The correlation of decrement in performance with plasma levels of THC after smoking one marijuana cigarette containing 100 μg/ kg (squares). (From Barnett, G., Licko, V., and Thompson, T., *Psychopharmacology*, 85, 51, 1985. With permission.)

from 25 ng/mℓ immediately after smoking to 2 ng/mℓ at 7 hr. While these tasks are widely used in laboratory evaluation of factors related to driving, there is no data to show predictive validity outside the laboratory. Therefore, even though impairment on laboratory tasks can be related to plasma THC levels, the extent to which it predicts driving impairment from smoking marijuana is not clear. Studies are needed to address such pharmacologic issues as drug tolerance and such behavioral issues as user experience in relation to performance.

V. CONCLUSIONS

It is clear that this complex drug still presents challenges to biomedical researchers in their efforts to discover and understand the various modes and mechanisms of action in humans. A review of the status of biomedical research on marijuana and its health-related effects on humans was recently completed by the Institute of Medicine of the National Academy of Sciences.[36] This extensive report summarizes results concerning effects on the nervous system and on behavior, the cardiovascular and respiratory systems, the reproductive system and on chromosomes, and effects on the immune system. Several pharmacokinetic studies have been reported in relation to the reproductive system.[37-39] However, it is clear that more work is needed in order to gain a full understanding of the broad range of psychological and biological effects that result from marijuana consumption. Recent reviews indicate that this is still an active area of research.[40-44]

REFERENCES

1. **Turner, C. E., El Sohly, M. A., and Boeren, E. G.,** Constituents of cannabis sativa L. XVII. A review of the natural constituents, *J. Nat. Prod.,* 43, 169, 1980.

2. **El Sohly, M. A., Holley, J. H., and Turner, C. E.,** Constituents of cannabis sativa L. XXVI. The delta-9-tetrahydrocannabinol content of confiscated marijuana, 1974—1983, in: *Marijuana '84',* Harvey, D. J., Ed., IRL Press, Oxford, 1985, 37.

3. **Garrett, E. R. and Hunt, C. A.,** Physicochemical properties, solubility, and protein binding of delta-9-tetrahydrocannabinol, *J. Pharm. Sci.,* 63, 1056, 1974.

4. **Widman, M., Agurell, S., Ehrnebo, M., and Jones, G.,** Binding of (+)-and (−)-delta-1-tetrahydro-cannabinols and (−)-7-hydroxy-delta-1-tetrahydrocannabinol to blood cells and plasma proteins in man, *J. Pharm. Pharmacol.,* 26, 914, 1974.

5. **Owens, S. M., McBay, A. J., Reisner, H. M., and Perez-Reyes, M.,** ^{125}I-Radioimmunoassay of delta-9-tetrahydrocannabinol in blood and plasma with a solid-phase second-antibody separation method, *Clin. Chem.,* 27, 619, 1981.

6. **Rosenthal, D. and Brine, D.,** Quantitative determination of delta-9-tetrahydrocannabinol in cadaver blood, *J. Forensic Sci.,* 24, 282, 1979.

7. **Hunt, C. A. and Jones, R. T.,** Tolerance and disposition of tetrahydrocannabinol in man, *J. Pharmacol. Exp. Ther.,* 215, 35, 1980.

8. **Lemberger, L., Silberstein, S. D., Axelrod, J., and Kopin, I. J.,** Marijuana: studies on the disposition and metabolism of delta-9-tetrahydrocannabinol in man, *Science,* 170, 1320, 1970.

9. **Lemberger, L., Axelrod, J., and Kopin, I. J.,** Metabolism and disposition of tetrahydrocannabinol in naive subjects and chronic marijuana users, *Ann. N.Y. Acad. Sci.,* 191, 142, 1971.

10. **Ohlsson, A., Lindgren, J.-E., Wahlen, A., Agurell, S., Hollister, L. E., and Gillespie, H. K.,** Single-dose kinetics of deuterium-labelled delta-1-tetrahydrocannabinol in heavy and light users, *Biomed. Mass Spectrom.,* 9, 6, 1982.

11. **Ohlsson, A., Agurell, S., Lindgren, J-E., Gillespie, H. K., and Hollister, L. E.,** Pharmacokinetic studies of delta-1-tetrahydrocannabinol in man, in *Pharmacokinetics and Pharmacodynamics of Psychoactive Drugs,* Barnett, G. and Chiang, C. N., Eds., Biomedical Publications, Foster City, Calif., 1985, 75.

12. **Wall, M. E., Sadler, B. M., Brine, D., Harold, T., and Perez-Reyes, M.,** Metabolism, disposition, and kinetics of delta-9-tetrahydrocannabinol in men and women, *Clin. Pharmacol. Ther.,* 34, 352, 1983.

13. **Harvey, D. J.,** Chemistry, metabolism and pharmacokinetics of cannabinoids, in *Marijuana in Science and Medicine,* Nahas, G. G. et al., Eds., Raven Press, New York, 1984, 38.

14. **Wall, M. E. and Perez-Reyes, M.,** The metabolism of delta-9-tetrahydrocannabinol and related canna-binoids in man, *J. Clin. Pharmacol.,* 21, 178s, 1981.

15. **Burstein, B.,** Biotransformation of the cannabinoids, in *Pharmacokinetics and Pharmacodynamics of Psychoactive Drugs,* Barnett, G. and Chiang, C. N., Eds., Biomedical Publications, Foster City, Calif., 1985, 396.

16. **Perez-Reyes, M.,** Pharmacodynamics of certain drugs of abuse, in *Pharmacokinetics and Pharmacodyn-amics of Psychoactive Drugs,* Barnett, G. and Chiang, C. N., Eds., Biomedical Publications, Foster City, Calif., 1985, 287.

17. **Widman, M., Halldin, M. M., and Agurell, S.,** Metabolism of delta-1-tetra-hydrocannabinol in man, in *Pharmacokinetics and Pharmacodynamics of Psychoactive Drugs,* Barnett, G. and Chiang, C. N., Eds., Biomedical Publications, Foster City, Calif., 1985, 415.

18. **Halldin, M. M., Andersson, L. K. R., Widman, M., and Hollister, L. E.,** Further urinary metabolites of delta-1-tetrahydrocannabinol in man, *Arzeimittelforschung,* 32, 1135, 1982.

19. **Halldin, M. M., Carlsson, S., Kanter, S. L., Widman, M., and Agurell, S.,** Urinary metabolites of delta-1-tetrahydrocannabinol in man, *Arzeimittelforschung,* 32, 764, 1982.

20. **Perez-Reyes, M., Timmons, M. S., Lipton, M. A., Christensen, H. D., Davis, K. H., and Wall, M. E.,** A comparison of the pharmacological activity of delta-9-tetrahydrocannabinol and its monohy-droxylated metabolites in man, *Experientia,* 29, 1009, 1973.

21. **Lemberger, L., Martz, R., Rodda, B., Forney, R., and Rowe, H.,** Comparative pharmacology of delta-9-tetrahydrocannabinol and its metabolite, 11-OH-delta-9-tetrahydrocannabinol, *J. Clin. Invest.,* 52, 2411, 1973.

22. **Ohlsson, A., Lindgren, J-E., Wahlen, A., Agurell, S., Hollister, L. E., and Gillespie, H. K.,** Plasma delta-9-tetrahydrocannabinol concentrations and clinical effects after oral and intravenous administration and smoking, *Clin. Pharmacol. Ther.,* 28, 409, 1980.

23. **Rowland, M. and Tozer, T. N.,** *Clinical Pharmacokinetics Concepts and Applications,* Lea & Febiger, Philadelphia, 1980.

24. **Chiang, C. N., Barnett, G., and Brine, D.,** Systemic absorption of delta-9-tetrahydrocannabinol after ophthalmic administration to the rabbit, *J. Pharm. Sci.,* 72, 136, 1983.

25. **Barnett, G., Chiang, C. N., Perez-Reyes, M., and Owens, S. M.,** Kinetic Study of smoking marijuana, *J. Pharmacokinet. Biopharm.,* 10, 495, 1982.

26. **Perez-Reyes, M., DiGuiseppi, S., Davis, K. H., Schindler, V. H., and Cook, C. E.,** Comparison of effects of marijuana cigarettes of three different potencies, *Clin. Pharmacol. Ther.,* 31, 617, 1982.

27. **Davis, K. H., Jr., McDaniel, I. A., Jr., Cadwell, L. W., and Moody, P. L.,** Some smoking characteristics of marijuna cigarettes. in *Cannabinoids: Chemical, Pharmacologic and Therapeutic aspects,* Agurell, S., Dewey, W. L., and Willette, R. E., Eds., Academic Press, New York, 1984, 97.

28. **Lindgren, J-E., Ohlsson, A., Agurell, S., Hollister, L. E., and Gillespie, H.,** Clinical effects and plasma levels of delta-9-tetrahydrocannabinol in heavy and light users of cannabis, *Psychopharmacology,* 74, 208, 1981.

29. **Chiang, C. N. and Barnett, G.,** Marijuana effect and delta-9-tetrahydrocannabinol plasma level, *Clin. Pharmacol. Ther.,* 36, 234, 1984.

30. **Cimbura, C., Lucas, D. M., Bennett, R. C., Warren, R. A., and Simpson, H. M.,** Incidence and toxicological aspects of drugs detected in 484 fatally injured drivers and pedestrians in Ontario, *J. Forensic Sci.,* 27, 855, 1982.

31. **Mason, A. P. and McBay, A. J.,** Ethanol, marijuana, and other drug use in 600 drivers killed in single-vehicle crashes in North Carolina, 1978—1981, *J. Forensic Sci.,* 29, 987, 1984.

32. **Williams, A. F., Peat, M. A., Crouch, D. J., Wells, J. K., and Finkle, B. S.,** Drugs in fatally injured young male drivers, *Public Health Rep.,* 100, 19, 1985.

33. **Chait, L. D., Fischman, M. W., and Schuster, C. R.,** ''Hangover'' effects the morning after marijuana smoking, *Drug Alcohol Depend.,* 15, 229, 1985.

34. **Yesavage, J. A., Leirer, V. O., Denari, M., and Hollister, L. E.,** Carry-over effects of marijuana intoxication on aircraft pilot performance: A preliminary report, *Am. J. Psychiatry,* 142, 1325, 1985.

35. **Barnett, G., Licko, V., and Thompson, T.,** Behavioral pharmacokinetics of marijuana, *Psychopharmacology,* 85, 51, 1985.

36. **Institute of Medicine,** National Academy of Sciences, Marijuana and Health, National Academy Press, Washington, D.C., 1982.

37. **Barnett, G. and Chiang, C. N.,** Effects of Marijuana on testostrone in male subjects, *J. Theor. Biol.,* 104, 685, 1983.

38. **Kolodny, R. C., Lessin, P., Toro, G., Masters, W. H., and Cohen, S.,** Depression of plasma testoterone with acute marijuana administration, in *The Pharmacology of Marijuana,* Braude, M. C. and Szara, S. Eds., Raven Press, New York, 1976, 217.

39. **Mendelson, J. H., Ellingboe, J. M., Keuhnle, J. C., and Mello, N. K.,** Effects of chronic marijuana use on integrated plasma testosterone and luteinizing hormone levels, *J. Pharmacol. Exp. Ther.,* 207, 611, 1978.

40. **Agurell, S., Halldin, M., Lindgren, J-E., Ohlsson, A., Widman, M., Gillespie, H., and Hollister, L.,** Pharmacokinetics and metabolism of delta-1-tetrahydrocannabinoids with emphasis on man, *Pharmacol. Rev.,* 38, 21, 1986.

41. **Dewey, W.,** Cannabinoid pharmacology, *Pharmacol. Rev.,* 38, 151, 1986.

42. **Hollister, L. E.,** Health aspects of cannabis, *Pharmacol. Rev.,* 38, 1, 1986.

43. **Martin, B. R.,** Cellular effects of cannabinoids, *Pharmacol. Rev.,* 38, 45, 1986.

44. **Razdan, R. K.,** Structure-activity relationships in cannabinoids, *Pharmacol. Rev.,* 38, 75, 1986.

Chapter 11

MARIJUANA ABUSE: ITS PHARMACOLOGY AND EFFECTS ON TESTICULAR FUNCTION

Syed Husain

I. INTRODUCTION

The various preparations of the plant *Cannabis sativa* constitute the most widely used illicit drugs throughout the world. In this country, during the past 2 decades, large-scale research was initiated to look into the pharmacology of marijuana because of the social and political concerns about its adverse effects as well as its therapeutic potentials. A wealth of information has emerged from these studies and is the subject of numerous books and reviews.[1-3] In some of these investigations, it was realized that Δ^9-tetrahydrocannabinol (THC), the active constituent of marijuana, has specific effects on the gonadal functions of various species, including man. For instance, Kolodny et al.[4] first demonstrated that acute as well as chronic administration of THC decreases plasma testosterone (T) levels, decreases sperm counts, and impairs potency in humans. Although conflicting reports have since been presented concerning these actions of THC, Dalterio et al.,[5] Burnstein et al.,[6] and Symons et al.[7] have confirmed these findings of Kolodny in mice and rats. Several other studies also indicate that various constituents of marijuana not only decrease plasma testosterone levels, but also cause regression of the testis, seminiferous tubules, prostate, and other reproductive organs.[8-10] Zimmerman et al.[11] investigated the effects of marijuana on sperm morphology and reported a higher incidence of abnormal sperms in mice treated with THC and cannabinol (CBN). Huang et al.[12] showed that apart from changing normal morphology, THC also decreased sperm motility and the number of sperms in marijuana smokers.

Since the time these effects of THC on gonadal functions were first reported, much research has been directed toward documenting these changes. However, in the last 5 years or so, attempts have also been made to explain the biochemical mechanism(s) which are responsible for these effects. These studies have yielded very valuable and interesting findings. For example, studies of Symons et al.[7] in rodents and of Smith et al.[13] in monkeys indicate that THC not only decreases plasma testosterone levels, but also reduces LH and FSH levels in the body. However, as we know, the release of LH and FSH is under the control of gonadotropin-releasing hormone (GnRH) from the hypothalamus. Therefore, other studies have suggested that the effects of THC on peripheral levels of LH and FSH are secondary to the THC-induced alterations in hypothalamic functions. These findings have led to the development of the concept that THC disrupts the integrity of the testis by indirectly acting through the hypothalamic-pituitary-gonadal axis (H-P-G axis).

Apart from these observations, different other studies have also been reported in literature which show a direct effect rather than a pituitary-mediated effect of marijuana on the testis. For example, Jakubovic and McGeer[14] showed a direct effect of THC on rat Leydig cells, whereby it causes a significant decrease in nucleic acid and protein synthesis in the testis. Similarly, Hembree et al.[15] examined the semen of 16 healthy, chronic marijuana smokers and found them to have significant oligospermia. In this oligospermia, there was no involvement of hormones, and they suggested this to be a direct effect of THC on the germinal epithelium of the testis.

It is obvious that at present, the exact mechanism or mechanisms by which THC interferes with testicular functions is not clear. In this paper, in vitro and in vivo data is presented which suggests a biochemical basis of the gonadal effects of THC and delineates the possible site(s) at which THC may have its effects.

II. MATERIALS AND METHODS

In all phases of in vitro studies, adult, male Sprague Dawley rats (275 ± 25 g) were used. On the other hand, for in vivo experiments, 55- to 60-day-old, young-adult, male rats (200 ± 25 g) were obtained. These animals had free access to rat chow and tap water. All chemicals used in this investigation were analytical grade. Glucose-6-^{14}C and fructose-U-

[14]C (Sp.Ac. 3 mCi/mmol each) were purchased from Amersham Corp., Arlington Heights, Ill. Pyruvate-2-^{14}C and ^{14}C-2-deoxy-D-glucose (Sp.Ac. 6.5 mCi/mmol and 337 mCi, mmol, respectively) were from New England Nuclear Corp., Boston, Mass. Other chemicals and enzymes used were β-NADH, β-NADP[+], EDTA, triethanolamine, glycerol-3-phosphate dehydrogenase (EC 1.1.1.8), triosephosphate isomerase (EC 5.3.1.1), aldolase (EC 4.1.2.13), glucose-6-phosphate dehydrogenase (EC 1.1.1.49), and phosphoglucose isomerase (EC 5.3.1.9). These chemicals were from Sigma Chemical Co., St. Louis, Mo. The National Institute on Drug Abuse (NIDA) kindly provided 95% pure THC in ethanolic solution.

A. Radiorespirometric Studies

To determine the in vitro effects of THC on energy metabolism in rat testicular tissue, [14]CO_2 production was followed from different ^{14}C-labeled substrates. For this purpose, rats were decapitated, their testes rapidly removed, decapsulated, and sectioned into several small pieces. The tissues were incubated in Warburg Flasks at 37°C for 100 min. These flasks contained modified Krebs-Ringer's bicarbonate Tris-buffered medium and the different radiolabeled substrates. THC was dissolved in ethanol, and the experimental tissues received different concentrations of THC in the medium prior to incubation. The control tissues received an equivalent amount of ethanol. The [14]CO_2 produced due to the catabolism of the labeled glucose, fructose, or pyruvate was trapped for 60 min in 3.5 N KOH placed in the center well of the Warburg flask. This was then counted and expressed as micromoles of [14]CO_2 produced per gram of dry tissue per 100 min incubation.

B. Analysis of Glycolytic Intermediates

To delineate the site(s) of THC action, the levels of glycolytic intermediates, such as dihydroxyacetone phosphate (DAP), fructose 1,6-diphosphate (F1,6-P_2), and glucose-6-phosphate (G6-P), were determined in testicular tissues exposed to THC. As usual, for this purpose, rat testes were sectioned in small pieces and placed in Warburg flasks containing Tris-buffered medium. The control flasks received 0.2 mℓ ethanol, and the experimental tissues were exposed to 0.3 mM THC in ethanol. After 100 min of incubation, tissues were freeze dried and their homogenates obtained after deproteinization. The pH of the homogenates was adjusted. F1,6-P_2 and DAP were determined in control and experimental samples by spectrophotometric technique of Michal and Beutler.[16] Similarly, G6-P was determined based on the enzymatic method of Lang and Michal.[17]

C. Uptake Studies with 2-Deoxy-D-glucose

To study the effects of THC on membrane uptake of glucose, a protocol similar to radiorespirometric studies was followed, except in this study, ^{14}C-2-deoxy-D-glucose was used as a substrate. After 100 min of incubation, tissues from control and experimental flasks were removed and digested for 4 hr in soluene-350 tissue solubilizer (Packard Instrument Co., Downers Grove, Ill.). It was then counted and tissue uptake of ^{14}C-2-deoxy-D-glucose was expressed as micromoles of glucose per gram of wet tissue per 100 min incubation.

D. In Vivo Acute and Chronic THC Effects on Glucose Metabolism in Testicular Tissue

To study the effects of acute treatment, groups of rats were administered 10 or 20 mg/kg, po THC in sesame oil. The respective controls received 2 mℓ/kg, po sesame oil. Similarly, for chronic study, groups of rats were treated for 15 days with 5, 10, or 20 mg/kg, po THC. In both treatment schedules, animals were sacrificed 2 hr after the last dose of THC. Testes from the acute and chronically treated rats were removed, decapsulated, and sectioned into several small pieces. These tissues were placed in separate Warburg flasks containing 2 mℓ Tris-buffered medium with 5.5 mM glucose. The flasks also contained 6-^{14}C-glucose as the tracer. Incubations were carried out for 100 min at 37° and the rates of $^{14}CO_2$ production in different groups of testicular tissue were determined in essentially the same manner as described earlier.

E. Uptake of 2-deoxy-D-glucose Following Acute and Chronic THC Treatment

To evaluate the effects of acute and chronic treatment on glucose uptake in the testis, rats were pretreated with respective doses of THC as described in the above section. Similarly, controls received 2 mℓ/kg, po sesame oil. Testicular tissues from different treatment groups were transferred in 20-mℓ Erlenmeyer flasks which contained Tris-buffered medium with 5.5 mM 2-deoxy-D-glucose and the radioactive tracer. After 100 min of incubation, tissues from control, acute, and chronically treated groups were removed from the incubation medium and digested for 4 hr in soluene-350 tissue solublizer. Radioactivity in the solublized testicular tissue was counted, and the tissue uptake of ^{14}C-2-deoxy-D-glucose was expressed as micromoles of glucose taken up per gram of wet tissue in 100 min of incubation.

F. Intratesticular Administration of THC

To study the in-vivo effects of THC after intratesticular (i.t.) administration, rats were given 5 μg THC dissolved in 10 μℓ of Tween® 80-ethanol-saline solution (1:1:8). The left testis of unanesthetized animals was immobilized by light pressure between the thumb and the first finger. Using a microliter syringe with a 30-gauge needle, THC was administered in the middle of the testis. In these rats, the right testis served as a control and received 10 μℓ injection of the vehicle. Animals were sacrificed 1 hr after the i.t. administration of THC. Testes were removed, decapsulated, and sectioned into six equal-size pieces. These control and THC-treated tissues were then subjected to radiorespirometric studies with 5.5 mM radiolabeled glucose as the substrate. In these control and treated tissues, micromoles of $^{14}CO_2$ produced per gram of dry tissue per 100 min incubation was compared to determine the effects of i.t. THC administration.

III. RESULTS AND DISCUSSIONS

Cellular energetics play a vital role in numerous biosynthetic processes of a cell and in maintenance of its functions. As described earlier, THC is shown to inhibit various cellular processes of the testis which include testosterone synthesis, nucleic acid synthesis, protein synthesis, sperm motility, as well as spermatogenesis. Since all these cellular processes require energy for their successful completion, it was hypothesized that THC produces its effects by blocking the utilization of energy-rich substrates in the testis. With this premise in mind, initially the effects of THC on energy metabolism in rat testicular tissue were studied by measuring in vitro production of $^{14}CO_2$ from different ^{14}C-labeled substrates.

At 0.1 mM concentration of THC which was dissolved in 3 μℓ of ethanol, a 15% inhibition was found in ^{14}CO production from 5.5 mM glucose, which was statistically significant. When testicular tissues were exposed to 0.2, 0.3, and 0.4 mℓ THC dissolved in 6, 9, and 12 μℓ ethanol, all these concentrations of THC produced a significant reduction in ^{14}CO production as compared to controls. This inhibition was dose related and caused a 18, 20, and 25% decrease in $^{14}CO_2$ production (Figure 1). In this study, a separate investigation with ethanol was conducted, since ethanol served as a vehicle for THC. These experiments revealed no significant effects of 3, 6, 9, or 12 μℓ of ethanol on glucose metabolism in the testis.

The capacity of THC to affect $^{14}CO_2$ production with different concentrations of glucose was then determined by incubating testicular tissues with various glucose concentrations in the presence of 0.3 mM THC. The dose of 0.3 mM THC was chosen because above this dose, THC forms a fine suspension in the medium and begins to precipitate. Therefore, in

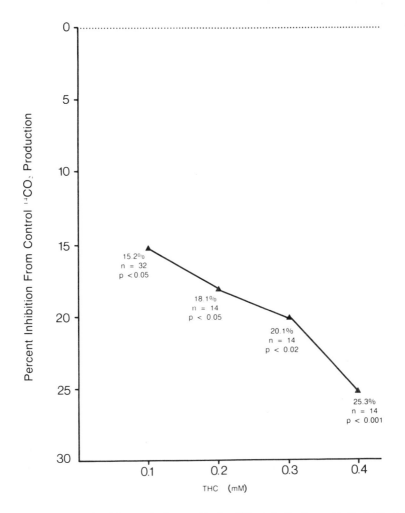

FIGURE 1.   Effects of Δ-9-tetrahydrocannabinol on CO_2 production from rat testicular tissue incubated in 5.5 mM glucose.

all subsequent experiments, a dose of 0.3 mM THC was used to investigate the effects of THC on testicular glycolysis. Exposure of testicular tissues to 0.3 mM THC in the medium with 1, 3, 5.5, and 10 mM glucose caused a 10, 24, 20, and 8% inhibition in $^{14}CO_2$ production, respectively (Figure 2). The decrease in $^{14}CO_2$ production with 3 and 5.5 mM glucose was statistically significant.

After noticing that THC produces a significant inhibition in glucose utilization, attempts were made to localize the site(s) of this inhibition. To do so, groups of testicular tissue were incubated in the medium containing different concentrations of pyruvate with 2-^{12}C pyruvate as the tracer. As usual, the control tissues received 9 $\mu\ell$ of ethanol. Unlike glucose, with pyruvate as a testicular substrate, there was no reduction in $^{14}CO_2$ production from tissues exposed to 0.3 mM THC. In these tissues, the control $^{14}CO_2$ production with 1.0 mM pyruvate was 3.50 μmol/g dry tissue per 100 min incubation. The presence of 0.3 mM THC in the incubation medium caused the $^{14}CO_2$ production to decrease to 3.2 μmol (Table 1). This was a 9% inhibition, which was not significant. Similarly, 2.5, 5.5, and 11.0 mM pyruvate showed no significant difference in $^{14}CO_2$ production between the control and the experimental tissues.

These observations with pyruvate were very meaningful. Thus far, it was observed that 0.3 mM THC significantly inhibited glucose conversion to $^{14}CO_2$. Pyruvate formation is an

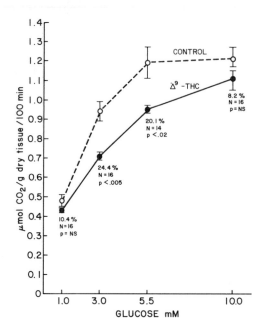

FIGURE 2.   Effects of 0.3 mM Δ-9-tetrahydrocannabinol on CO_2 production from rat testicular tissue incubated in different concentrations of glucose. (From Husain, S. and Lamé, M., *Pharmacology*, 23, 102, 1981. With permission)

intermediate step in this conversion. However, when pyruvate was used as a substrate, it was observed that its conversion to $^{14}CO_2$ was not blocked by THC. These observations led us to conclude that THC produces its inhibitory effects on glucose metabolism at a level above pyruvate entry into the glycolytic scheme.

To further delineate the site(s) of this inhibition and to substantiate our conclusions, other groups of testicular tissue were then incubated in different concentrations of fructose with U-^{14}C fructose as the tracer. Figure 3 shows the effects of 0.3 mM THC on $^{14}CO_2$ production from different concentrations of fructose. THC was able to inhibit $^{14}CO_2$ production from all concentrations of fructose. This inhibition was highly significant. This was important because (1) it fortified our previous observations and (2) because fructose is a sugar which is present in high concentrations in the testis and is a readily available substrate for the energy needs of the testis.

At this stage, to investigate the site(s) of this inhibition further, the levels of glycolytic intermediates, such as dihydroxyacetone phosphate (DAP), fructose 1,6-diphosphate (F1,6-P_2), and glucose-6-phosphate (G6-P), were determined in testicular tissues exposed to THC. Analysis of glycolytic intermediates further narrowed the sites of THC action. Table 2 shows the levels of these intermediates in control and THC exposed testicular tissues. As DAP, F1,6-P_2, and G6-P were all inhibited significantly with 0.3 mM THC, it confirmed our previous findings and limited the steps of THC action to hexokinase and/or membrane uptake step.

In studying the effects of THC on membrane uptake of glucose, it was found that except 0.033 mM THC, all other concentrations of THC significantly inhibited the uptake of 2-deoxy-D-glucose into testicular tissue (Table 3).

Although the data so far strongly supported our hypothesis, it was critical to determine if similar effects occur in animals which are treated acutely or chronically with different concentrations of THC. It is critical because assumptions of in vitro studies are challenged, as they may not prove valid when studied in live animals. Therefore, both acute and chronic

Table 1

EFFECTS OF Δ^9 – TETRAHYDROCANNABINOL ON CO_2 PRODUCTION FROM RAT TESTICULAR TISSUE INCUBATED IN DIFFERENT CONCENTRATIONS OF PYRUVATE[a]

PYRUVATE (mM)	CONTROL[b] (μmol CO_2/g dry tissue /100 min)	Δ^9 – THC	INHIBITION (%)	P
1.0	3.50 ± 0.18 (8)[c]	3.18 ± 0.17 (8)	9.1	N.S.
2.5	3.01 ± 0.12 (8)	2.88 ± 0.29 (8)	4.03	N.S.
5.5	6.87 ± 0.44 (8)	6.26 ± 0.31 (8)	8.87	N.S.
11.0	6.94 ± 0.53 (8)	7.06 ± 0.31 (8)	-1.72	N.S.

[a] Rat testicular tissues were exposed in vitro to 0.3 mM Δ^9 – THC with different concentrations of pyruvate and $2-^{14}C$-pyruvate (6.5 mCi/mmol) as a tracer in the medium.

[b] Controls received 9 μl of 95% ethanol per 2 ml of incubation medium.

[c] Values are expressed as mean μmol CO_2/gram dry tissue /100 min incubation ± SEM. The number of experiments is placed in parentheses.

From Husain, S. and Lamé, M., *Pharmacology*, 23, 102, 1981. With permission.

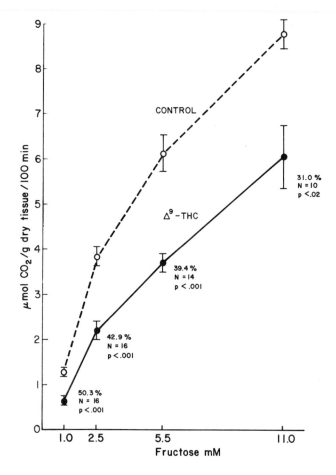

FIGURE 3.   Effects of 0.3 mM Δ-9-tetrahydrocannabinol on CO_2 production from rat testicular tissue incubated in different concentrations of fructose. (From Husain, S. and Lamé, M., *Pharmacology*, 23, 102, 1981. With permission.)

studies were conducted. For this study, the selection of the acute and chronic doses of THC was based on personal observations and information from the literature which indicates that 10 mg/kg, po dose of THC in rats corresponds to about 1.4 mg/kg oral dose in humans. This is equivalent to about five marijuana cigarettes containing 1% THC.[18] Both acute and chronic treatment of rats with THC led to a significant reduction in testicular production of $^{14}CO_2$ from 5.5 mM glucose (Tables 4 and 5). When rats were treated chronically for 15 days with 5 mg/kg, po THC, it caused a 29% inhibition in testicular utilization of glucose (Table 5). This inhibition was comparable to the effects produced by a 10-mg/kg acute dose of THC (Table 4). The maximum decrease in glucose utilization was with a 20-mg/kg, acute dose, whereas 10- and 20-mg/kg chronic doses of THC had lesser but highly significant reduction in glucose utilization (Table 4 and 5). Development of tolerance to the chronic doses of THC may be responsible for this decreased effect. THC is a highly lipophilic drug and shows great propensity for its storage in gonadal fat.[19] It is, therefore, highly desirable to measure and correlate these effects with the testicular levels of THC. The observations of this study, however, lend support to our in vitro data which suggests that cellular energetics are involved in the gonadal effects of THC.

Results obtained from 2-deoxy-D-glucose experiments indicated that acute treatment of rats with THC (10 and 20 mg/kg, po) had no significant effects on the uptake of six carbon sugars (Table 6). An inhibitory trend, however, was observed when rats were treated chron-

Table 2

LEVELS OF GLYCOLYTIC INTERMEDIATES IN RAT TESTICULAR TISSUE EXPOSED TO 0.3 mM Δ^9 -TETRAHYDROCANNABINOL

GLYCOLYTIC INTERMEDIATES	CONTROL[a] (nmol/g frozen tissue/100 min)	Δ^9-THC	INHIBITION (%)	P
DIHYDROXYACETONE PHOSPHATE	163.64 ± 4.37(6)[b]	126.45 ± 3.91(6)	22.7	< 0.001
FRUCTOSE - 1,6 - DIPHOSPHATE	173.03 ± 8.24(6)	120.14 ± 7.69(6)	30.5	< 0.001
GLUCOSE - 6 - PHOSPHATE	41.85 ± 1.52(6)	29.62 ± 0.97(6)	29.2	< 0.001

[a] Control tissues received 200 µl of ethanol (95%) for 44.4 ml of incubation medium which contained 5.5 mM glucose.

[b] Values are mean nmol/gram frozen tissue/100 min incubation ± SEM for the number of experiments in parentheses.

From Husain, S. and Lamé, M., *Pharmacology*, 23, 102, 1981. With permission.

Table 3

EFFECTS OF Δ^9-TETRAHYDROCANNABINOL ON THE MEMBRANE UPTAKE OF 2-DEOXY-D-GLUCOSE BY RAT TESTICULAR TISSUES[a]

Δ^9-THC (mM)	CONTROL[b] (μmol 2-deoxy-D-glucose/gram wet tissue/100 min)	Δ^9-THC (μmol 2-deoxy-D-glucose/gram wet tissue/100 min)	INHIBITION (%)	P
0.033	7.97 ± 0.33 (8)[c]	7.80 ± 0.33 (8)	2.1	N.S.
0.1	8.64 ± 0.42 (8)	6.41 ± 0.22 (8)	25.8	<.001
0.2	7.89 ± 0.25 (8)	4.54 ± 0.08 (8)	42.4	<.001
0.3	8.00 ± 0.24 (13)	4.59 ± 0.15 (13)	42.6	<.001
0.4	8.11 ± 0.35 (8)	4.37 ± 0.16 (8)	46.1	<.001

[a] The incubation medium contained 5.5 mM 2-deoxy-D-glucose with ^{14}C-2-deoxy-D-glucose (specific activity, 337 mCi/mmol) as a tracer.

[b] Controls received, in each case, an equivalent amount of 95% ethanol used to introduce Δ^9-THC into test flasks. For 0.033, 0.1, 0.2, 0.3 and 0.4 mM doses of Δ^9-THC, the equivalent amounts of ethanol were 1 μl, 3 μl, 6 μl, 9 μl and 12 μl, respectively, for 2 ml of incubation medium.

[c] Values are expressed as mean μmol 2-deoxy-D-glucose/gram wet tissue/100 min incubation ± SEM. The number of experiments is placed in parenthesis.

From Husain, S. and Lamé, M., *Pharmacology*, 23, 102, 1981. With permission.

Table 4

In-Vivo Effects Of Acute Δ⁹-Tetrahydrocannabinol (THC) Treatment On Glucose Metabolism In The Rat Testis

THC[a] (mg/kg)	Glucose Metabolism[b] (μmol CO_2 /g dry tissue/100min)	Percent Inhibition	Significance[c]
0	3.65±0.11 (26)		
10	2.59±0.13 (22)	29	<0.001
0	3.62±0.20 (12)		
20	1.62±0.15 (15)	55	<0.001

[a] Rats were treated acutely with respective oral doses of THC in sesame oil. Controls received 2 ml/kg, po sesame oil.

[b] Testes were removed from control and THC treated rats 2 hr following THC administration. Testicular tissues were incubated with 5.5 mM glucose containing glucose 6-¹⁴C as the tracer (specific activity 2.96 mCi/mmol).

[c] Significance determined by students' t-test.

From Harvey, D. J., Ed., *Marihuana '84*, Proc. Oxford Symp. on Cannabis, IRL Press, Oxford, 1985. With permission.

Table 5

In-Vivo Effects Of Chronic Δ⁹–Tetrahydrocannabinol (THC) Treatment On Glucose Metabolism In The Rat Testis

THC[a] (mg/kg)	Glucose Metabolism[b] (μmol CO /g dry tissue/100min)	Percent Inhibition	Significance[c]
0	3.75±0.27 (21)		
5	2.64±0.20 (21)	29	<0.005
0	3.65±0.28 (20)		
10	2.35±0.27 (20)	35	<0.005
0	4.02±0.15 (17)		
20	2.52±0.28 (17)	37	<0.001

[a] Rats were treated chronically for 15 days with respective oral doses of THC in sesame oil. Controls received 2 ml/kg, po sesame oil.

[b] Testes were removed from control and THC treated rats 2 hr following THC administration. Testicular tissues were incubated with 5.5 mM glucose containing glucose 6–^{14}C as the tracer (specific activity 2.96 mCi/mmol).

[c] Significance determined by students' t–test.

From Harvey, D. J., Ed., *Marihuana '84*, Proc. Oxford Symp. on Cannabis, IRL Press, Oxford, 1985. With permission.

Table 6

Uptake Of 2-Deoxy-D-Glucose In Rat Testicular Tissue After Acute Treatment With Δ⁹-Tetrahydrocannabinol (THC)

THC[a] (mg/kg)	Uptake[b] (μmol/g wet tissue/100min)	Percent Change from Control	Significance[c]
0	4.24±0.32 (5)		
10	4.70±0.35 (5)	+10.8	N.S.
0	5.33±0.10 (5)		
20	5.65±0.26 (5)	+6.0	N.S.

[a] Rats treated acutely with respective oral doses of THC in sesame oil. Controls received 2 ml/kg, po sesame oil.

[b] Testicular tissues from control and THC treated rats were incubated with 5.5 mM 2-deoxy-D-glucose containing ^{14}C-2-deoxy-D-glucose (specific activity 282 mCi/mmol) as a tracer in the medium.

[c] Significance determined by a paired t-test.

From Harvey, D. J., Ed., *Marihuana '84*, Proc. Oxford Symp. on Cannabis, IRL Press, Oxford, 1985. With permission.

ically with 5, 10, or 20 mg/kg, po THC. A significant inhibition of 2-deoxy-D-glucose uptake (22%) was observed with a 20-mg/kg dose (Table 7).

In experiments with i.t. administration of 5 μg THC, it was found that THC had a significant in vivo effect on glucose metabolism in the testis. As compared to controls, the THC-treated testes showed a 12.4% decrease in [14]CO production (Table 8).

On the basis of these in vitro and in vivo observations, we conclude that besides the specific H-P-G axis effects, THC also disrupts many synthetic gonadal functions by inhibiting the cellular energetics of the testis. Furthermore, the sites of this inhibition seem to be at the membrane uptake step and/or at the hexokinase step.

ACKNOWLEDGMENTS

This research was supported by NIDA grant DA 03593. Technical assistance of Vickie Bauer is also acknowledged.

Table 7

Uptake Of 2-Deoxy-D-Glucose In Rat Testiclar Tissue After Chronic Treatment With Δ⁹-Tetrahydrocannabinol (THC)

THC[a] (mg/kg)	Uptake[b] (μmol/g wet tissue/100min)	Percent Change from Control	Significance[c]
0	5.63±0.17 (10)		
5	5.55±0.22 (10)	−1.4	N.S.
0	5.88±0.36 (9)		
10	5.84±0.18 (9)	−0.7	N.S.
0	7.06±0.57 (9)		
20	5.50±0.30 (9)	−22.1	<0.025

[a] Rats treated chronically for 15 days with respective oral doses of THC in sesame oil. Controls received 2 ml/kg, po sesame oil.

[b] Testicular tissue from control and THC treated rats were incubated with 5.5 mM 2-deoxy-D-glucose containing ¹⁴C-2-deoxy-D-glucose (specific activity 282 mCi/mmol) as a tracer in the medium.

[c] Significance determined by a paired t-test.

From Harvey, D. J., Ed., *Marihuana '84*, Proc. Oxford Symp. on Cannabis, IRL Press, Oxford, 1985. With permission.

Table 8
IN VIVO EFFECTS OF INTRATESTICULAR Δ⁹-TETRAHYDROCANNABINOL (THC) ON GLUCOSE METABOLISM IN THE RAT TESTIS

Treatment[a]	Glucose metabolism[b] (μmol CO_2/g dry tissue/100 min)	Percent inhibition	Significance[c]
Control	4.61 ± 0.52 (34)		
THC	4.04 ± 0.43 (32)	12.41	<0.001

[a] Left testis of the rats received intratesticular injection of 5 μg THC dissolved in 10 $\mu\ell$ of Tween® 80-ethanol-saline solution. The right testis received 10 $\mu\ell$ of the vehicle.

[b] Control and THC-treated testes were removed from the rats one hr after THC administration. Testicular tissues were incubated with 5.5 mM glucose containing glucose 6-^{14}C as the tracer (specific activity 2.96 mCi/mmol).

[c] Significance determined by Student t test.

REFERENCES

1. **Marihuana and Health,** National Academy of Science Press, Washington, D. C., 1982.
2. **Agurell, S., Dewey, W. L. and Willette, R. E., Eds.,** *The Cannabinoids: Chemical, Pharmacologic and Therapeutic Aspects,* Academic Press, New York, 1984.
3. **Harvey, D. J., Ed.,** *Marihuana '84,* Proc. Oxford Symp. on Cannabis, IRL Press, Oxford, 1985.
4. **Kolodny, R. C., Masters, W. H., Kolodner, R. M., and Toro, G.,** Depression of plasma testosterone levels after chronic intensive marihuana use, *N. Engl. J. Med.,* 290, 872, 1974.
5. **Dalterio, S., Bartke, A., Roberson, C., Watson, D., and Burstein, S.,** Direct and pituitary mediated effects of Δ⁹-tetrahydrocannabinol on the testis, *Pharmacol. Biochem. Behav.,* 8, 673, 1978.
6. **Burstein, S., Hunter, S. A., Shoupe, T. S., Taylor, P., Bartke, A., and Dalterio, S.,** Cannabinoid inhibition of testosterone synthesis by mouse Leydig cells, *Res. Commun. Chem. Pathol. Pharmacol.,* 19, 557, 1978.
7. **Symons, A. M., Teale, J. D., and Marks, V.,** Effects of Δ⁹-tetrahydrocannabinol on the hypothalamic-pituitary gonadal system in maturing male rat, *J. Endocrinol.,* 68, 43P, 1976.
8. **Ditix, V. P., Sharma, V. N., and Lohiya, N. K.,** The effects of chronically administered cannabis extract on the testicular function of mice, *Eur. J. Pharmacol.,* 26, 111, 1974.
9. **Dixit, V. P. and Lohiya, N. K.,** Effects of cannabis extract in the response of accessory sex organs of adult male mice to testosterone, *Indian J. Physiol. Pharmacol.,* 19, 98, 1975.
10. **Marks, B. H.,** Δ¹-tetrahydrocannabinol and leutinizing hormone secretion, *Prog. Brain Res.,* 39, 331, 1973.
11. **Zimmerman, A. M., Zimmerman, S., and Raj, A. Y.,** Effects of cannabinoids on spermatogenesis in mice, in *Marihuana—Biological Effects, Analysis, Metabolism, Cellular Responses, Reproduction, and Brain,* Proc. 7th Int. Congr. Pharmacology, Nahas, G. G., and Paton, W. D., Eds., Pergamon Press, Oxford, 1979, 407.
12. **Huang, H. F. S., Nahas, G. G., and Hembree, W. C.,** Effects of marihuana inhalation on spermatogenesis of the rat, in *Marihuana—Biological Effects, Analysis, Metabolism, Cellular Responses, Reproduction, and Brain,* Proc. 7th Int. Congr. Pharmacology, Nahas, G. G. and Paton, W. D., Eds., Pergamon Press, Oxford, 1979, 419.
13. **Smith, C. G., Besch, N. F., and Asch, R. H.,** Effects of marihuana on the reproductive system, in *Advances in Sex Hormone Research,* Thomas, J. A. and Singhal, R. L., Eds., Urban & Schwarzenberg, Baltimore, 1980, 273.
14. **Jakubovic, A. and McGeer, P. L.,** In vitro inhibition of protein and nucleic acid synthesis in rat testicular tissue by cannabinoids, in *Marihuana: Chemistry, Biochemistry, and Cellular Effects,* Nahas, G. G., Ed., Springer-Verlag, New York, 1976, 223.
15. **Hembree, W. C., Zeidenberg, P., and Nahas, G. G.,** Marihauna's effects on human gonadal function, in *Marihuana: Chemistry, Biochemistry and Cellular Effects,* Nahas, G. G., Ed., Springer-Verlag, New York, 1976, 521.

16. **Michal, G. and Beutler, H. O.,** D-fructose-1,6-diphosphate, dihydroxyacetone phosphate and *d*-glyceraldehyde-3-phosphate, in *Methods of Enzymatic Analysis, Vol. 3, 3rd. ed.,* Bergmeyer, H. U., Ed., Verlag Chemie, Weinheim, West Germany, 1974, 1314.
17. **Lang, G. and Michal, G.,** D-Glucose-6-phosphate and *d*-fructose-6-phosphate, in *Methods of Enzymatic Analysis, Vol. 3, 3rd., Ed.,* Bergmeyer, H. U., Ed., Verlag Chemie, Weinheim, West Germany, 1974, 1238.
18. **Rosenkrantz, H. and Braude, M. C.,** Comparative chronic toxicities of delta-9-tetrahydrocannabinol administered orally or by inhalation in rat, in *The Pharmacology of Marihuana, NIDA Mongr. Ser.,* Braude, M. C. and Szara, S., Eds., Raven Press, New York, 1976, 571.
19. **Rawitch, A. B. and Rohrer, R.,** Delta-9-tetrahydrocannabinol uptake by adipose tissue: preferential accumulation in gonadal fat organs, *Gen. Pharmacol.,* 10, 525, 1979.

Chapter 12

MARIJUANA: ANALYSIS AND DETECTION OF USE THROUGH URINALYSIS

Mahmoud A. ElSohly and Hala N. ElSohly

TABLE OF CONTENTS

I. INTRODUCTION

Cannabis sativa L. is one of the oldest plants known to medicine and one of the most thoroughly studied plants today. The history of the use of *Cannabis* and its preparations can be documented back to 2737 B.C. in the first known pharmacy textbook *Pen Tsao* or *The Great Herbal*.[1] The plant and its preparations have been indicated for a wide variety of ailments including gout, rheumatism, malaria, beriberi, cholera, neuralgia, constipation, absent-mindedness, asthma, epilepsy, insomnia, skin infections, tetanus, hydrophobia, convulsions, pain, hysteria, anxiety, insanity, anorexia, uterine hemorrhage, and physical stress.[2,3] It was not until 1920 when limited nonmedical use of marijuana began, and in 1937 the Marijuana Tax Act (a federal law in the U.S.) prohibited the nonmedicinal use of the drug while still recognizing its therapeutic value.[4] In 1942, however, the drug was not admitted in the USP, indicating no acceptable medical use in the U.S.

To date, the crude drug marijuana obtained from *Cannabis* is the most widely used illicit drug in the world, especially in North America and Western Europe. It is because of this widespread use of the drug, particularly among young people, that investigators all over the world have concentrated their efforts to study the chemistry and biological activities of the plant.

Even though the plant has been known and used in medicine for thousands of years, the correct chemical structure of the major psychologically active component was not elucidated until 1964.[5] The number of research publications on the subject has since steadily increased. Between 1964 and 1974, there were 3045 scientific citations,[6] and the number of publications up to 1980 was 6149.[7] During the following 2 to 3 years, there were over 1300 published reports in the literature.[8] Today there are over 400 different chemicals belonging to 18 different classes of compounds known to exist in cannabis,[9] as shown in Table 1. However, the most studied component is delta-9-THC (delta-9-tetrahydrocannabinol or THC). The concentration of THC, the most psychologically active component, is used to describe the potency of a given marijuana sample. Analysis of confiscated marijuana over the last 10 years showed that the THC concentration has been on the rise since 1975.[10] At that time, THC was less than 1% and reached an average of approximately 4% in 1984. The average THC concentration in confiscated marijuana in 1985 was slightly less than the preceding year (see Figure 1). Whether this decline in potency represents a new trend remains to be seen.

II. URINALYSIS AS A MEANS OF DETECTING MARIJUANA USE

The last few years have witnessed an ever-increasing campaign against the use of illicit drugs. The statistics presented in other chapters of this book regarding drug use in our society are certainly alarming and cause concern. As a result, many government agencies (particularly the military) and private corporations have embarked on drug testing programs designed to identify drug users through urinalysis. The extent of testing and the number of drugs tested differ from place to place. However, invariably, all drug testing programs include testing for marijuana use since this is the most widely used illicit drug.

Drug testing for marijuana is based on the detection of metabolites of THC in urine. Several metabolites of THC have been reported in human urine.[11-13] 11-Nor-delta-9-tetrahydrocannabinol-9-carboxylic acid (THC–COOH) is the most abundant urinary metabolite present either in the free or conjugated (glucuronide) form.[13-15]

In urinalysis drug testing programs, urine specimens are often screened by a rapid and less specific method, and those samples presumed positive are confirmed by a more specific method. The most widely used methods for screening urine specimens for THC–COOH have been radioimmunoassays (RIA) and enzyme immunoassays (EIA), while the method of choice for confirmation is GC/MS.

Table 1
CLASSES OF CHEMICAL CONSTITUENTS
IDENTIFIED IN *CANNABIS SATIVA*

Compound	Number known
Cannabinoids	61
Cannabigerol (CBG)	6
Cannabichromene (CBC)	4
Cannabidiol (CBD)	7
Delta-9-tetrahydrocannabinol (delta-9-THC)	9
Delta-8-tetrahydrocannabinol (delta-8-THC)	2
Cannabicyclol (CBL)	3
Cannabielsoin (CBE)	3
Cannabinol (CBN)	6
Cannabinodiol (CBND)	2
Cannabitriol (CBT)	6
Miscellaneous types	9
Other cannabinoids	4
Nitrogenous compounds	20
Quarternary bases	5
Amides	1
Amines	12
Spermidine alkaloids	2
Amino acids	18
Proteins, glycoproteins, and enzymes	9
Sugars and related compounds	34
Monosaccharides	13
Disaccharides	2
Polysaccharides	5
Cyclitols	12
Aminosugars	2
Hydrocarbons	50
Simple alcohols	7
Simple aldehydes	12
Simple ketones	13
Simple acids	20
Fatty acids	12
Simple esters and lactones	13
Steroids	11
Terpenes	103
Monoterpenes	58
Sesquiterpenes	38
Diterpenes	1
Triterpenes	2
Miscellaneous compounds of terpenoid origin	4
Noncannabinoid phenols	16
Flavanoidglycosides	19
Vitamins	1
Pigments	2

From Turner, C. E., ElSohly, M. A., Boereu, E. G., *J. Nat. Products*, 43(2), 169, 1980. With permission.

A variety of chromatographic techniques have been used to assay for THC–COOH in urine, including thin-layer chromatography (TLC),[16-21] gas chromatography (GC),[22,23] gas chromatography/mass spectrometry (GC/MS),[24-26] high-performance liquid chromatography (HPLC),[27] HPLC/GC,[28] and HPLC/radioimmunoassay (HPLC/RIA).[29-32] However, RIA[33-36] and enzyme-multiplied immunoassay (EMIT)[37,38] are procedures used to screen urine samples for the THC metabolites.

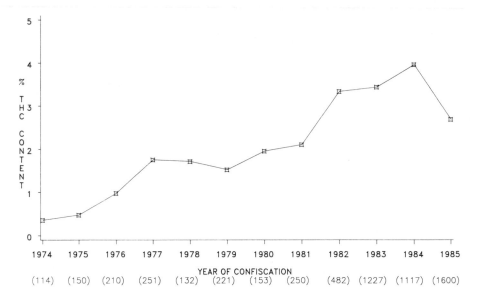

FIGURE 1.   Normalized percentage of delta-9-tetrahydrocannabinol vs. year of confiscation (number of seizures in parentheses).

In this review we will elaborate on the work done in our laboratory concerning urinalysis and the use of different methodologies to screen and confirm marijuana use.

III. IMMUNOASSAYS AND THEIR USE IN SCREENING URINE SPECIMENS FOR CANNABINOIDS

Immunoassay procedures, both RIA and EIA, are being widely used to screen for recent marijuana use by analyzing urine samples for the presence of THC–COOH.

Using commercially available kits we have evaluated a radioimmunoassay (Abuscreen® radioimmunoassay for cannabinoids, denoted by RIA-I in Tables 2 and 3) in which the potential cross-reactivity of a series of selected compounds has been determined.[36] The compounds evaluated included cannabinoids and some noncannabinoid phenolic constituents of *Cannabis*. The potential for cross-reactivity of these compounds was examined by determining the concentration in urine which would yield a response equivalent to a standard supplied by the manufacturer (Roche Diagnostic Systems). In the spring of 1984, the manufacturer reformulated its product using an antibody raised against a different antigen. The results of an evaluation of this new antibody (denoted by RIA-II in Tables 2 and 3) along with a summary of the previous results are given.[39] In addition, the results of a similar evaluation of the cross-reactivity potential of an antibody employed in an EIA are presented.

The pool of test compounds has been expanded to include some noncannabinoid related materials that may appear in a normal urine sample.

A summary of the results of the analysis of the spiked urine samples in the three immunoassay systems appears in Table 2. The compounds are ranked in order of decreasing percent cross-reactivity with respect to RIA-II.

Examination of these results shows that from all compounds tested only 16 possess ≥20% cross-reactivities in at least one of the assays (see Table 3). This represents 12, 15, and 9 compounds for EIA, RIA-I, and RIA-II, respectively, with two of the compounds in the RIA data having not been evaluated in the EIA system. At the 50% level, these numbers are reduced to 10, 9, and 4 for EIA, RIA-I, and RIA-II, respectively.

The observations on the cross-reactivity potential of this series of compounds can be summarized as follows:

Table 2
SUMMARY OF CROSS-REACTIVITY DATA

Test compound	Percent cross-reactivity		
	EIA	RIA-I[a]	RIA-II
11-nor-HHC-9-beta-COOH	125	125	152
11-nor-delta-9-THC-9-COOH	84	95	97
11-nor-delta-8-THC-9-COOH	84	135	93
11-OH-delta-8-THC	88	179	62
11-OH-delta-9-THC	71	161	39
11-nor-HHC-9-alpha-COOH	47	41	31
10-alpha-OH-delta-9(11)-THC	—[b]	22	23
10-alpha-OH-delta-8-THC	—	27	20
8-alpha,9-alpha-Epoxy-HHC	74	80	14
beta-HHC	11	13	14
delta-9(11)-THC	8.2	29	13
8-beta-OH-delta-9-THC	81	10	12
8-beta,11-diOH-delta-9-THC	90	21	10
delta-8-THC	8.2	33	9.8
8-alpha-OH-delta-9-THC	115	244	9.4
8-alpha-11-diOH-delta-9-THC	63	116	7.7
9-alpha,10-alpha-Epoxy-HHC	38	74	7.4
alpha-HHC	4.5	8.3	6.4
delta-9-THC	6.0	13	4.0
delta-9-THC acetate	<4.7[c]	6.9	3.9
Cannabitriol	<0.9	10	2.9
11-nor-CBN-9-COOH	15	6.1	1.8
delta-9-THC-acid A/delta-8-THC-acid A (mixture 65:35)	1.3	1.8	1.4
11-nor-9-oxy-10-alpha-OH-HHC-diacetate	—	1.6	<1.3
Cannabigerol	<1.0	<1.3	<1.3
Cannabispiran	<0.9	<1.3	<1.3
Cannabielsoin	1.7	<1.3	<1.3
3′,4′,5′-Trinor-delta-9-THC-2′-COOH	<0.9	<1.3	<1.3
2′,3′,4′,5′-Tetranor-delta-9-THC-1′-COOH	<0.9	<1.3	<1.3
1′,2′,3′,4′,5′-pentanor-delta-9-THC-3-COOH	<0.9	<1.3	<1.3
Nabilone	<0.9	<1.3	<1.3
Levonantradol	<0.9	<1.3	<1.3
delta-9-THC-acid B	<0.9	<1.3	<1.3
Cannabinol	2.9	<1.1	<1.1
beta-Cannabispiranol	<0.8	<1.0	<1.0
Cannabicyclol	<0.8	<1.0	<1.0
Canniprene	<0.8	<1.0	<1.0
Dehydrocannabispiran	<0.8	<1.0	<1.0
Cannabitetrol	1.7	<1.0	<1.0
Cannabicitran	<0.8	<1.0	<1.0
Cannibichromene	<0.7	<1.0	<1.0
Cannabidiol	<0.7	<1.0	<1.0
5-beta-Pregnane-3-alpha, 20-alpha-diol	—	<1.5	<1.5
Rutin	—	<1.3	<1.3
5-OH-Indole-2-carboxylic acid	<0.3	<0.3	<0.3
5-OH-Indole-3-acetic acid	<0.3	<0.3	<0.3
3-Indolebutyric acid	<0.3	<0.3	<0.3
Indole-3-acetic acid	<0.3	<0.3	<0.3

[a]   Data from Jones et al.[3]
[b]   Compound not tested.
[c]   Based on maximum concentration tested.

From Jones, A. B., ElSohly, H. N., and ElSohly, M. A., in *Marihuana '84*, Proc. Oxford Symp. on Cannabis, Harvey, D. J., Ed., IRL Press, Oxford, 1985. With permission.

Table 3
COMPOUNDS WITH CROSS-REACTIVITIES ≥20% IN ANY OF THE SYSTEMS

Test compound	Percent cross-reactivity		
	EIA	RIA-I	RIA-II
11-nor-HHC-9-beta-COOH	125	125	152
11-nor-delta-9-THC-9-COOH	84	96	97
11-nor-delta-8-THC-9-COOH	84	135	93
11-OH-delta-8-THC	88	176	62
11-OH-delta-9-THC	71	161	39
11-nor-HHC-9-alpha-COOH	47	41	31
10-alpha-OH-delta-9(11)-THC	—	22	23
10-alpha-OH-delta-8-THC	—	27	20
8-alpha,9-alpha-Epoxy-HHC	74	80	14
delta-9(11)-THC	8.2	29	13
8-beta-OH-delta-9-THC	81	10	12
8-beta,11-diOH-delta-9-THC	90	21	10
delta-8-THC	8	33	9.8
8-alpha,OH-delta-9-THC	115	244	9.4
8-alpha,11-diOH-delta-9-THC	63	95	7.7
9-alpha,10-alpha-Epoxy-HHC	74	38	7.40

From Jones, A. B., ElSohly, H. N., and ElSohly, M. A., in *Marihuana '84*, Proc. Oxford Symp. on Cannabis, Harvey, D. J., Ed., IRL Press, Oxford, 1985. With permission.

1.   All compounds showing cross-reactivity are of the dibenzopyran-type structure (related to delta-9-THC, delta-8-THC, or HHC), but not all dibenzopyran-type structures are cross-reactive. The opening of the pyran ring results in the loss of binding to all antibodies (e.g., cannabidiol is less than 1% cross-reactive in all systems). Some degree of unsaturation or some degree of oxygenation is required in the 8, 9, 10, or 11 position(s) for appreciable cross-reactivity to occur. For example, cannabinol (with an aromatic ring) has no appreciable cross-reactivity as compared to delta-8-THC or delta-9-THC. Similarly, 11-nor-CBN-9-COOH shows little cross-reactivity as compared to the corresponding delta-8-THC, delta-9-THC, or HHC acid derivatives. Some stereospecificity is seen with EIA and RIA-I, 8-alpha-OH-delta-9-THC is highly cross-reactive in both systems when compared to the corresponding beta-isomer (8-beta-OH-delta-9-THC). However, this stereospecificity is not observed with RIA-II.

2.   The following structural modification reduces the binding potentials of the resulting compounds to the antibodies:
     a. Substitution of the phenolic ring on the 2 and 4 positions (e.g., delta-9-THC acid A and delta-9-THC acid B vs. delta-9-THC).
     b. Derivatization of the phenolic OH (e.g., delta-8-THC-acetate vs. delta-8-THC).
     c. Oxidation of the aliphatic side chain to a carboxylic acid (e.g., the 3-COOH, 1'-COOH, or 2'-COOH derivatives of delta-9-THC vs. delta-9-THC itself).

3.   The other compounds unrelated chemically to the cannabinoids included in the screen do not bind to the antibodies. These are 5-beta-pregnane-3-alpha-20-alpha-diol (a steroid found in some urine samples), rutin (a flavanoid found in the cannabis plant), and the indoles (5-OH-indole-3-acetic acid and 5-OH-indole-2-carboxylic acid) which are chemically related to melanin metabolic products which might be normal constituents of some urine samples.

It is thus concluded that the antibodies used in the most widely employed methods for screening (RIA and EMIT) urine for marijuana have very good specificity for cannabinoids (THC and metabolites).

IV. CONFIRMATION METHODS

Although GC/MS is the method of choice for confirming the use of marijuana, other procedures are also used. For the purpose of this review, we will only discuss three methods — namely HPLC, GC/ECD, and GC/FID.

A. HPLC

An HPLC procedure was developed for the analysis of 11-nor-delta-9-tetrahydrocanna-binol-9-carboxylic acid (THC–COOH) in urine.[27] Hydrolyzed urine samples were cleaned up using Bond-Elut® columns. 11-Nor-cannabinol-9-carboxylic acid (CBN–COOH) was used as internal standard. The analysis was carried out using a C_8 reversed-phase column with acetonitrile:50 mM phosphoric acid (65:35) as the eluting solvent. Detection was done by ultraviolet detector at 214 nm. The minimum detectable level of THC–COOH was 25 ng/mℓ.

This procedure offers a rapid and reproducible method for the analysis of the major metabolite of THC in urine samples. Hydrolysis of the urine was found essential since the majority of the THC–COOH in most urine samples existed in the conjugated form.[13-15] It has been found[15,22] that base hydrolysis under the conditions described was more efficient and reproducible than either acid or enzyme hydrolysis. The hydrolyzed urine was then subjected to a clean-up procedure utilizing a proprietary bonded-phase silica gel (Bond-Elut®, Analytichem International). This clean-up procedure offered many advantages over partitioning. For example, there was no solvent evaporation or concentration using Bond-Elut® columns, especially when used in conjunction with the HPLC analysis. The final eluate from Bond-Elut® columns resulted in much cleaner samples for analysis (as compared with acid-base partitioning). When this procedure was used for the analysis of blank urine samples (five different individuals) no interfering peaks were observed under either the metabolite THC–COOH or the internal standard (CBN–COOH). Typical chromatograms of urine samples analyzed by this method are shown in Figure 2A.

HPLC could be used as an alternative to GC, with the advantage that no derivatization is required.

A calibration curve was prepared using blank urine spiked with THC–COOH at concentration ranging from 10 to 200 ng/mℓ. A linear relationship ($4 = 0.989$) was obtained (plotting peak height ratio of THC–COOH/CBN–COOH vs. concentration). However, when the peak heights of THC–COOH were plotted against concentration, a linear relationship was also observed ($r = 0.997$). This indicates that the procedure could be used for the analysis of urine samples by measuring the peak heights of THC–COOH without the use of internal standard. However, it is always preferable and more accurate to use internal standard. The percent recovery of THC–COOH from urine samples over the concentration range studied was determined to be $\geq 90\%$. The reproducibility of the method was measured by the analysis of five replicates of two urine samples assayed to contain 100.4 ng/mℓ and 31.0 ng/mℓ of THC–COOH. The coefficient of variation of the high-concentration sample was 3.6% and that of the low-concentration sample was 12.9%.

B. GC/FID

A gas chromatographic procedure with a flame ionization detector (GC/FID) was developed in our laboratory.[40] Different columns, packed (3% OV-17) and capillary (DB-5 and DB-1) types were used (Figures 2B, C, and D). However, because of the poor sensitivity of FID, these methods necessitated the use of large volumes of urine, elaborate cleanup

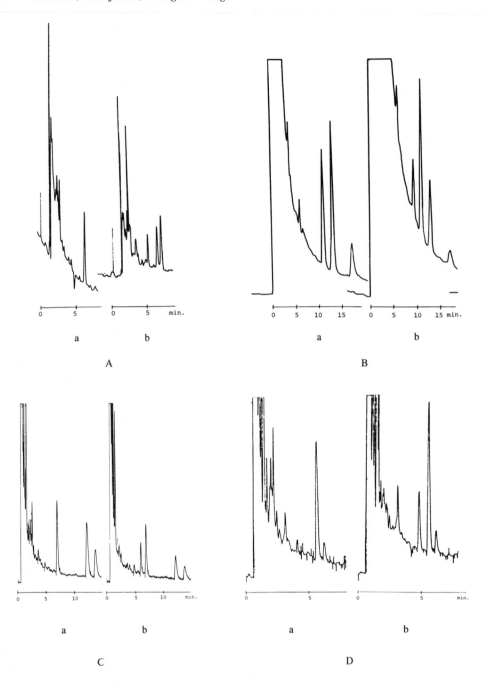

FIGURE 2.   Representative chromatograms from different methods used for the analysis of urine samples for THC–COOH(I) using 75 ngdimℓ of CBN–COOH(II) as internal standard. (A) HPLC C_8 column; (B) GC/FID 3% OV-17 packed column; (C) GC/FID DB-1 capillary column; (D) GC/FID DB-5 capillary column; (E) GC/ECD 2% OV-25 packed column; and (F) GC/MSD DB-1 capillary column. Chromatogram(a) is a blank and (b) is blank urine spiked with 25 ng/mℓ of I. (From Jones, A. B., ElSohly, H. N., and ElSohly, M. A., in *Marihuana '84*, Proc. Oxford Symp. on Cannabis, Harvey, D. J., Ed., IRL Press, 1985. With permission.)

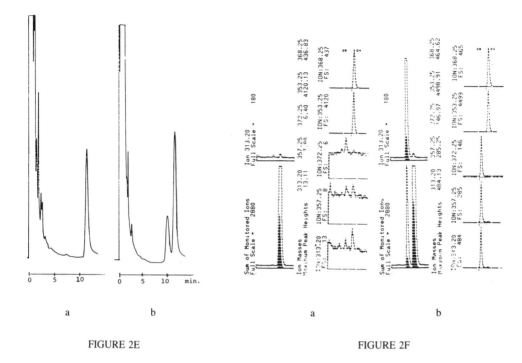

FIGURE 2E   FIGURE 2F

procedures, tremendous sample concentration ($\times 500$) and injection of a large proportion of the sample (25%) into the GC.

C. GC/ECD

A gas chromatographic/electron capture detection procedure was developed for the analysis of THC–COOH, which requires only a small volume of urine (1 mℓ or less).[23] Hydrolyzed urine samples were extracted by a simple acid-base partitioning step. The extracted metabolite was derivatized with pentafluorobenzyl bromide in a biphasic system using benzyltributyl-ammonium hydroxide as a phase transfer catalyst. CBN–COOH was used as I.S. A linear relationship was observed between the peak height ratio of the metabolite/internal standard and the concentration of the metabolite (r = 0.9996) and between the peak height and concentration of the metabolite (r = 0.9995). The coefficient of variance (CV) was found to be 7.1% and 2.6% at concentration of 10 and 100 ng/mℓ respectively (n = 5). Concentration of 5 ng/mℓ of metabolite in urine resulted in a peak-to-noise ratio of 4:1; however, concentration down to 1 to 2 ng/mℓ could be determined. Data for the calibration curve were collected by analyzing urine samples prepared by spiking blank urines with various concentrations of THC–COOH(I) (5 to 200 ng/mℓ) and 50 ng/mℓ of CBN–COOH (II) as I.S. A typical chromatogram is shown in Figure 2E.

Table 4 shows points of comparison between FID and ECD.

Different solvents, including methylene chloride, hexane, hexane saturated with aceto-nitrile, and 5% methylene chloride in hexane, were examined for carrying out this reaction. It was found that methylene chloride, hexane saturated with acetonitrile, and 5% methylene chloride in hexane were of comparable efficiency. However, the chromatograms resulting from the use of methylene chloride as solvent for derivatization of urine extracts had more extraneous peaks and a larger solvent front. Hexane, on the other hand, although showing much cleaner chromatograms, gave a low yield of the derivatized products. Thus, for the purpose of this work, hexane with 5% methylene chloride was chosen as the most appropriate solvent for derivatization.

Table 4

**COMPARISON OF VARIOUS PARAMETERS IN
THE GC/FID[a] AND GC/ECD PROCEDURES
WHERE SIGNIFICANT DIFFERENCES EXIST[b]**

Parameter	GC/FID	GC/ECD
Vol. of sample required	10 mℓ	1 mℓ or less
Vol. of base required	2 mℓ	0.2 mℓ
Vol. of additional solvents required	44 mℓ organic	5 mℓ organic
	10 mℓ aqueous	0.2 mℓ, aqueous
Final vol. of sample	20 $\mu\ell$	100 $\mu\ell$
Total sample concentrating factor	$\times 500$	$\times 10$
Vol. injected into GC	5$\mu\ell$	1 $\mu\ell$
Overall analysis time	120 min	35 min
Minimum detectable concentration in urine	~ 25 ng/mℓ	~ 2 ng/mℓ

[a]   As described in Reference 22.
[b]   For one sample.

From ElSohly, M. A., Arafat, E. S., and Jones, A. B., *J. Anal. Toxicol.*, 8, 7, 1984. With permission. Copyright 1984 Preston Publications.

D. GC/MS

GC/MS is the method of choice for confirming marijuana use. It offers the advantage of providing a means of identifying the peak in the chromatogram. The most commonly used MS method involves the use of selected ions monitoring (SIM) technique whereby one or three ions are monitored. These ions represent major fragmentations of the molecule in the ion source of the mass spectrometer. Where multiple ions are monitored, the ion ratios in a given specimen are compared to those of a standard analyzed at the same time as a means of confirming the identity of the peak in question. For THC–COOH, the most commonly used derivative is the methyl ether, methyl ester. The derivatization results in major ions at m/z 372 (M$^{+\cdot}$), 357 (M–CH$_3$)$^{+\cdot}$, and 313 (M–COOCH$_3$)$^{+\cdot}$. The intensity of the ion ratios 372/313 and 357/313 in an unknown specimen should be within $\pm 20\%$ of those of the standard THA–COOH derivative.

V. COMPARISON OF HPLC, GC/FID, GC/ECD, AND GC/MS

Very few studies have been conducted with the purpose of correlating results obtained by several cannabinoid urine assays. Irving et al.[44] reported on a comparative study evaluating immunoassays for cannabinoids in urine. GC/FID and GC/MS were used for confirmation of all specimens found positive by any of the immunoassays and confirmation rates of each method were reported.

In our laboratory, Jones et al.[42] conducted a comparative study for the analysis of the major urinary metabolite of THC using RIA, EMIT, HPLC, GC/ECD, and GC/MS. The study was carried out using different extraction procedures, and the analyses were undertaken at different times.

Table 5 shows the results of the analyses of 29 urine samples by five different methods. The analyses using RIA, EIA, HPLC, and GC/ECD were carried out simultaneously. After a storage period of 2 months (freezer, $-18°C$) from the original analysis, the samples were

Table 5
SUMMARY OF RESULTS FROM THE ANALYSIS OF 29
URINE SAMPLES BY 5 METHODS

Sample code	RIA[a]	EIA[b]	HPLC[c]	GC/ECD[c]	GC/ECD-1[d]	GC/MS[d]
P-22	85	26	NA[e]	16,18	11	11,11
P-23	98	77	34	35,33	17	24,23
P-24	>100	>100	45	55,52	39	38,38
P-25	>100	>100	36	43,42	27	28,27
P-26	91	62	13,16	78,42,57	41	32,32
P-27	94	>100	36,37	23,25	16	17,16
P-28	>100	77	46	42,43	30	29,27
P-29	>100	>100	NA	176,180	107	109,88
P-30	>100	>100	91,64	127,114	37	66,93
P-31	>100	>100	NA	63,57	49	66
P-32	92	77	57	40,41	12	27
P-33	77	41	25	27,26	23	16,19
P-34	90	31	25,20	15,18	9	15
P-35	77	30	NA	19,16	7	16,15
P-36	>100	75	30	27,19	20	21,18
P-37	>100	100	70	72,78	64	70,66
P-38	>100	100	114	97,130	113	NA
P-39	>100	>100	66	68,58	57	60,65
P-40	>100	>100	NA	175,148	173	205,198
P-41	>100	92	45	32,37	11	38,36
P-42	81	75	24	20,19	15	18,17
P-43	96	88	40	38,32	50	57,54
P-44	86	72	21	22,25	21	26,24
P-45	>100	>100	178	133,152	74	195,232
P-46	89	69	NA	16,24	10	19
P-47	89	96	NA	24,21	6	20,19
P-48	>100	>100	122	131,129	73	127,144
P-49	59	39	18	22,23	15	12,13
P-50	91	68	NA	30,34	NA	29

Note: Replicate entries represent values obtained when multiple aliquots were analyzed.

[a] Concentration expressed in equivalent ng 11-nor-delta-9-THC-9-COOH per mℓ based on calibration curve generated at the time of the analysis.
[b] Concentration expressed in equivalent ng 11-nor-delta-9-THC-9-COOH per mℓ and estimated from responses obtained with 20 and 75 ng/mℓ standards supplied by the manufacturer with the reagents.
[c] Concentration expressed in ng 11-nor-delta-9-THC-9-COOH per mℓ obtained from calibration data.
[d] After 2 months storage at $-18°C$ after original by RIA, EIA, HPLC, and GC/ED.
[e] NA — Not analyzed due to insufficient volume of sample.

From Jones, A. B., ElSohly, H. N., Arafat, E. S., and ElSohly, M. A., *J. Anal. Toxicol.,* 8, 249, 1984. With permission. Copyright 1984 Preston Publications.

thawed to room temperature and aliquots were withdrawn and reanalyzed by GC/ECD (designated GC/ECD-I in Table 5) and by GC/MS. Because of the limited urine volume, some samples were not analyzed by the HPLC procedure which required 10-mℓ aliquots.

Quantitative estimates were obtained by the immunoassay procedures using calibration curves when the level of metabolites in urine was ≤100 ng/mℓ. These estimates were, as expected, higher than those found by the other procedures which are specific for THC–COOH(I).

Table 6
CORRELATION OF
COEFFICIENTS (r)[a]

Procedures	r
GC/ECD — replicates	0.9779
GC/MS — replicates	0.9838
HPLC vs. GC/ECD	0.9071
HPLC vs. GC/ECD-I	0.7614
GC/ECD vs. GC/MS	0.9684
GC/ECD vs. GC/ECD-I	0.8704
GC/ECD vs. GC/MS	0.8843
GC/ECD-I vs. GC/MS	0.8523

[a] Calculated from the data in Table
5 which showed significance at p
$= 0.001$.[12] All other correlations
were nonsignificant at $p = 0.05$.

From Jones, A. B., ElSohly, H. N.,
Arafat, E. S., and ElSohly, M. A.,
J. Anal. Toxicol., 8, 249, 1984. With
permission. Copyright 1984 Preston
Publications.

Other metabolites of delta-9-THC are reported to cross-react with the antisera of both immunoassay procedures.[43,44] Comparison of the data obtained by GC/ECD and by RIA and EIA shows that the concentration of I in urine could be estimated to be about 31.0% of the value obtained by RIA (SD $\pm$ 11.7, n = 16) and about 48.9% of the value obtained by EIA (SD $\pm$ 19.2, n = 17). Comparisons were made between the data obtained by GC/ECD, HPLC, and GC/MS. Correlation coeffcents for any combination of these procedures and within the replicates of any given procedure were calculated and given in Table 6.

These correlation coefficients were found to be significant to the 0.001 level.[45] The high degree of reproducibility of the GC/ECD and GC/MS methods was demonstrated when duplicate samples were analyzed (r = 0.9779 and 0.9838, respectively). The correlation coefficients between the various methods ranged from 0.7614 to 0.9684. The lower r values in Table 5 were observed when correlations were carried out at different times. This is attributed to the apparent change in the metabolite upon storage, primarily because of its low solubility in the urine aqueous matrix. This phenomenon was also observed by other investigators.[46] The r value for any two procedures carried out at the same time, however, was always better than 0.85.

It is thus concluded that (1) the HPLC[27] and GC/ECD[23] methods reported for the analysis of I are reliable and have a high correlation with GC/MS,[26] (2) the analysis of urine samples for the metabolite I using HPLC, GC/ECD, or GC/MS will always show a lower value than that obtained by any immunoassay procedure, and (3) storage of urine samples, even under freezer conditions, could result in a different value for the concentration of THC–COOH upon reanalysis.

When a urine specimen is submitted to different laboratories for analysis, disagreement in the results usually occurs. This could be explained on the basis of the differences in extraction procedures and internal standards used, the differences in the time lapse between submission and analysis, and the mere fact that different aliquots were used.

A recent study was designed to compare several methods and control all the above variables. One urine aliquot was withdrawn, the internal standard added, the sample extracted after hydrolysis, and the same extract was then subjected to analysis using various techniques.

Table 7
RETENTION TIME (Rt, MIN) AND RELATIVE RETENTION TIME (RRt) DATA ON DELTA-9-THC-COOH AND DELTA-8-THC-COOH RELATIVE TO CBN–COOH (I.S.)

	delta-9-THC-COOH Rt ± SD	CBN–COOH(II) Rt ± SD	(I/II) RRt ± SD	delta-8-THC-COOH(III) Rt	delta-8-THC-COOH(III) RRT (III/II)
HPLC	6.64 ± 0.13	6.98 + 0.15	0.92 + 0.01	5.80	0.85
ECD,OV-25	9.96 + 0.13	11.49 + 0.06	0.87 + 0.01	11.10	0.96
FID,OV-17	9.33 + 0.13	10.19 + 0.02	0.92 + 0.01	9.40	0.92
FID,DB-5	6.12 + 0.04	7.06 + 0.04	0.87 + 0.03	6.01	0.85
FID,DB-1	4.84 + 0.03	5.59 + 0.03	0.87 + 0.01	4.72	0.85
MSD,DB-1	3.26 + 0.03	3.76 + 0.03	0.87 + 0.01	3.18	0.85

From Jones, A. B., ElSohly, H. N., and ElSohly, M. A., in *Marihuana '84*, Proc. Oxford Symp. on Cannabis, Harvey, D. J., Ed., IRL Press, Oxford, 1985. With permission

The methods used in this study included HPLC, where no derivatization was necessary, GC/ECD, where the pentafluorobenzyl derivatives were prepared, and GC/FID and GC/MS, where the methyl derivatives were made. GC/FID analysis was carried out on three different columns, namely a packed 3% OV-17 column, a capillary DB-5 column, and a capillary DB-1 column.

Table 7 shows a list of retention times (Rt and RRt) of delta-9-THC-COOH and delta-8-THC-COOH under the experimental conditions used for the different methods. CBN–COOH served as a suitable internal standard since it partitioned similar to THC–COOH with baseline resolution in all cases. The concentration of CBN–COOH was selected at 75 ng/mℓ so that a reasonable detector response could be observed with all methods. However, concentrations of 25 ng/mℓ or less could be easily used with GC/MS or GC/ECD.

Urine samples were base-hydrolyzed after addition of internal standard, acidified to pH 2 to 3, then passed over Bond-Elut® columns. The extraction procedure used was that adopted in the HPLC method with minor modification in order for the final extract to be suitable for analysis by all methods. It was found essential to wash the column with 25 mℓ acetonitrile/water (1:9) instead of acetonitrile:50 mM phosphoric acid prior to elution with 1.5 mℓ acetonitrile. The residual acidity in the final extract apparently interfered with the derivatization of the extract, particularly the methylation reaction.

The percent recovery of THC–COOH at 25 ng/mℓ through the extraction process was found to be 83 to 98% with an average of 90%. This was carried out by comparing the absolute THC–COOH responses of urine specimens spiked prior to extraction with those of spiked extracts of blank urines. Calibration curves were generated using blank urines spiked with concentrations of 10 to 150 ng/mℓ THC–COOH and 75 ng/mℓ CBN–COOH. Additional points from 5 ng/mℓ THC–COOH samples were included in the GC/ECD and GC/MS curves. In all cases, the peak areas for THC–COOH and CBN–COOH peaks were calculated. In the case of the GC/MS method, the analysis was carried out using the SIM program. Three ions were monitored for THC–COOH — namely m/z 372, 357, and 313 — and two ions were monitored for CBN–COOH (m/z 368 and 353). For quantitation, the area ratio (313/353) was used. The ion ratios (372/313, 357/313, and 353/368) were calculated for the calibration standards as well as for all specimens analyzed and was used as a means for identifying the THC–COOH and CBN–COOH peaks. There was close agreement between the ion ratios of the standards and the specimens analyzed throughout the study ($< \pm 5\%$).

Table 8
CALIBRATION CURVE DATA,[a] LIMIT OF DETECTION, AND COEFFICIENT OF VARIANCE FOR THE ANALYSIS OF URINE SAMPLES USING DIFFERENT METHODS

Method	Slope	Y-Intercept	Corr. Coeff. (r)	Detection limit (LOD K = 3) ng/mℓ	CV(%)[b] at 25 ng/mℓ
HPLC	0.032	−0.083	0.9974	7.0	6.5
ECD OV-25	0.015	−0.019	0.9910	2.0	15.6
FID OV-17	0.014	−0.014	0.9891	12.0	12.0
FID DB-5	0.012	−0.021	0.9929	14.0	11.0
FID DB-1	0.015	+0.001	0.9955	11.0	6.0
MSD DB-1	0.005	−0.034	0.9954	1.0	11.0

[a]   Peak height ratio was plotted vs. concentration.
[b]   n = 7.

From Jones, A. B., ElSohly, H. N., and ElSohly, M. A., in *Marihuana '84,* Proc. Oxford Symp. on Cannabis, Harvey, D. J., Ed., IRL Press, Oxford, 1985. With permission.

Table 8 shows the calibration data for all methods where a linear relationship existed between peak area ratio (THC–COOH/CBN–COOH) and concentration of THC–COOH. The correlation coefficients (r) ranged from 0.9891 to 0.9974.

The coefficients of variance (CV) of the different methods of 25 ng/mℓ THC–COOH is shown in Table 8 and ranged from 6.0 to 15.6% (n = 7). Table 8 also contains the limit of detection of each assay.[47] the GC/MS and GC/ECD were at comparable sensitivity of 1 and 2 ng/mℓ. The HPLC method was of medium sensitivity (7 ng/mℓ), while the GC/FID methods were the least sensitive (11 to 14 ng/mℓ).

Figure 2 shows representative chromatograms of each of the analytical methods described here. The lack of interfering peaks in normal human urine was evidenced in all cases by extracting and analyzing a variety of blank urines. At the 25-ng/mℓ level of spiked urine the chromatograms (Figure 2) were of high quality.

The different analytical techniques were then used to determine the concentration of THC–COOH in urine specimens provided by Brooks Air Force Base Drug Testing Laboratory. The specimens were screened by Abuscreen® RIA prior to analysis for THC–COOH concentration. Table 9 shows the results of the analysis by the different methods using the same extract obtained from a single aliquot of each specimen. The specimens are arranged in Table 9 in a decreasing order of their response in the RIA screen. Since the GC/MS method was the most sensitive and definitive, all other methods were compared to it.

Correlations were made between the results obtained by GC/MS vs. HPLC, GC/ECD, GC/FID (OV-17), GC/FID DB-5, and GC/FID DB-1. The correlation coefficients were found to be 0.92, 0.98, 0.96, 0.90, and 0.92, respectively. Although there was a high degree of correlation between the GC/MS and HPLC methods (r = 0.92), it is noted from Table 8 that the observed concentration of THC–COOH was generally lower using the HPLC method. This could be explained if there was another cannabinoid metabolite with the same retention time as CBN–COOH. Therefore, a second aliquot of urine specimen code #235 was extracted without the addition of the internal standard (CBN–COOH). HPLC analysis of the extract showed that, indeed, there is a small peak under the internal standard which accounts for the lower value observed by the HPLC analysis of this specimen.

The significance of the data shown in Table 8 is that none of the analytical methods employed showed any significantly higher values for THC–COOH than the GC/MS values. In addition, all urines which had no or low concentrations of the acid metabolite by GC/

Table 9
CONCENTRATION OF 11-NOR-DELTA-9-THC-9-COOH IN HUMAN URINE (ng/mℓ) USING DIFFERENT ANALYTICAL METHODS

Code	MSD DB-1	FID DB-1	FID DB-5	FID OV-17	ECD OV-25	HPLC C-8	RIA
233	44	47	41	47	36	35	108
235	(35)[a]	(34)	(34)	(33)	(28)	(24)	(102)
238	24	20	(X)[b]	21	20	18	102
239	33	26	25	29	32	23	98
236	33	29	(X)	31	28	25	94
241	29	31	22	23	24	25	89
242	30	24	(X)	27	23	22	81
240	(38)	(36)	40	(33)	(30)	(20)	79
244	(30)	(23)	(28)	(27)	(22)	(18)	77
251	13	—[c]	—	—	13	9	75
250	14	—	—	14	14	17	62
247	10	—	—	—	13	9	52
246	11	—	—	13	13	12	50
245	15	—	—	15	11	12	48
249	9	—	—	—	11	8	46
237	10	—	—	—	9	7	40
252	(5)	(—)	(—)	(—)	(7)	—	36
234	4	—	—	—	8	—	35
248	4	—	—	—	5	—	26
243	(—)	(—)	(—)	(—)	(—)	(—)	17

[a] Values in parentheses denote average of duplicate analyses.
[b] —: Negative.
[c] X: Rejected because of poor chromatography.

From Jones, A. B., ElSohly, H. N., and ElSohly, M. A., in *Marihuana '84,* Proc. Oxford Symp. on Cannabis, Harvey, D. J., Ed., IRL Press, Oxford, 1985. With permission.

MS analysis (<15 ng/mℓ) were either negative or showed concentrations which were comparable to the GC/MS values.

It is concluded, therefore, that methods other than GC/MS could be reliably used to analyze for THC–COOH in urine specimens.

REFERENCES

1. **Martin, F.,** *Abnormal Psychology. Clinical and Scientific Perspectives,* Holt, Rinehart & Winston, New York, 1977, 507.
2. **Wood, G. B. and Bache, F.,** *The Dispensary of the United States of America 1851,* Lippincott & Grambo, Philadelphia, 1851, 310.
3. **Brecher, E. M.,** in *Licit and Illicit Drugs 1972,* Little, Brown, Boston, 1972, 403.
4. **Solomon, L. D.,** *The Marijuana Papers,* Bobbs, Merrill, New York, 1966, 426.
5. **Gaoni, Y. and Mechoulam, R.,** Isolation, Structure, and partial synthesis of an active constituent of hashish, *J. Am. Chem. Soc.,* 86, 1646, 1964.
6. **Waller, C. W., Johnson, J. J., Buelke, J., and Turner, C. E.,** *Marihuana: An Annotated Bibliography 1976,* Macmillan, New York, 1976.

7. **Waller, C. W., Nair, R. S., McAllister, A. F., Urbanek, B., and Turner, C. E.,** *Marihuana: An Annotated Bibliography,* Vol. 2, Macmillan New York, 1982; and **Waller, C. W., Baran, K., Urbanek, B., and Turner, C. E.,** *Marihuana: An Annotated Bibliography 1980 Supplement,* University of Mississippi Press, University, Mississippi, 1983.

8. **Waller, C. W., Urbanek, B., and Turner, C. E.,** *Marihuana: An Annotated Bibliography, 1980 Supplement,* University of Mississippi Press, University, Mississippi, 1983.

9. **Turner, C. E., ElSohly, M. A., and Boeren, E. G.,** Constituents of *Cannabis sativa* L. XVII. A review of the natural constituents, *J. Nat. Products,* 43, 169, 1980.

10. **ElSohly, M. A., Holley, J. H., and Turner, C. E.,** Constituents of *Cannabis sativa* L. XXIV. The delta-9-tetrahydrocannabinol content of confiscated marijuana, 1974—1983, *Marihuana '84: Proc. Oxford Symp. on Cannabis,* Harvey, D. J., Ed., IRL Press, Oxford, 1985, 37.

11. **Halldin, M. M., Carlsson, L, K. P., Kanter, S. L., Widman, M., and Agurell, S.,** Urinary metabolites of delta-1-tetrahydrocannabinol in man, *Drug Res.,* 32, 764, 1982.

12. **Halldin, M. M., Anderson, U. K. R., Widman, M., and Hollister, L. E.,** Further urinary metabolites of delta-1-tetrahydrocannabinol in man, *Drug Res.,* 32, 1135, 1982.

13. **Halldin, M. M. and Widman, M.,** Glucuronic acid conjugate of delta-1-tetrahydrocannabinol identified in the urine of man, *Drug Res.,* 33, 177, 1983.

14. **Wall, M. E. and Perez-Reyes, M.,** The metabolism of delta-9-tetrahydrocannabinol and related cannabinoids in man, *J. Clin. Pharmacol.,* 21, 1978s, 1981.

15. **Williams, P. L. and Moffat, A. C.,** Identification in human urine of delta-9-tetrahydrocannabinol-11-oic acid glucuronide: a tetrahydrocannabinol metabolite, *J. Pharm. Pharmacol.,* 32, 445, 1980.

16. **Kanter, S. L., Hollister, L. E., and Musumeici, M.,** Marijuana metabolites in urine of man: identification of marijuana use by detection of delta-9-tetrahydrocannabinol-11-oic-acid using thin-layer chromatography, *J. Chromatogr.,* 234, 201, 1982.

17. **Kanter, S. L., Hollister, L. E., and Zamora, J. U.,** Marijuana metabolites in urine of man. XI. Detection of unconjugated and conjugated delta-9-tetrahydrocannabinol-11-oic acid by thin-layer chromatography, *J. Chromatogr.,* 235, 507, 1982.

18. **Schermann, J. M., Hollinger, H., Nam, N. H., Boudet, L., Kichon, J., and Thang, D. C.,** Detection and quantitation of cannabinoids in biological fluids: specificity and kinetics after smoking, *Clin. Toxicol.,* 18, 565.

19. **Kogan, M. J., Newman, E., and William, N. J.,** Detection of marijuana metabolite 11-nor-delta-9-tetrahydrocannabinol-9-carboxylic acid in human urine by bonded-phase adsorption and thin-layer chromatography, *J. Chromatogr.,* 306, 441, 1984.

20. **Nakamura, G. P., Stall, W. J., Folen, V. A., and Masters, R. G.,** Thin-layer chromatography/mass spectrometric identification of 11-nor-delta-9-tetrahydrocannabinol-9-carboxylic acid, *J. Chromatogr.,* 264, 336, 1983.

21. **Wilson, N. J., Kogan, M. J., Pierson, D. J., and Newman, E.,** Confirmation of EMIT cannabinoid assay results by bonded phase adsorption with thin-layer chromatography, *J. Toxicol. Clin. Pharmacol.,* 20, 1465, 1983.

22. **Whiting, J. D. and Manders, W. W.,** Confirmation of a tetrahydrocannabinol metabolite in urine by gas chromatography, *J. Anal. Toxicol.,* 6, 49, 1982.

23. **ElSohly, M. A., Arafat, E. S., and Jones, A. B.,** Analysis of the major metabolite of delta-9-tetrahydrocannabinol in urine. III. A GC/ECD procedure, *J. Anal. Toxicol.,* 8, 7, 1984.

24. **Nordquist, M., Lindgren, J. E., and Agurell, S.,** A method for the identification of acid metabolites of tetrahydrocannabinol (THC) by mass-fragmentography, in Cannabinoid Assays in Humans, NIDA Res. Monogr. No. 7, Willette, R. E., Ed., Department of Health, Education and Welfare, Washington, D.C., 1976, 64.

25. **Karlsson, K., Jonsson, J., Aburg, K., and Roos, C.,** Determination of delta-9-tetrahydrocannabinol-11-oic-acid in urine as its pentaflouropropyl, partafluoropropionyl derivative by GC/MS utilizing negative ion chemical ionization, *J. Anal. Toxicol.,* 7, 198, 1983.

26. **Foltz, R. L., McGinnis, J. M., and Chinn, D. M.,** Quantitative measurement of delta-9-tetrahydrocannabinol and two major metabolites in physiological specimens using capillary column gas chromatography negative ion chemical ionization mass spectrometry, *Biomed. Mass Spectrom.,* 10, 316, 1983.

27. **ElSohly, M. A., ElSohly, H. N., Jones, A. B., Dimson, P. A., and Wells, K. E.,** Analysis of the major metabolite of delta-9-tetrahydrocannabinol in urine. II. An HPLC procedure, *J. Anal. Toxicol.,* 7, 262, 1983.

28. **Karlsson, L. and Roos, C.,** Combination of liquid chromatography with ultraviolet detection and gas chromatography with electron capture detection for the determination of delta-9-tetrahydrocannabinol-11-oic acid in urine, *J. Chromatogr.,* 306, 183, 1984.

29. **Williams, P. L., Moffat, A. C., and King, L. J.,** Combined high-performance liquid chromatography and radioimmunoassay method for the analysis of delta-9-tetrahydrocannabinol metabolites in human urine, *J. Chromatogr.,* 186, 595, 1979.

30. **Williams, P. L. and Moffat, A. C.,** Identification in human urine of delta-9-tetrahydrocannabinol-11-oic acid glucoronide: a tetrahydrocannabinol metabolite, *J. Pharm. Pharmacol.,* 32, 445. 1980.

31. **Law, B., Mason, P. A., Moffat, A. C., and King, L. J.,** Confirmation of *Cannabis* use by the analysis of delta-9-tetrahydrocannabinol metabolites in blood and urine by combined HPLC and RIA, *J. Anal. Toxicol.,* 8, 19, 1984.

32. **Peat, M. A., Peyman, B. A., and Johnson, J. R.,** High performance liquid chromatography immunoassay of delta-9-tetrahydrocannabinol and its metabolites in urine, *J. Forensic Sci.,* p. 110, 1984.

33. **Cook, C. E.,** Radioimmunoassay of cannabinoids, in: *Cannabinoid Analysis in Physiological Fluids,* ACS Symp. Ser. No., Vinson, J. A., Ed., American Chemical Society, Washington, D.C., 1979, 137.

34. **Teale, J. D., Forman, E. J., King, L. J., and Marks, V.,** Radioimmunoassay of cannabinoids in blood and urine, *Lancet,* 2, 553, 1974.

35. **Chase, A. R., Kelly, P. R., Taunton-Rigby, A., Jones, R. T., and Harwood, T.,** Quantitation of cannabinoids in biological fluids by radioimmunoassay, in Res. Monogr. No., Willette, R. E., Ed., Department of Health, Education and Welfare, Washington, D.C., 1978.

36. **Jones, A. B., ElSohly, H. N., and ElSohly, M. A.,** Analysis of the major metabolite of delta-9-tetrahydrocannabinol in urine. V. Cross-reactivity of selected compounds in a radioimmunoassay, *J. Anal. Toxicol.,* 8, 252, 1984.

37. **Rowley, G. L., Armstrong, T. A., Crowe, C. P., Eimstad, W. M., Hu, W. M., Kam, J. K., Rodgers, R., Ronald, R. C., Rubenstein, K. E., Shelton, B. G., and Ullman, E. F.,** Determination of THC and its metabolites, in Cannabinoid Assays in Humans, NIDA Res. Monogr. Ser. *No.* 7, Willette, R. E., Ed., U.S. Department of Health, Education and Welfare, Washington, D.C., 1976, 28.

38. **Rodgers, R., Crowe, C. P., Eimstad, W. M., Hu, W. M., Kam, J. K., Ronald, R. C., Rowley, G. I., and Ullman, E. F.,** Homogenous enzyme immnoassay for cannabinoids in urine, *Clin. Chem.,* 24, 95, 1978.

39. **Jones, A. B., ElSohly, H. N., and ElSohly, M. A.,** Cross-reactivity of selected compounds in urine immunoassays for the major metabolite of delta-9-tetrahydrocannabinol, *Marihuana '84:* Proc. Oxford Symp. on cannabis, Harvey, D. J., Ed., IRL Press, Oxford, 1985, 169.

40. **ElSohly, M. A., ElSohly, H. N., Stanford, D. F., Evans, M. G., and Jones, A. B.,** Analysis of human urine for 11-nor-delta-9-tetrahydrocannabinol-9-carboxylic acid. A comparison between HPLC, GC/ECD, GC/FID, and GC/MS methods, *Marihuana '84:* Proc. Oxford Symp. on Cannabis, Harvey, D. J., Ed., IRL Press, Oxford, 1985, 137.

41. **Irving, J., Leed, B., Foltz, R. L., Cook, C. E., Bursey, J. T., and Willette, R. E.,** Evaluation of immunoassays for cannabinoids in urine, *J. Anal. Toxicol.,* 8, 192, 1984.

42. **Jones, A. B., ElSohly, H. N., Arafat, E. S., and ElSohly, M. A.,** Analysis of the major metabolite of delta-9-tetrahydrocannabinol in urine. IV. A comparison of five methods, *J. Anal. Toxicol.,* 6, 249, 1984.

43. **Abuscreen, Radioimmunoassay for Cannabinoids (^{125}I),** Roche Diagnostic Systems, Division of Hoffman-LaRoche, Inc., Nutley, N.J. Package insert issued January, 1983.

44. **EMIT d.a.u. Cannabinoid Urine Assay,** Syva Corporation, Palo Alto, Calif., Package insert issued November, 1981.

45. **Goldstein, A.,** *Biostatistics,* McMillian, New York, 1967, 144.

46. **Wall, M. E.,** personal communication.

47. **Long, G. L. and Winefordner, J. D.,** Limit of detection. A closer look at the IUPAC definition, *Anal. Chem.,* 55, 712A, 1983.

Chapter 13

DESIGNER DRUGS: AN OVERVIEW

Gene Barnett and Rao S. Rapaka

TABLE OF CONTENTS

I. INTRODUCTION

"To conquer disease and achieve a surcease from pain, man has ransacked the entire earth for drugs. And what he could not find in nature the chemist created in his laboratory. But many of these useful drugs are like the finger of God — they can heal and they can smite."[1] The misuse of drugs has played a role in society at least as far back as Hippocrates and was reflected in the vocabulary of the times: *pharmakon* — a drug, medicine, or poison; *pharmacopeus* — a purveyor of toxic substances; *pharmakopoloi* — traveling quack doctor; *pharmakoi* — condemned criminal.[2] The problems of drug use and misuse are still of concern, and health hazards posed by the availability of designer drugs is a major focus today.[3]

"Designer drugs are analogs, or chemical cousins, of controlled substances that are designed to produce effects similar to the controlled substances they mimick. By slightly altering the chemical formula of a controlled substance....a new drug is created which will produce the high or euphoria the user wants." This definition was given during Congressional hearings[4] on designer drugs in 1985 where the illicit drug trade was estimated to be a $110 billion per year industry in the U.S., which is about three times the total sales of the U.S. pharmaceutical industry.[5] The illicit importation was an estimated 10 tons of heroin, 85 tons of cocaine, and 15,000 tons of marijuana. Further, "The production of illicit drugs abroad continues unabated, and in our own country illicit marijuana has become a major cash crop."[4] The designer drug portion of the illicit market is estimated at $1 billion and primarily in opiate-type and phenylisopropylamine-type street drugs at the current time.[3]

Why is there drug abuse? Why do people consume designer drugs or other illicit drugs? The answer commonly given: because it feels good. The drugs that are so used are psychoactive drugs, ones that produce effects on thought, feeling, mood, self-perception, and give a sense of "high" or intoxication. Self-administration of drugs for nonmedical, indeed, recreational purposes can be a hazard as it may lead to compulsive or addictive use. Drugs from the illicit marketplace have the additional hazard of containing impurities or untested chemicals that can be toxic and life threatening. Efforts to understand why opiates and hallucinogens are self-administered yields the following descriptions. Intravenous use of an opiate produces warm flushing of the skin and sensations in the lower abdomen described by addicts as similar in intensity and quality to sexual orgasm. Consumption of a hallucinogen drug, or other central nervous system sympathomimetic drugs, such as cocaine, produces a heightened awareness of sensory input, often with an enhanced sense of clarity, and the user receives vivid and unusual sensory experiences, attention is focused inward with a sense of union with the cosmos or mankind. The phenomenon of drug abuse has become a sophisticated and relatively new area of study of the human being from perspectives of physiology and psychology, where concern is given to such issues as tolerance and cross tolerance, dependence and addiction, and induced behavioral reinforcement that will certainly lead to a better understanding of the human organism.[6]

The design of new drugs often utilizes basic principles of the chemistry laboratory whereby the structure of a drug molecule is slightly altered in order to alter the pharmacological activity. This principle of structure-activity relationships, known as SAR, has been applied to many medically approved drugs that are in the marketplace. For the opiates, SAR studies have been pursued in the search for a nonaddicting analgesic for the treatment of pain. Slight structural changes have produced new drugs with altered receptor-binding properties and altered potency or activity. Basic research on the opiates during the last decade has lead to important scientific discoveries of multiple opiate receptors, the endogenous opiods, and renewed interest in the structure and function of polypeptides.[7] The hallucinogen family of drugs are not as well understood as the opiates. A 1978 conference on quantitative SAR studies of the opiates and hallucinogens found detailed discussions on opiate receptor binding and sophisticated arguments as to the existence of multiple opiod receptors with different pharmacologic properties, while discussions on the hallucinogens were in a relatively early stage of development.[8] There are substantial benefits to be gained from a basic understanding of how drugs of this family, many of which can be classified as sympathomimetic drugs together with cocaine, interact and/or interfere with the chemical messengers or neurotransmitters of the autonomic nervous system.

Clandestine production of drugs, so called street drugs, is intended to avoid federal regulation and control. The result is availability of unknown substances of unknown purity that may have the potential to cause serious toxicity with potentially dangerous health consequences for the naive drug user. A review of illicit drugs and analogues produced by the clandestine pharmaceutical industry concludes that the quality of personnel involved in drug synthesis ranges from cookbook amateurs to highly skilled chemists. And quite surprisingly, "most of these new analogs have been previously reported in the literature with animal data that suggest they would be reasonably active and have similar pharmacological effects to the lead compound in the series."[9]

II. REGULATORY EFFORTS AT DRUG CONTROL

For various reasons, governments have been attempting to control the sale and use of drugs for many years at both the national and international levels. Efforts to provide a legal framework in order to guide and coordinate the nations in the control of psychoactive drugs began in 1909 with an international commission to control the opium poppy plant. In 1961 control efforts extended to the coca bush and the marijuana plant, and finally in 1971 to synthetic substances. Within the world community, the 1961 Single Convention on Narcotic Drugs, together with the amending Protocol of 1972, and the 1971 Convention of Psychotropic Substances are the primary pieces of international legislation that set up the mechanisms for coordinated control of dependence-producing and mind-altering drugs. A list of these treaties is present in Table 1.[10]

The U.S. government has established a series of legislative controls on drug use and production in order to safeguard the public. These efforts are extended over both control of drug misuse or abuse and over the production of new drugs for medical therapeutic use to improve the quality of life. The various legislative acts are listed in Table 2. Throughout the legislative history there was an obvious concern for pure drugs that are safe and effective. The creation of the Food and Drug Administration (FDA) has provided for a more rational manner of discovery and development of new chemical entities for medical use. It is instructive to briefly review the FDA procedures in order to be aware of the extensive efforts that are required in order to assure, as much as is possible, that a drug is safe before it is permitted for general use by the public.

The U.S. imposed special restrictions on those drugs with potential for abuse under the Comprehensive Drug Abuse Prevention and Control Act of 1970, which is commonly referred to as the Controlled Substances Act. Under this legislation the Drug Enforcement Agency (DEA) has designated and classified all drugs with abuse potential. There are five schedules of controlled substances known as Schedules I, II, III, IV, V, and within each schedule are lists of specific drugs including narcotics, stimulants, hallucinogens, and depressants. The drugs in Schedule I are those that have a high abuse potential and include heroin, marijuana, and the hallucinogens. These are drugs that have no currently accepted medical use, thus a physician will have no concern with Schedule I unless he is involved in conducting research. For Schedule II drugs, which also have a high abuse potential, the physician cannot give telephone prescriptions nor refills. Schedule III drugs, which are classified as having a lower abuse potential than drugs in I or II, are limited such that medical prescriptions must be rewritten after 6 months or 5 refills. The drugs listed in Schedule IV, classified as moderate potential for abuse, have the same restrictions as those in III except that the penalty for

Table 1
INTERNATIONAL DRUG CONTROL TREATIES

1909—The Shanghai International Opium Commission
The first international body concerned with narcotic drugs
1912—The Hague International Opium Convention
Established international cooperation in the control of narcotic drugs
1925—International Opium Convention
Established a system of import and export requirements for trade in narcotic drugs
1931—Convention Limiting the Manufacture and Distribution of Narcotic Drugs
Limited manufacturing to meet medical and scientific needs
1936—Convention on Suppression of Illicit Traffic in Dangerous Drugs
Set up punishment for illicit drug traffickers
1946—Protocol
Transferred to the United Nations functions previously held by the League of Nations
1948—Protocol
Brought under control selected synthetic substances that were dependence producing
1953—Opium Protocol
Further restricted the amounts of opium for trading and those nations which were permitted do so
1961—Single Convention on Narcotic Drugs
Modernized systems of multilateral treaties on control
Formed the International Narcotics Control Board
Extended controls to include the coca bush and marijuana plant
Prohibited opium smoking and eating, coca leaf chewing, and cannabis smoking
Provided for medical treatment and rehabilitation of abusers
1971—Convention on Psychotropic Substances
Extended the Single Convention of 1961 to control central nervous system stimulants, sedative-hypnotics, and
  hallucinogens
Introduced provisions for prevention and treatment of drug abuse
1972—Protocol Amending the Single Convention on Narcotic Drugs
Intensified efforts to prevent illicit production, traffic in, and use of narcotic drugs; emphasized prevention
  through information and education; emphasized need for measures for treatment, rehabilitation, and social
  reintegration of abusers
Strengthened role of International Narcotics Control Board in reducing demand, supply production, manufacture,
  traffic, and use
1981—International Drug Abuse Control Strategy
Adopted Global Plan for strategy and 5-year program for action to deal with the growing drug abuse problem.

illegal possession is less severe. Schedule V drugs have a low abuse potential and may be dispensed without a prescription unless otherwise specified by state law. The list and classification of substances is in accord with the international conventions for psychotropic drugs. The FDA routinely evaluates those new drug candidates that may have a possible potential for producing dependence in order to determine abuse liability.

III. ROLE OF THE FOOD AND DRUG ADMINISTRATION

The Food and Drug Administration (FDA) became the administrative body to oversee drug evaluation and give official approval to market new drug products within the U.S. In order to begin studies in humans it is first necessary to file an Investigational Exemption for a New Drug (IND) with the FDA. The IND includes detailed information on the composition and source of the drug, manufacturing information, data from animal studies to determine possible acute toxicity, and clinical plans for the studies to be done. Once the IND is granted, clinical studies may be initiated in order to obtain sufficient data to submit a New Drug Application (NDA) to the FDA to gain approval for marketing. Such studies, which are extremely time consuming and costly, are carried in three phases. In Phase 1, clinical trials are done to establish dose-effect relationships in a small number of healthy volunteer subjects. Usually, chronic animal studies are also initiated at this time to establish

Table 2
NATIONAL DRUG CONTROL LEGISLATION

1906—Pure Food and Drug Act
Prohibited mislabeling and adulteration of drugs
1909—Opium Exclusion Act
Prohibited the importation of opium
1912—Amendment to the Pure Food and Drug Act
Prohibited false and midleading advertising
1914—Harrison Narcotics Act
Established regulations for the use of opium, opiates, and cocaine
1937—Amendment to the Harrison Narcotics Act
Established regulations for the use of marijuana
1938—Food, Drug, and Cosmetic Act
Required that new drugs be safe as well as pure
1952—Durham-Humphrey Act
Gave power to the FDA to determine which products could be sold without prescription
1962—Kefauver-Harris Amendment to the Food, Drug, and Cosmetic Act
Gave power to the FDA to require proof of efficacy for new drugs
Established guidelines for reporting information on adverse reactions, clinical testing, and advertising of new drugs
1970—Controlled Substances Act
Established DEA authority to classify drugs according to abuse potential and to control their distribution
1984—National Narcotics Act
Provided authority for quickly adding new controlled substance analogues to Schedule of Controlled Substances

drug safety and possible toxicities due to long-term use. Phase 2 studies are then carried out with patients, those that have the disease to be treated, in order to establish safety and efficacy in this special population. Phase 3 studies are finally carried out in large numbers of patients in the expected clinical setting to be encountered. In Phase 1 both the investigators and volunteer subjects are aware of the drug treatment being given. Phase 2 studies are usually done with a single-blind protocol where the physicians are aware of the treatments given, but the patients are unaware of what dose is being given or whether they are receiving a placebo (no drug control) or an older known successful drug treatment (a positive control) for comparision purposes. In Phase 3 clinical trials both the physician and patient are unaware of which treatment is being given, a double-blind treatment protocol, in an effort to minimize uncertainty in determining drug efficacy and possible toxic side effects. When these studies are successfully completed and a careful review and evaluation of the data has been carried out, the FDA will grant approval of the NDA and the new chemical entity can be marketed for sale. At this time the new drug enters Phase 4 where postmarketing surveillance is done to obtain further data on the safety and efficacy of the drug once it is in general use. With an extremely large number of subjects it is then hoped to detect as soon as possible any as yet unobserved harmful properties of the new drug.

IV. THE STRUCTURE-ACTIVITY RELATIONSHIP (SAR)

Chemical strategies to design new drugs have a long and successful history in medical chemotherapeutics. Many useful new drugs or modifications to older drugs have clearly resulted in improved health care for countless persons throughout the world. A good example may be that of Valium® and the benzodiazepine family of drugs. This group of widely used Schedule IV drugs, known as sedative-hypnotic or antianxiety agents in medical treatment, act on the central nervous system.[11]

Selected benzodiazepine drugs with their molecular structures and chemical names are listed in Figure 1 and present a good example of SAR concepts. The diagram drawn at the top of the figure is the chemist's symbolic method of representation for the general family

BENZODIAZEPINES: NAMES AND STRUCTURES

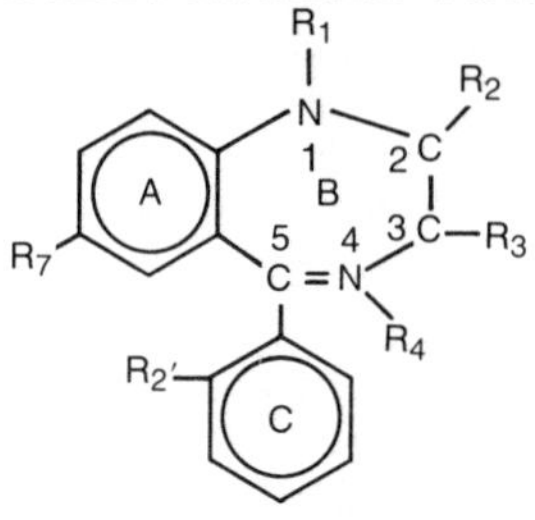

Benzodiazepine	R_1	R_2	R_3	R_7	$R_{2'}$
Chlordiazepoxide	(—)	—NHCH$_3$	—H	—Cl	—H
Clonazepam	—H	=O	—H	—NO$_2$	—Cl
Clorazepate	—H	=O	—COO$^-$	—Cl	—H
Demoxepam	—H	=O	—H	—Cl	—H
Diazepam	CH$_3$	=O	—H	—Cl	—H
Flurazepam	—CH$_2$CH$_2$N(C$_2$H$_5$)$_2$	=O	—H	—Cl	—F
Halazepam	—CH$_2$CF$_3$	=O	—H	—Cl	—H
Lorazepam	—H	=O	—OH	—Cl	—Cl
Nitrazepam	—H	=O	—H	—NO$_2$	—H
Nordazepam	—H	=O	—H	—Cl	—H
Oxazepam	—H	=O	—OH	—Cl	—H
Prazepam	—CH$_2$—CH$_2$$\underset{CH_2}{\overset{CH_2}{<}}$	=O	—H	—Cl	—H
Temazepam	—CH$_3$	=O	—OH	—Cl	—H

FIGURE 1.   The chemical names and structures are given for some drugs of the benzodiazepine type. See text for explanation of the table. Note that there is no substituent at position R_4, except for chlordiazepoxide and demoxepam which are *N*-oxzides. (From Harvey, S. C., in *The Pharmacological Basis of Therapeutics,* 7th ed., Gilman, A. G., Goodman, L. S., Rall, T. W., and Murad, F., Eds., Macmillan, New York, 1985, chap. 17. With permission.)

of drugs that belong to the benzodiazepine class of molecules. The general structure consists of three rings denoted by the letters A, B, C, together with a number of locations on the drug molecule where specific atoms or groups of atoms are introduced at the sites labeled $R_1 R_2, R_3, R_7, R_2'$. For example Valium® has the chemical name diazepam, and the molecular structure is designated by replacing R1 by the atoms CH3, called a methyl group by the chemist, replacing R_2 with =O, a keto oxygen atom, replacing both R_3 and R_2' with a hydrogen atom H, and replacing R_7 with Cl, a chlorine atom.

Slight alterations in the substituents at the R sites result in new molecular structures, giving different drugs that have different pharmacological activities; thus, the term structure-activity relationship. In the case of diazepam or Valium®, a change in R_1 from CH$_3$ to H results in the drug nordiazepam. Then a second change in R_3 from H to OH, the hydroxy group, results in the drug oxazepam or Serax®. And continuing further, a change at R_2' from H to Cl results in the drug lorazepam or Ativan®. Similarly, changing nordiazepam at R_7 from Cl to NO$_2$, the nitro group, gives nitrazepam or Mogadon. Further, a change at site R_2' from H to Cl gives the drug clonazepam or Clonopin®. In medical treatment each drug has a different recommended dosage for safe and effective use. Likewise, each drug has its own dose-effect relationship, as shown schematically in Figure 2.[12]

It is not a simple task to carry out the types of changes on the structures of molecules as the above reading might imply. Alterations of molecules depend on complex procedures for chemical synthesis, availability and purity of chemical solvents and reagents, the use of high-vacuum systems, sophisticated considerations of molecular stereochemistry, physico-chemical properties of solvents and solutes, the reproducibility of tests for biological activity,

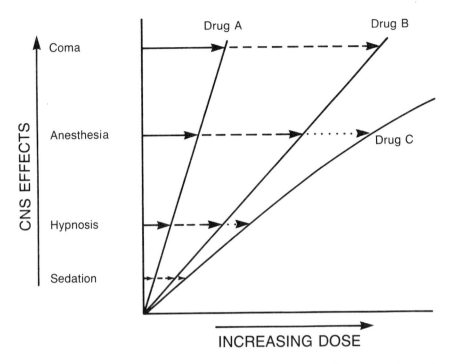

FIGURE 2. Schematic dose-effect curves for sedative-hypnotic drugs. (From Trevor, A. J. and Way, W. L., in *Basic and Clinical Pharmacology*, Katzung, B. G., Ed., Lange Medical Publications, Los Altos, Calif., 1984, chap. 20. With permission.)

the nature of the mechanism of drug action, and all the unforseen problems and challenges that invariably occur during basic scientific research and development.

V. OPIUM AND THE OPIATES

It is clear from legislative efforts that opium has a long colorful history of use in many societies dating back many hundreds of years. In the beginning, opium use was well accepted, but as the liabilities of chronic usage became increasing apparent, the drug fell into disfavor.[13] Opium is obtained from the seeds of the opium poppy plant which contains over 25 alkaloid-type chemical compounds. Morphine is the principle opiate alkaloid present in the plant, about 10%, and codeine is present at about 0.5%. Two nonopiod alkaloids found in the plant, thebaine and papaverine, have turned out to be useful in the synthesis of other drugs. The extraction of morphine from crude opium at the beginning of the 19th century began the modern era of drug treatment. This isolation of a pure and powerful compound allowed reproducible and quantitative drug treatment in humans in place of the unreliable results obtained from ‘natural unextracted sources. Synthetic drug development began in the mid 19th century, ›rimarily in Germany, while development of a modern technological drug industry in the U.S. began after World War I. By the 1940s the technology was so developed as to permit highly specific molecular modification of compounds in order to alter potency and toxicity of the new synthetic drugs.

The chemical structures for examples from the major classes of opiate drugs are shown in Figure 3. Morphine is a phenanthrene type of molecular structure, while methadone, a synthetic drug used in the treatment of opiate addiction, is a member of the phenylheptylamine class of opioid compounds and meperidine, a synthetic drug known as Demerol®, is of the phenylpipridine class. These chemicals are all in Schedule II as they have medical use and a high potential for abuse that can lead to addiction. The use of slight structure changes to

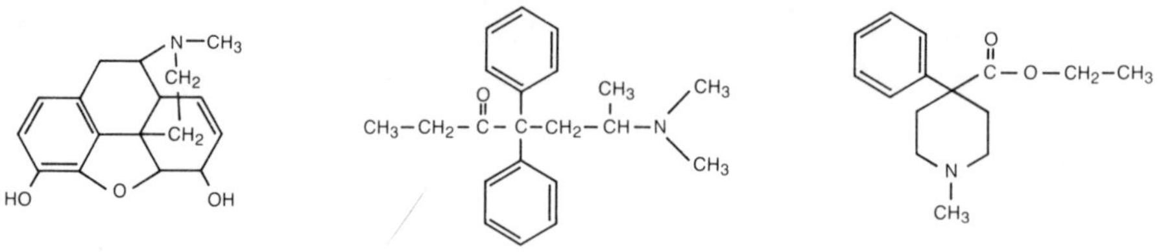

FIGURE 3.   Molecular structures for the opiate drugs morphine, methadone, and meperidine.

alter pharmacological activity applies to the opiate drugs perhaps more dramatically than for the benzodiazepines. Extensive research has yielded a large number of narcotic agonists and antagonist molecules with a wide range of pharmacological properties as part of the ongoing search for a nonaddicting analgesic drug.

A slight change in the structure of the morphine molecule results in a great change in activity. Simply by replacing one of the H atoms of the CH_3 group shown in the top right portion of structure in Figure 3 with the group $CH=CH_2$, the morphine molecule, which produces a strong analgesic effect, is transformed into the nalorphine molecule which is a strong antagonist that completely blocks the effects of morphine. Replacement of the H atoms of the two OH groups by acetyl groups, CH_3CO, gives the structure of heroin. With this slight change in the molecular structure the drug is more lipophilic than morphine and thus, crosses the blood-brain barrier more easily into the brain and produces an enhanced pharmacologic effect that is readily recognized by experienced opiate users. In a similar manner for methadone, a synthetic opiate used in replacement therapy for treatment of heroin addiction, a slight change to the structure produces the widely used drug propoxyphene or Darvon®. Such slight changes produce what are often called look-alike drugs.

Meperidine, shown in Figure 3, is a Schedule II controlled substance that has been a template for the design of a look-alike drug not on the controlled substances list. A slight change in the structure gives the drug known as MPPP, a Demerol® look-alike drug which is known on the streets as synthetic heroin. The structure differs from meperidine only in that the group bonded to the ring, –COO, is altered to –OCO in MPPP. It is now known that MPPP usually includes an impurity MPTP that has been found to produce permanent brain damage that creates the symptoms of Parkinson's disease.[14] Extensive research has lead to a full understanding of the lethal results of consuming this street drug. The detailed story of the scientific pursuit and identification of the cause and the manner in which this occurs is the topic of Chapter 15.

Another opiate that has created serious health hazards on the streets is fentanyl, or Sublimaze®, which is a potent, extremely fast-acting narcotic analgesic that subsequently has a high abuse liability. It is approximately 100 times more potent than morphine and has been a template for many look-alike drugs for the clandestine chemist to synthesize new uncontrolled substance analogues. Figure 4 shows the molecular structures for fentanyl and the analogues alpha-methyl-fentanyl, 3-methyl-fentanyl, and para-fluoro-fentanyl. While it is clear that the structural changes are very slight, the change in pharmacologic activity is dramatic. On the basis of classic animal tests to evaluate relative potencies, the analogue para-fluoro is 100, alpha-methyl is 900, and 3-methyl is 1100 times more potent than morphine. Statistics gathered by the DEA suggest that drug overdose deaths associated with fentanyl-like drugs has increased steadily over the last 5 years, with a total of 50 deaths reported from California alone.[15] The National Narcotic Act of 1984 has been invoked to rapidly classify a number of these new compounds as controlled substance analogues of fentanyl.

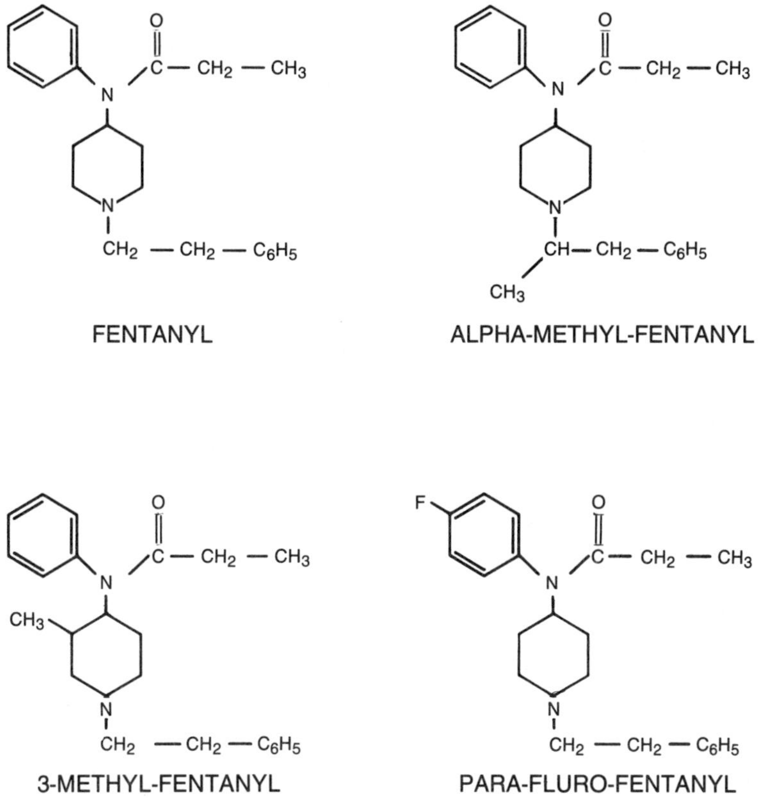

FIGURE 4. Molecular structures for fentanyl and the chemical analogues alpha-methyl-fentanyl, 3-methyl-fentanyl, and para-fluoro-fentanyl.

VI. THE HALLUCINOGENS

It may be appropriate that two of the popular street drugs of this type go by such names as ''Adam'' and ''Eve'' since they produce pharmacological effects by interfering with the basic neurotransmitter system for the autonomic nervous system which regulates bodily function and response. Unlike the opiates, where there is substantial understanding of the biological receptors involved in opiod pharmacological response, there is much less understanding of the catecholamines and receptors for the sympathetic nervous system. There is detailed knowledge about the molecular nature of the chemical transmitters, however, and structure-activity studies are providing information about receptor structure and function as well.

Amino acids are used by the body to synthesize dopamine which is then transported into the nervous system neuronal vesicles where it undergoes biotransformation to form norepinephrine, the basic adrenergic neurotransmitter involved in the control and regulation of such cardiovascular and peripheral functions as heart rate, blood flow, blood vessel dilation and contraction, and muscle constriction and relaxation. Figure 5 shows the chemical structures for dopamine, norepinephrine, and epinephrine, another of the neurotransmitters. These three compounds are all natural or endogenous compounds which, when administered as a treatment drug, produce pharmacological effects by direct interaction with adrenergic neuron receptors. The synthetic drug isoproterenol, also shown in Figure 5, is also a direct-acting catecholamine. The three catecholamine compounds — norephinephrine, ephinephrine, and isoproterenol — have clinical use based on their actions on bronchial smooth muscle, blood

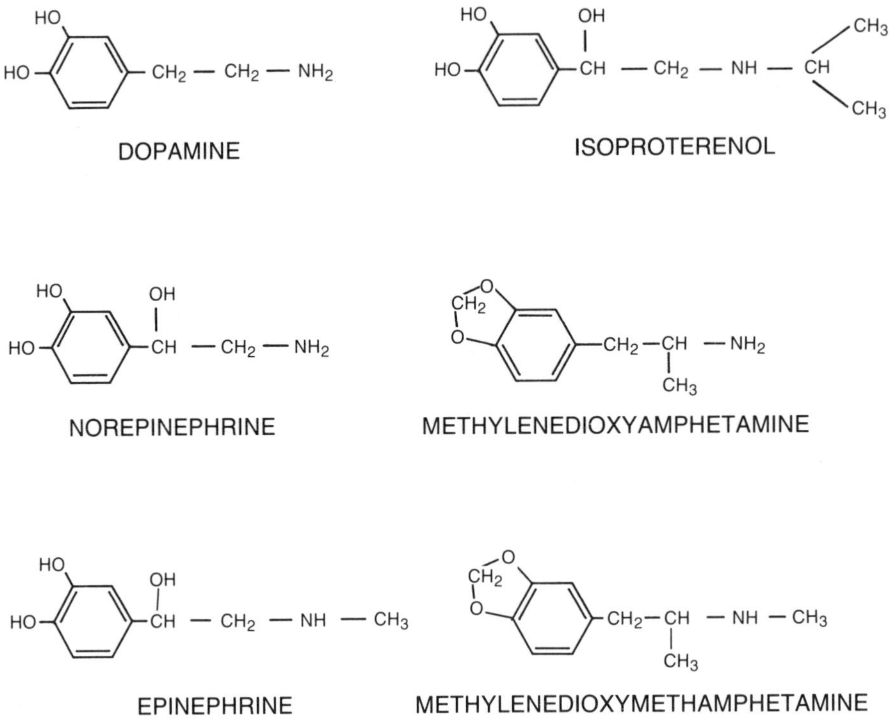

FIGURE 5.   Molecular structure for dopamine, norepinephrine, epinephrine, isoproterenol, methyl-enedioxyamphetamine (MDA), and methylenedioxymethamphetamine (MDMA).

vessels, and the heart. Because of their cardiovascular and central nervous system actions they can also have serious side effects if used improperly. Also shown in Figure 5 are the chemical structures for methylenedioxyamphetamine or MDA and methylenedioxymetham-phetamine or MDMA. They clearly have similarities in chemical structure to the catechol-amines and probably have similarities in pharmacological actions as well.

To explore briefly the complexity of action of this type of drugs, some amphetamine-type drugs are presented in Figure 6 which are closely related to the catecholamine class. It is known that amphetamine does not act directly on the adrenergic receptor, but is taken up into the neuronal vesicle where it displaces norepinephrine. This indirect-acting drug elicits sympathomimetic effects on the central nervous system, stimulation or mood elevation, and on the peripheral vasculature, increased blood pressure and heart rate. All the drugs in Figure 6, except phenylephrine, are indirect-acting agents due to the fact that their action depends on displacement of stored norepinephrine. When the mechanism of action is in this indirect fashion, the pharmacologic response under repeated administration of a given dose produces tachyphylaxis, which is a gradually diminishing response to the drug stimulus also called drug tolerance. The slight structural difference between amphetamine and metham-phetamine, which is seen in Figure 6 as the replacement of an H with a CH_3 on the nitrogen center, is sufficient to allow the latter to cross the blood-brain barrier more easily and elicit a stronger central nervous system stimulus, while also having a weaker peripheral action. Therefore, the ratio of central-to-peripheral action is altered by the slight change in the structure of the drug molecule. Ephedrine, with the added hydroxy group OH, also has a different ratio of central-to-peripheral action than amphetamine as its central effect is weaker, while its peripheral action is prolonged in duration. Phenylpropranolamine and hydroxyam-phetamine, which also have slight structural alterations from amphetamine, are similar in structure to the direct-acting catecholamines, but are indirect-acting drugs. Both are less

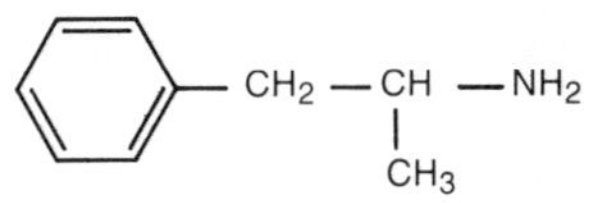

AMPHETAMINE

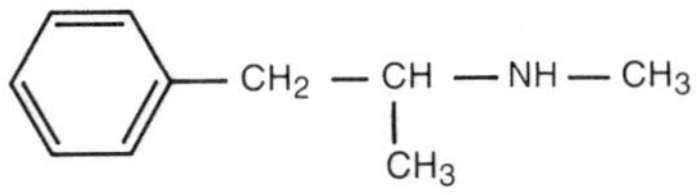

METHAMPHETAMINE

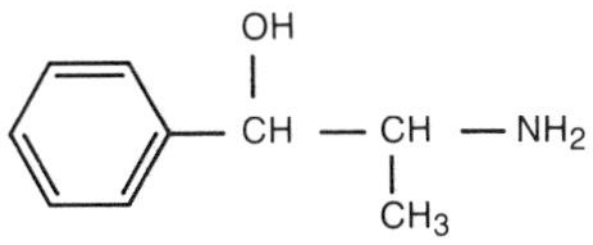

PHENYLPROPRANOLAMINE

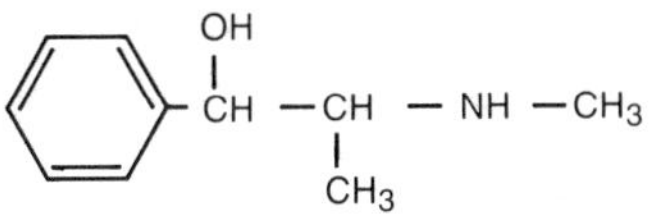

EPHEDRINE

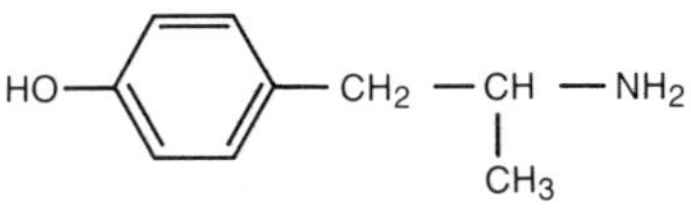

HYDROXYAMPHETAMINE

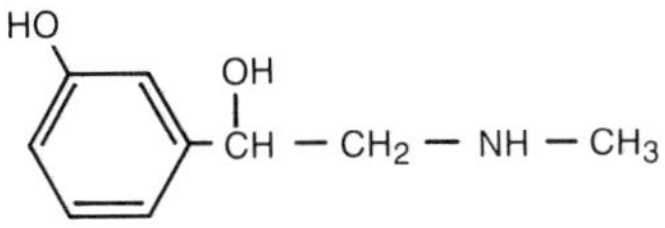

PHENYLEPHRINE

FIGURE 6. Molecular structures for amphetamine, methamphetamine, phenylpropranolamine, hydroxyamphetamine, ephedrine, and phenylephrine.

potent central nervous system stimulants than ephedrine, while they have a marked effect on peripheral blood vesicles. The time course of effect for phenylpropranolamine is probably biphasic in nature as it first causes vasoconstriction which is then followed by vasodilation, thus producing first a pressor and then a depressor action on mean blood pressure. To further stress the complexity of this class of drugs, phenylephrine is a direct-acting sympathomimetic drug, but it has very little central action.

It should be clear that this general class of drugs are extremely complex as to the nature of their pharmacological effects in the human body.[16] As with all drugs, they can also produce adverse effects. This toxicity for drugs that act on the cardiovascular and central nervous system can produce a suddenly life-threatening crises, especially for persons that have a predisposition or an undetected vulnerability.

MDA has been a Schedule I drug since the Controlled Substances Act of 1970, while MDMA was put on the controlled substances list in 1985 by the emergency provisions of the 1984 National Narcotics Act. This was a move that caused controversy as there are claims that MDMA has value in psychotherapy and research will be greatly impeded by Schedule I classification. A detailed consideration of MDMA, its pharmacology, and related issues is presented in Chapter 14.

VII. CONCLUSIONS

For the street drug there is no assurance of proper preparation of pure drug and there is no information available on controlled clinical studies of their safety. Furthermore, persons consuming such drugs are probably not adequately aware of the potential risks produced by the pharmacological action to their body. Therefore, the unknown consequences of consumption must truly be considered a hazard to health. The recent report that MDMA may be related to deaths due to heart-related causes must be seriously considered.[17] And the new arrival to the street scene of methylenedioxyethamphetamine or MDEA, alias "Eve", just one more new drug on the street, again demands that we reflect on the nature of our social condition. What are the reasons for the popularity of chemical escape from reality? It cannot be as simplistic an answer as "because it feels good". We must find out why there are among us so many humans for whom it is considered a necessary ingredient to life. Attempts to control the supply of illicit drugs will not solve the problem. In a nation where pharmaceutical sales are in the billion-dollar range, one must conclude that drugs have a prominent position in society, for treatment as well as for recreation/abuse. the lack of general knowledge of the populus concerning the basic concepts of pharmacology is widely prevelant and dangerous. To provide basic education and information on how the body handles a drug and how the drug effects the body will provide a positive step of great import towards informed consent and awareness before drug consumption, thus assuring better medical therapy and perhaps less drug abuse.

REFERENCES

1. **Krantz, J. C., Jr.,** *Historical Medical Classics Involving New Drugs,* Williams & Wilkins, Baltimore, 1974, 121.
2. **LaWall, C. H.,** *Four Thousand Years of Pharmacy,* Lippincott, Philadelphia, 1927, chap. 1.
3. **Ziporyn, T.,** A growing industry and menace: makeshift laboratory's designer drugs, *J. Am. Med. Assoc.,* 256, 3061, 1986.
4. **Rangel, C. B.,** Statement, Designer Drugs, Hearing before the Committee On the Budget, United States Senate, Washington, D.C., July 18, 1985, 6.
5. **Pharmaceutical Manufacturers Association,** Annual Report, Washington, D.C., 1986.
6. **Jaffe, J. H.,** Drug addiction and drug abuse, *The Pharmacological Basis of Therapeutics,* 7th ed., Gilman, A. G., Goodman, L. S., Rall, T. W., and Murad, F., Eds., New York, MacMillan, 1985, chap. 23.
7. **Rapaka, R. S., Barnett, G., and Hawks, R., Eds.,** *Opioid Peptides: Medicinal Chemistry,* National Institute on Drug Abuse, Rockville, Md., 1986.
8. **Barnett, G., Trsic, M., and Willette, R.,** Eds., *QuaSAR: Quantitative Structure Activity Relationships of Analgesics, Narcotic Antagonists, and Hallucinogens,* National Institute on Drug Abuse, Rockville, Md., 1978.
9. **Soine, W. H.,** Clandestine drug synthesis, *Med. Res. Rev.,* 6,41,1986.
10. **Rexed, B., Edmondson, K., Khan, I., and Samsom, R. J., Eds.,** *Guidelines for the Control of Narcotic and Psychotropic Substances* World Health Organization, Geneva, 1984.
11. **Harvey, S. C.,** Hypnotics and Sedatives, in *The Pharmacological Basis of Therapeutics,* 7th ed., Gilman, A. G., Goodman, L. S., Rall, T. W., and Murad, F., Eds., Macmillan, New York, 1985, chap. 17.
12. **Trevor, A. J. and Way, W. L.,** Sedative hypnotics, in *Basic and Clinical Pharmacology,* Katzung, B. G., Ed., Lange Medical Publications, Los Altos, Calif., 1984, chap. 20.
13. **Way, E. L.,** History of opiate use in the Orient and the United States, in "Opioids in Mental Illness: Theories, Clinical Observations, and Treatment Possibilities", Verebey, K., Ed., *Ann. N.Y. Acad. Sci.,* 398, 12, 1982.
14. **Snyder, S. H., and D'Amato, R. J.,** MPTP: a neurotoxin relevant to the pathophysiology of Parkinson's disease, *Neurology,* 36, 250, 1986.
15. **Henderson, G.,** Statement in Designer Drugs, Hearing before the Committee On The Budget, United States Senate, Washington, D.C., July 18, 1985, 22.
16. **Robinson, R. L.,** Sympathomimetic drugs, in *Modern Pharmacology,* Craig, C. R. and Stitzel, R. E., Eds., Little, Brown, Boston, 1982, 23.
17. **Dowling, G. P., McDonough, E. T., III, and Bost, R. O.,** "Eve" and "Ecstasy": a report of five deaths associated with the use of MDEA and MDMA, *J. Am. Med. Assoc.,* 257, 1615, 1987.

Chapter 14

SUBSTITUTED AMPHETAMINE CONTROLLED SUBSTANCE ANALOGUES

David E. Nichols

TABLE OF CONTENTS

I. INTRODUCTION

First and foremost, drug abuse is a social problem rather than a physiological one. It is not entirely clear that any solutions can be found by focusing attention on the drugs themselves, rather than on the societal conditions that lead to drug abuse. Therefore, it seems appropriate to consider some of the broader issues, rather than to deal exclusively with the chemistry or structure-activity relationships of hallucinogenic amphetamine derivatives.

The task is made doubly difficult by this author's belief that although controlled substance analogues of the hallucinogenic amphetamine type possess the potential for nearly unimaginable tragedy, at the same time, research with these substances holds hope for future advances in psychiatric medicine.

On the one hand, if hallucinogenic drugs can be seen as useful substances, they may serve as a potentially rich source of new psychotherapeutic compounds, which could catalyze a revolution in psychiatry and psychotherapy. However, virtually no approved clinical research is being carried out with hallucinogens, and this appears to be a continuing situation in the forseeable future. And, while there may be no clinical research, "recreational" use of hallucinogenic controlled substance analogues continues pretty much unabated.

II. SOCIAL ISSUES

"It is becoming clear that a drug-free Eden, if it ever existed, will never return. The days when youth had no access or interest in the bewildering array of consciousness-transforming drugs will, in all likelihood, not be seen again."[1] For some reason, the notion seems to be developing today that we can somehow achieve a "drug-free society". However, Cohen's opinion seems to be a more realistic assessment of the present state of affairs. As long as psychoactive drugs are available, young people will experiment with them. From 1962 to 1980, the number of 18- to 25-year-olds who had ever tried illicit drugs (other than marijuana) increased more than tenfold, from 3 to 33%. These data at first seem frightening, but are they really meaningful? Is it cause for serious alarm if a majority of young adults have "ever used" some illicit drug? Adolescence is a period of exploratory, risk-taking, sensation-seeking behavior, and in a highly technological society such as ours, chemical exploration now seems to be a part of that world. As Cohen has pointed out, a distinguishing feature of drug abuse is whether or not people go on to use drugs dysfunctionally.

Despite growing concern over drug abuse, any connections between illicit drug use and the social ills attributed to it are hard to prove. An excellent analysis of prospective studies of drug use concluded that, "few unfavorable outcomes of drug use, especially marijuana use, have been identified."[2]

The real issue is this: how can one come of age in America without becoming a casualty of the acute or chronic use of drugs that affect mood, thinking, and sensing in the process? When is a young person capable of making decisions about drugs that can impact on his or her health and future? Obviously, this will never occur unless sufficient accurate information about the drug is acquired. The approach that seems most reasonable is one of education.

As a society, we should believe that when facts are presented in an objective way, and if real dangers exist, that this information will be accepted. However, one should be wary of "crying wolf". For example, during the years of peak LSD use, one report suggested that LSD caused chromosome damage.[3] This research was widely reported by the media. However, we now know that LSD does not have such an effect.[4,5] The danger of genetic damage was disproven, no additional physiological hazards have been demonstrated, and use of this drug continues today.

When misinformation is supplied, this will eventually become evident. If the supplying of misinformation is seen as a "scare tactic" to keep persons away from drug use, the drug-using subculture will tend to ignore any real warnings of a genuine toxicity problem as just another repeat of earlier misinformation. How many young persons heard that smoking marijuana led inevitably to heroin use, only to discover for themselves that this was not the case? The movie *Reefer Madness* was originally produced to illustrate the destructiveness of marijuana, yet is not factual and today is viewed by marijuana users as a comedy. With such a past history of providing "educational" information, how seriously do marijuana-using persons take the warnings that marijuana can suppress the immune system or that marijuana smoke is heavily laden with carcinogenic hydrocarbons?

It is imperative that misinformation about drugs not be propagated. The *less* people know about the effects of recreational drugs, the more dangerous they consider the drugs to be.[6,7] However, the perception of danger is a motivating factor in risk-taking behavior. It is extremely important that when dangers associated with illegal drug use are identified, that the potential users have a complete understanding of the danger so as to avoid misusing those materials. Incredibly, this author has heard individuals who believe that anyone who uses illegal drugs is a societal menace and deserves any consequent health damage that occurs. It would be wise for those persons to consider that there must be millions of individuals who are now in highly responsible positions that at one time or another have experimented with drugs. As a nation, we should feel lucky that these persons did not suffer health damage as a result of their experimentation.

In some ways the recent concern over "designer drugs" parallels the situation that occurred with marijuana. While use of marijuana was confined to blacks and the lower socioeconomic classes in the U.S., it received little notice. It was not until marijuana was widely used by adolescents of the "middle class" during the 1960s that it was perceived to be a "problem". Similarly, although large numbers of opiate addicts suffer injuries related to intravenous administration of street drugs, it took the introduction of highly potent fentanyl analogues, and the resulting increase in overdose deaths, and MPTP-induced Parkinsonian symptoms to focus attention on this problem. Likewise, the popularity of MDMA was seen as a serious problem when college students and young professionals began to use it.

We know that to have the potential for abuse, a drug must have desirable pharmacological properties. Perhaps it is appropriate to discuss what it is about hallucinogenic drugs that makes them so attractive. Hallucinogens are an unusual class of drugs. The drug-induced state can be so like a spontaneous transcendental experience that an overwhelming feeling of significance accompanies it. The experience seems to have a value in its own right, which the nonuser can neither share nor understand.[8] There has been, and will probably continue to be, a good deal of human experimentation with hallucinogenic drugs. If one considers descriptions in the *Rig Veda* of the use of SOMA, there is evidence that these types of substances have been used for at least 4 millenia. It is the overwhelming sense of meaningfulness of the experience that causes these drugs to be rediscovered every few decades and leads people to coalesce around the idea that something of spiritual importance derives from their usage.[1]

Is the solution proscription and prosecution for use? As much as we as a society would like to believe that all the individual's needs can be provided by our system and our way of life, drug abuse is found at all socioeconomic levels.

It seems to be reasonably well documented that humans are particularly curious to experience altered states of consciousness.[9,10]

There are some who argue that this is a relatively recent phenomenon and that drug users "embrace a constellation of attitudes and values that reflect an openness to deviant behavior and nonconformity with respect to social institutions."[11] However, the preponderance of evidence shows that drug abuse exists at every level of the society, and that virtually every society has found ways to alter human consciousness both with and without the use of chemical catalysts.

The conclusion that the occasional need to alter one's state of consciousness is one of man's basic drives seems inescapable.[10] Whether this state be obtained as the result of a formalized religious service, in the form of a "runner's high", through a variety of relaxation or meditative techniques, through the use of alcohol or marijuana, or any of a number of other methods, there is some driving force that leads humans to desire altered states of consciousness. There seem to be two different approaches to this. Some "...commend the sober mind...," with the admonition that with sufficient training, it (the mind) can achieve even that which is inconceivable.[1] The alternate approach seems to be to admit that all humans simply do not have the motivation or dedication to satisfy these needs through some form of mental discipline.

Misinformation and "scare tactics" have not proven to be adequate deterrents to drug abuse. Furthermore, research with hallucinogens suggests that they have therapeutic value.[12-14] Also of importance are the results of an early pilot study with prison inmates, where hallucinogens were employed in *successful* rehabilitation efforts.[8] Rather than using evidence of illicit use or abuse of these drugs to assess their value or therapeutic potential, further formalized and systematic research is needed.

III. HALLUCINOGENIC AMPHETAMINE ANALOGUES

Since most hallucinogenic amphetamine derivatives were synthesized in efforts to understand the mechanism of action and structure-activity relationships of this class, rather than to circumvent the law, this author greatly prefers the term "controlled substance analogues" to the one adopted by the media, "designer drugs". This is especially true in the present case. Even though a few of these compounds have become popular as recreational substances, they were all outgrowths of legitimate research, and were not "designed" in clandestine laboratories by "renegade chemists" in some attempt to thwart the drug laws.

The current problem with the growth and spread of socially unacceptable uses of drugs was anticipated more than 10 years ago by Shulgin,[15] in an article entitled "Drugs of Abuse in the Future". Although most of the discussion in that paper was directed toward potential stimulants and opiate-type drugs, Shulgin noted that the hallucinogenic agents that are the most likely candidates for future abuse are those that are totally synthetic and have a sufficiently simple structure for synthesis. He identified three potential types of compounds: tryptamines and carbolines, phenethylamines, and choline analogues related to atropine and scopolamine. The latter group of compounds are more properly classified as deliriants and have not proven to be popular; hence, the tryptamines and phenethylamines shall be the focus of our present attention.

As it happens, there are relatively few tryptamines with significant biological activity, when compared with the variety of possible phenethylamine derivatives. First, the tryptamines are sensitive to ring substitution, with activity being limited to an unsubstituted indole, a methoxy in the 5-position, or a hydroxy in the 4-position. Other substituents, or other substitution locations, give compounds that lack hallucinogenic activity. Within these constraints, activity seems to lie within a fairly narrow range of amine substitutions, including *N,N*-dimethyl, diethyl, diisopropyl, di-*n*-propyl, or methylisopropyl.[16]

However, perhaps even more important to this issue is the fact that substituted indoles, the required precursors to tryptamines, are generally difficult to synthesize, and require a high level of skill on the part of the chemist. It appears that novel synthetic tryptamines with biological activity that would make them attractive for abuse generally will not be economical to manufacture. These compounds are unlikely to appear as serious drug abuse problems. The carbolines are prepared from tryptamines, so the possibility is even more remote that these will appear as problems.

On the other hand, phenethylamine derivatives are relatively easy to synthesize. Mescaline serves as the prototype of this variety of analogue. Although mescaline is a naturally occurring alkaloid, it possesses relatively low potency. Thus, it is only very rarely that mescaline has been seen on the illicit market, and then only at a high price. It is simply not economical to manufacture mescaline. However, a fairly wide range of structural variation within the phenethylamine class leads to compounds possessing psychoactive properties. Ring substitutions at the 4-, 2,4-, 2,4,6-, 3,4-, 3,4,5-, and 2,4,5-positions can all give rise to active compounds.

Either a two-carbon (''phenethylamine'') or three-carbon (''phenylisopropylamine'') side chain leads to activity. The latter type of structure is referred to as a ''substituted amphetamine hallucinogen''.

For a drug to gain popularity on the illicit market, at least two criteria must be fulfilled. First, and most fundamentally, the drug must have some pharmacological property that is considered desirable to potential users. Second, it must be economical for manufacture by clandestine laboratories. Generally, this means that the compound must have a fairly high potency. One might assume, for example, that if the active dose of mescaline was 10 mg, rather than 300 mg, then mescaline would have become a very popular drug on the illicit market.

Also included in this latter consideration are not only cost, but the ease of obtaining starting materials. Thus, while some phenethylamines can be prepared from commercially available benzaldehydes or benzoic acids, others require a tedious multistep synthesis from some accessible precursor. Whether or not this starting material has a low cost, unless the final compound is extremely potent, substances that require complicated synthetic schemes are unlikely to attract the attention of clandestine laboratories.

As a result of research over the past 20 years, a great deal is known about which compounds have desirable properties, which are easy to synthesize, and which ones could likely prove to be problems in the future. It is fortunate that the structure-activity relationships are fairly restrictive, as contrasted, for example, with drugs that have opiate-type activity.

IV. TOXICITY

The typical hallucinogens have rarely caused death. Lethal overdoses of LSD and mescaline and chronic organ toxicity are unknown. When death does occur, it is most often accidental and usually associated with the drug-induced mental aberrations, (see for example Reference 18). Suicides have occurred during the postdrug state when depression or fear of remaining psychotic may occur. Very few homicides have been reported.[1]

Adverse reactions to typical hallucinogens usually are treated by support, reassurance, and a quiet environment in the company of family or hospital staff members. However, most hallucinogenic experiences never receive medical attention.

In contrast to the opiate-type drugs, which produce genuine physical dependence and addiction, hallucinogens do not have this capability. Whereas chronic use of opiates produces a pharmacological "need" for the drug, hallucinogens are typically not used on a chronic basis, since repeated use leads to rapid development of tolerance and reduced drug effect.

The National Commission on Marijuana and Drug Abuse[19] suggested that drug use can be divided into five classes. Experimental use is defined as trying a drug once or twice to find out what it is like. Recreational-social use is the pattern of ordinary social drinkers or marijuana users, and also that of many nonaddicted heroin users. Situational use is use for special but nonmedical purposes. This would include the use of stimulants for work or study, tranquilizers for public speaking, and psychedelic drugs for religious or personal insight. Most people are probably capable of using these types of drugs only in these ways, which produce relatively little harm. The other two categories, intensive use and compulsive use, cause most of the "drug problem",[20] yet are rarely associated with use of hallucinogenic drugs.

The difference between usage patterns of opiates and hallucinogens has another practical consequence. One can imagine that toxicological problems will be more readily apparent with opiates, stimulants, or other drugs that are typically used on a frequent or chronic basis. For example, if a particular opiate analogue has some subtle toxicological property, this effect is more likely to become manifest, or amplified, in a population of drug users who administer that drug on a continuing, chronic basis.

It needs to be kept in mind that it is not just "designer drugs" that are the problem. Rather, it is simply the fact that users of illicit drugs obtain "street drugs". Such clandestinely manufactured materials typically are not pure and contain a variety of impurities that may in themselves be toxic. The recent tragedy with an MPTP-contaminated meperidine analogue would not have occurred had the drug been purified and freed of the MPTP contaminant. So the problem is not just with controlled substance analogues, but is a more general hazard associated with street drug use.

There are two types of toxicity that can be expected with hallucinogenic amphetamine analogues, or with any drug for that matter. The first is acute toxicity. With opiate analogues, the most serious form of acute toxicity would be death due to severe respiratory depression. Alone in this situation, an individual would become a casualty. However, hallucinogenic amphetamine overdose would not typically lead to rapid death. First, this type of substance, while it can be administered intravenously like the opiates, is more often taken orally. The pharmacokinetics of oral administration allow more time for medical intervention if it is apparent that an overdose has been taken. Hallucinogenic amphetamines do not cause respiratory depression, and do not typically lead to loss of consciousness.

The two analogues of this class that have caused the most deaths are paramethoxyamphetamine (PMA)[21] and 3,4-methylenedioxyamphetamine (MDA).[22] The toxic manifestations reported in overdose with these drugs include restlessness, agitation, sweating, rigidity, convulsions, high blood pressure, tachycardia, and extreme hyperpyrexia, all suggestive of excessive CNS stimulation. With these obvious symptoms the overdose victim or his companions are more likely to recognize that a problem exists and have more time to seek medical assistance than in an opiate overdose. Although there is presently no antidote recognized for poisoning with these agents, Davis et al.[23] have shown chlorpromazine to be effective against a lethal dose of MDA in dogs.

Vascular spasm has been associated with excessively high doses of the hallucinogenic amphetamine 2,5-dimethoxy-4-bromoamphetamine (DOB). One case report describes effects of a dose of 75 mg of DOB that led to severe peripheral vascular spasm which was apparently improperly treated and eventually resulted in bilateral above-the-knee amputations.[24] Appropriate medical intervention can prevent such severe consequences.[25] Of course, a 75-mg dose of DOB must be considered massive, since the psychoactive effects of this drug can be detected in the submilligram range. Death due to DOB overdose has also been reported.[26]

The second type of toxicity that can occur is chronic. This is a toxicity that would be manifest over a long period of use. There are no toxicological studies with hallucinogenic amphetamines that would suggest what form such toxicity might take, since most hallucinogenic amphetamines are not used over long periods of time, or on a chronic or daily basis. Therefore, these concerns have not been addressed in the scientific literature.

Yet the dangers of hallucinogenic amphetamine use are real and present. Consider the consequences of the following scenario. A new drug hits the illicit market in large quantities. Its chemical structure is very simple and the starting material is present in most chemistry laboratories. One can envision widespread usage of the drug and, probably, a sort of cottage industry that would develop to manufacture the drug locally by persons with relatively little chemical expertise. Thus, not only would the drug proliferate, but much of the available drug would be impure or might not be the advertised drug at all. Suppose further that the drug or a common contaminant had a toxic effect that was not immediately evident, but was only manifest much later. It might be a neurotoxic action, for example, suggested as a possibility for MDA[27] or MDMA,[28] or it perhaps might be a carcinogenic agent. In any event, large numbers, perhaps millions, of persons might have experimented with the drug before the toxic effect was observed. This would be a tragedy of a magnitude never previously encountered. This possibility should generate sufficient concern to force a serious search for ways to forestall such an occurrence.

To quote a statement made in 1978, "We cannot afford to wait until an enterprising illicit drug manufacturer successfully markets some new drug, one which might receive enthusiastic public acceptance. We need to be prepared to recognize the symptoms which might be seen in acute intoxication involving such a new drug."[29]

Certain means have been suggested to remedy this situation.[29] First of all, ethical considerations should be reexamined with respect to psychoactive drug studies. It has also been suggested that a set of human research standards be developed for the study of drugs in acute trials, with specific focus on the mind-altering properties of these drugs. Clearly, the ethics of self-experimentation and informed consent need to be readdressed for such studies. In other words, the issues that presently discourage clinical studies with hallucinogenic drugs should be reexamined.

V. MDMA

I have so far only alluded to the substance MDMA, also known as Ecstasy, which became popular in the past few years as a recreational substance. While hallucinogenic amphetamines have been used for many years, it was the sudden popularity of 3,4-methylenedioxy-methamphetamine, MDMA, that brought to a focus concerns about controlled substance analogues of the hallucinogenic amphetamine type.

MDMA was patented in 1914, but was never marketed. In the 1970s it was rediscovered to be a mild psychoactive agent, which did not produce the striking changes in mental states that are characteristic of powerful hallucinogenic agents such as LSD or mescaline.[29] Sometime subsequent to this, MDMA was employed by a number of therapists as an adjunct to psychotherapy. George Greer,[30] a psychiatrist practicing in New Mexico, privately published a report of 29 case studies where he concluded that MDMA was beneficial to his patients.

In contrast, a study by Ricaurte et al.,[29] found that MDA, a structurally related compound, produced serotonin nerve terminal degeneration in rat brain. When MDMA was openly sold, and flagrantly advertised as "a legal drug", it was inevitable that government action had to be taken. With the power that Congress had recently granted to the Drug Enforcement Agency (DEA) to curb the tide of new, controlled substance analogues, the study by Ricaurte et al. was presented as evidence for the dangers of MDMA use, and the DEA invoked its emergency scheduling powers to place MDMA into Schedule I of the Controlled Substances Act of 1970.

Interestingly, although MDMA is chemically related to the hallucinogenic amphetamines, it is not itself hallucinogenic.[29,31]   In rats, MDMA has pharmacological properties similar to both amphetamine and to hallucinogens. However, in man it has a psychoactive effect that seems distinct from other known classes of compounds. It has been suggested that MDMA, and substances with a similar pharmacology, are representatives of a completely new pharmacologic class that has been named "entactogens".[32] One of the more powerful arguments for this new classification is the fact that it is the (+)-isomer of MDMA that is more biologically potent, while it is the (−)-isomer of the hallucinogenic amphetamine analogues that is more active.

It is not clear whether many other MDMA-like compounds will appear on the illicit market. At present, it appears that the 3,4-methylenedioxy aromatic ring substituent is required for MDMA-like pharmacology. In addition to the *N*-methyl derivative, MDMA, the *N*-ethyl derivative MDE has been available on the illicit market. Only one additional compound is presently known with an MDMA-like effect. This is the homologue where the alpha-methyl in the side chain of MDMA has been replaced with an alpha-ethyl. It is somewhat less potent in humans than MDMA.[32]

The acute toxicity of MDMA would appear to be low. However, a major concern developed after publication of the study by Ricaurte et al.,[27] where administration of the chemically related compound MDA to rats caused serotonin nerve terminal degeneration. It is not known if this toxicity occurs in man, or if it does, what the consequences are. This issue will probably have to be resolved before extensive clinical research to study the therapeutic potential of MDMA can be approved.

VI. RESEARCH CONCERNS

There are no convincing arguments that it is a good idea to categorize hallucinogenic drug analogues with addictive or acutely toxic substances such as heroin or fentanyl analogues. While there are real dangers, there is no evidence that they are of the same magnitude as those associated with abuse of opiates, cocaine and other stimulants, or sedative-hypnotics (all of which are dwarfed, of course, by the public health costs of alcohol and tobacco use.) Indeed, Nicholi[11] did not even treat the subject of hallucinogens when he considered the problem of nontherapeutic use of psychoactive drugs.

It is quite possible to develop psychoactive chemicals that could be safely used in a recreational context. Whether or not our society would accept the use of such substances is quite another matter. Certainly no drugs can be viewed as either "good" or "evil" in and of themselves; it is the context of drug use that must be viewed as positive or negative. Huxley, in his article "Criteria for a Socially Sanctionable Drug",[10] has even discussed what pharmacological properties a drug must have that would allow it to be socially acceptable.

However, even though the evidence from many cultures suggests that humans need to experience altered states of awareness, the notion that drugs can or should be used by "well" people seems repugnant to our society. Nevertheless, enforcement has not succeeded in controlling recreational use of hallucinogens. Therefore, it is not clear how increased penalties for the use of hallucinogens will abolish the human desire to experiment with these drugs.

Indeed, it seems axiomatic that making a substance illegal, and prohibiting its use, can actually encourage its use, engendering a sort of adventurism.

In the attempts to control the black market use of hallucinogenic drugs, a massive "overkill" in legislation has occurred. While the drugs are still widely available on the street, clinical investigators face a formidable array of paperwork and approvals to obtain them, one result being a disincentive to carry out research on hallucinogens. Although some readers may violently disagree with this supposition, a quote from a paper written by Szara, in 1967,[33] is still relevant:

> "Finally, there is a situation I feel compelled to comment upon. I am referring to the nonmedical use or abuse of hallucinogenic drugs. There is an obvious need for regulating the use of these powerful and potentially dangerous agents. However, we should not throw the baby out with the bath water. The recent run of unfavorable publicity in newspapers and national magazines has forced the Sandoz Company to stop manufacturing LSD in the United States, and the company has turned over its LSD supply to the NIMH as of April 15, 1966.
>
> This publicity pressure threatens serious scientific research not only with LSD but with the entire class of hallucinogenic drugs. We cannot put blame on the drugs; we can only put blame on the manner and the ways they are being used. It is my belief that it would be most unfortunate if we were to permit undue hysteria to destroy a valuable tool of science and evaporate an eventual hope for the many hopeless."

What now exists is a situation where there is a real need for research with psychedelic and hallucinogenic substances, but society and its regulatory agencies refuse to permit clinical research to occur. Instead, one finds self-experimentation, with results that are unpublished and unavailable to the scientific community, with reports of drug effects that are anecdotal, anonymous, and completely unreliable. When a drug such as MDMA surfaces and gains popularity, it merely strengthens the resolve of enforcement agencies to proscribe any use, under any circumstances, of these compounds. This situation may be justified with opiate analogues, since nonmedical use of these substances does not constitute "research" and is rarely experimentation. These drugs have their representatives in the armamentarium of clinical medicine. The same can be said of CNS stimulants, which are widely abused, but which are also pharmacologically well-defined. It is only with hallucinogens that the situation seems unique. At present, no clinical counterpart exists, and no research is occurring to study them further.

While governmental agencies proclaim their desire to see more clinical research done, there is no suitable protocol for study of these drugs. Without widely recognized medical benefit, the benefit/risk ratios are perceived to be infinitesimally small. Without a significant benefit/risk ratio, no studies will be allowed. Even when an acceptable benefit can be demonstrated, the regulations are so cumbersome that they restrict research. I recall the story related by Dr. George Greer, concerning a patient of his in his 70s who had crushed vertebra secondary to multiple myeloma and was in severe chronic pain. Prior to the scheduling of MDMA, the only treatment that had given this patient significant and long-lasting relief was MDMA-assisted therapy. After MDMA was placed into Schedule I, Greer attempted to obtain a compassionate Investigational Exemption for a New Drug (IND) for this patient, in order to conduct another MDMA session. In spite of the fact that MDMA had been used recreationally on a widespread basis with no known significant adverse health consequences, and in spite of the continuing chronic pain of this patient, his age and terminal prognosis, approval of Greer's IND was postponed for lack of sufficient preclinical animal data. Apparently, informed consent of the patient to utilize this experimental treatment was of no consequence. The patient has subsequently died, in pain, with his physician powerless to relieve his suffering.

It would seem that the use of hallucinogens or related psychoactive drugs to facilitate psychotherapy is just as valid a technique as any of the approximately 400 other forms of therapy that are currently available, none of which is superior to the others.[34] As long as the patient is properly informed as to the nature of the drug effect and possible adverse psychological consequences, his desire to use these treatments should be respected. The wishes of the terminal patient referred to above, who was in severe chronic pain, were ignored by the procedures that currently govern clinical drug studies.

Most classes of drugs are developed to be used daily, over a long period of time. By contrast, research with hallucinogens suggests that, if they found a place in medicine, they would be used intermittently and infrequently, as therapeutic catalysts to bring about some psychological transformation. Protocols for Phase I studies are not designed for drugs that are to be used episodically in this way.

Because of disincentives for research, scientists and clinicians who began research with LSD were unable to complete their efforts. Although feeling that they had gained an initial understanding of how to use LSD in a proper therapeutic context, so as to derive maximum benefit for their patients, clinical research with LSD, for all practical purposes, is now completely dead. Why? Because Schedule I classification is very restrictive, making it difficult even for medical treatment of the terminally ill. One hears time and again from regulatory officials how Schedule I classification is no impediment to research; yet if this is so, where is the clinical research with LSD today? The facts speak for themselves.

One hears the standard retorts that LSD was proven dangerous, or had no value, or was too tricky to use. There are many clinical reports to the contrary.[12-14] Like any new technology, it takes time to learn what can and cannot be done, and how to most effectively use new tools. Psychotherapeutic approaches using hallucinogens were just being developed when scheduling occurred and researchers pulled out of the field. However, LSD was found to be safe when used under appropriate clinical conditions[35] and is probably one of the safest drugs known in terms of physiological toxicity. Nonetheless, there seems to be minimal interest on the part of government agencies to fund this sort of research, and clinical scientists are either afraid of the controversy that continues to surround LSD, or are unsure how to go about getting approval and funding to work with it. As a result, there is a whole new generation of uninformed clinical scientists who have dismissed any possible therapeutic value of LSD.

This author has commented extensively on the need for discovery of new types of psychoactive drugs, many of which, like MDMA, might arise from research with hallucinogenic amphetamine analogues.[36] Presently, regulations on clinical studies appear likely to thwart the discovery of such novel mind-altering substances. Unless there is a change in philosophy, psychiatric practice will remain limited by the *types* of psychoactive drugs which are now in use.

In order to assess properly both the potential for abuse and the therapeutic value of hallucinogens, research must be allowed, indeed, must be encouraged. It is *only through education*, armed with factual research results, that we can hope to control the use of hallucinogenic drugs. In our haste to control these substances, it is to be hoped that we will not, again, "throw the baby out with the bath water."

REFERENCES

1. **Cohen, S.**, *The Substance Abuse Problems*, Vol. 2, Haworth Press, New York, 1985.
2. **Kandel, D. B.**, Convergences in prospective longitudinal surveys on drug use, *Longitudinal Research on Drug Use*, Kandel, D. B., Ed., John Wiley & Sons, New York, 1978.

3. **Cohen, M. M., Marinello, M. J., and Back, M.,** Chromosomal damage in human leukocytes induced by lysergic acid diethylamide, *Science,* 155, 1417, 1967.

4. **Dishotsky, N. I., Loughman, W. D., Mogar, R. E., and Lipscomb, W.R.,** LSD and genetic damage, *Science,* 172, 431, 1971.

5. **Long, S. Y.,** Does LSD induce chromosomal damage and malformations? A review of the literature, *Teratology,* 6, 75, 1972.

6. **Glaser, D. and Snow, M.,** Public Knowledge and Attitudes on Drug Abuse, New York State Addiction Control Commission, New York, 1969.

7. **Swisher, J. D.,** Drug education: pushing or preventing? *Peabody J. Educ.,* p. 68, 1971.

8. **Clark, W. H.,** Ethics and LSD, *J. Psychoact. Drugs,* 17, 229, 1985.

9. **Weil, A.,** *The Natural Mind,* Houghton Mifflin, Boston, 1972.

10. **Huxley, M.,** Criteria for a socially sanctionable drug, *Interdiscip. Sci. Rev.,* 1, 176, 1977.

11. **Nicholi, A. M., Jr.,** The nontherapeutic use of psychoactive drugs. A modern epidemic, *N. Engl. J. Med.,* 308, 925, 1985.

12. **Pahnke, W. N., Kurland, A.A., Unger, S., Savage, C., and Grof, S.,** The experimental use of psychedelic (LSD) psychotherapy, *J. Am. Med. Assoc.,* 212, 1856, 1970.

13. **Grof, S.,** *LSD Psychotherapy,* Hunter House, Pomona, Calif., 1980.

14. **Brandrup, E. and Vanggaard, T.,** LSD treatment in a severe case of compulsive neurosis, *Acta Psychiatr. Scand.,* 55, 127, 1977.

15. **Shulgin, A. T.,** Drugs of abuse in the future, *Clin. Toxicol.,* 8, 405, 1975.

16. **Repke, D. B., Grotjahn, D. B., and Shulgin, A. T.,** Psychotomimetic *N*-methyl-*N*-isopropyltryptamines. Effects of variation of aromatic oxygen substituents, *J. Med. Chem.,* 28, 892, 1985.

17. **Nichols, D. E. and Glennon, R. A.,** Medicinal chemistry and structure-activity relationships of hallucinogens, *Hallucinogens: Neurochemical, Behavioral, and Clinical Perspectives,* Jacobs, B. L., Ed., Raven Press, New York, 1984, 95.

18. **Reynolds, P. C. and Jindrich, E. J.,** A mescaline associated fatality, *J. Anal. Toxicol.,* 9, 183, 1985.

19. National Commission on Marijuana and Drug Abuse, Drug Use in America: Problem in Perspective, U.S. Government Printing Office, Washington, D. C., 1973.

20. **Bakalar, J. B. and Grinspoon, L.,** *Drug Control in a Free Society,* Cambridge University, Press, New York, 1984.

21. **Cimbura, G.,** PMA deaths in Ontario, *Can. Med. Assoc. J.,* 110, 1263, 1974.

22. **Cimbura, G.,** 3,4-Methylenedioxyamphetamine (MDA). Analytical and forensic aspects of fatal poisoning, *J. Forensic Sci.,* 17, 329, 1972.

23. **Davis, W. M., Catravas, J. D., and Waters, I. W.,** Effects of an i.v. lethal dose of 3,4-methylenedioxyamphetamine (MDA) in the dog and antagonism of chlorpromazine, *Gen. Pharmacol.,* 17, 179, 1986.

24. **Eichorn, G.,** DOB—on the street, *San Francisco Bay Area Reg. Poison Cent. Newsl.,* 3, 3, 1981.

25. **Bowen, J. S.,** Davis, G. B., Kearney, T. E., and Bardin, J., Diffuse vascular spasm associated with 4-bromo-2,5-dimethoxyamphetamine ingestion, *J. Am. Med. Assoc.,* 249, 1477, 1983.

26. **Winek, C. L., Collom, W. D., and Bricker, J. D.,** A death due to 4-bromo-2,5-dimethoxyamphetamine, *Clin. Toxicol.,* 18, 261, 1981.

27. **Ricaurte, G., Bryan, G., Strauss, L., Seiden, L., and Schuster, C.,** Hallucinogenic amphetamine selectively destroys brain serotonin nerve terminals, *Science,* 222, 986, 1985.

28. **Schmidt, C. J., Wu, L., and Lovenberg, W.,** Methylenedioxymethamphetamine: a potentially neurotoxic amphetamine analog, *Eur. J. Pharmacol.,* 124, 175, 1986.

29. **Shulgin, A. T. and Nichols, D. E.,** Characterization of three new psychotomimetics, *The Psychopharmacology of Hallucinogens,* Stillman, R. C. and Willette, R. E., Eds., Pergamon Press, New York, 1978, 74.

30. **Greer, G.,** MDMA: a new psychotropic compound and its effects in humans, Copyright by George Greer, 333 Rosario Hill, Santa Fe, N.M. 87501.

31. **Anderson, G. M., III, Braun, G., Braun, U., Nichols, D. E., and Shulgin, A. T.,** *Absolute Configuration and Psychotomimetic Activity,* NIDA Res. Monogr. No. 22, National Institute on Drug Abuse, Rockville, Md., 1978.

32. **Nichols, D. E., Hoffman, A. J., Oberlender, R. A., Jacob, P., III, and Shulgin, A. T.,** Derivatives of 1-(1,3-benzodioxo-5-yl)-2-butanamine. Representatives of a novel therapeutic class, *J. Med. Chem.,* 29, 2009, 1986.

33. **Szara, S.,** Hallucinogenic drugs—curse or blessings?, *Am. J. Psychiatry,* 123, 1513, 1967.

34. **Karasu, T. B.,** The specificity versus nonspecificity dilemma: toward identifying therapeutic change agents, *Am. J. Psychiatry* 143, 687, 1986.

35. **Strassman, R.,** Adverse reactions to psychedelic drugs, *J. Nerv. Ment. Dis.,* 172, 577, 1984.

36. **Nichols, D. E.,** The discovery of novel psychoactive drugs: has it ended? *J. Psychoact. Drugs,* 1986, in press.

Chapter 15

PHARMACOLOGY AND TOXICOLOGY OF MPTP: A NEUROTOXIC BY-PRODUCT OF ILLICIT DESIGNER DRUG CHEMISTRY

Anthony Trevor, Neal Castagnoli, Jr., and Thomas P. Singer

TABLE OF CONTENTS

I. INTRODUCTION

The identification of MPTP (1-methyl, 4-phenyl, 1,2,3,6-tetrahydropyridine, I) as the cause of a parkinsonian syndrome in man, very similar in its neuropathological profile to idiopathic Parkinson's disease, has provoked an extraordinarily intense research effort directed towards understanding the chemistry, pharmacology, and toxicology of this molecule. There are many reasons for this interest, perhaps foremost being the possibility that elucidation of the molecular mechanisms involved in the selective neurotoxic actions of MPTP on nigrostriatal dopaminergic neurons may provide clues to the presently obscure etiology of a disease that afflicts a significant proportion of our mature population. Certainly, an understanding of the cause(s) of the naturally-occurring disease offers opportunities for the institution of possible preventive measures and for the development of therapeutic agents more effective than those currently available. A prominent theme underlying research interest in MPTP, in this regard, is that of the possibility of an environmental etiology for Parkinsonism, since pyridine-containing compounds structurally related to MPTP are abundant in the environment.

MPTP is clearly of great interest to researchers in the drug abuse field. The devastating neurotoxic effects of MPTP provide a painful but graphic illustration of the dangers inherent to clandestine "designer drug" chemistry. An account of the identification of MPTP as a nigrostriatal toxin has all the elements of a detective story by P.D. James. The compound is first mentioned in the scientific literature in the 1950s when it was tested for analgesic activity and, believe it or not, for possible "antiparkinson" effects, both with negative results. In 1977, a young drug abuser living in Bethesda was hospitalized and ultimately diagnosed as suffering from a parkinsonian syndrome, responsive to L-dopa. Researchers at the National Institute of Mental Health (NIMH)[1] established that he had illicitly synthesized a meperidine congener, MPPP (1-methyl-4-propionoxy-4-phenylpyridine, II) for his own intravenous use and, by the application of mass spectrometric analytical methods, were able to detect traces of this compound, the precursor chemicals used and MPTP in the glassware that he had used for his chemistry "homework". These compounds were prepared and tested in laboratory rats, mixtures of MPPP and MPTP causing profound catatonia acutely, but failing to produce chronic neurotoxic effects. We now appreciate that the rat is remarkably resistant to the neurotoxic effects of MPTP. The choice of this species for assessing the potential toxicity of MPTP was unfortunate, since it discouraged further laboratory investigations on the neurotoxin by the NIMH researchers for some time. The young man who had inadvertently initiated this chain of inquiry subsequently died from a drug overdose and an autopsy revealed substantial cell loss in the substantia nigra, similar to that which occurs in idiopathic Parkinson's disease. A major "clue" pointing to an association between MPTP and Parkinsonism was revealed in 1982 by investigators in California.[2] Four young drug abusers were identified who had developed parkinsonian symptoms after intravenous use of an illicit "street heroin". Analysis of available drug samples led to the identification of both MPPP and MPTP, with higher amounts of the former compound in samples used by the patients that were less severely afflicted. Interestingly, during the course of their investigations the California researchers discovered that the original scientific report of synthesis of MPPP had been very neatly excised from a journal in the Lane Library of the Stanford University Medical School! The local "entrepreneur" involved in the illicit synthesis of MPPP appears to have been a poor chemist, since MPTP represents a side product formed through inadequate control of temperature and/or acidity of the reaction (see Figure 1). The scientific detective work pursued by two groups of investigators, 3000 mi apart, both implicated MPTP as the likely causative agent of the parkinsonian symptoms observed in these young drug abusers. The direct proof of the neurotoxicity of MPTP came from administration of the compound to the rhesus monkey, a sensitive species, which resulted in a parkinsonian

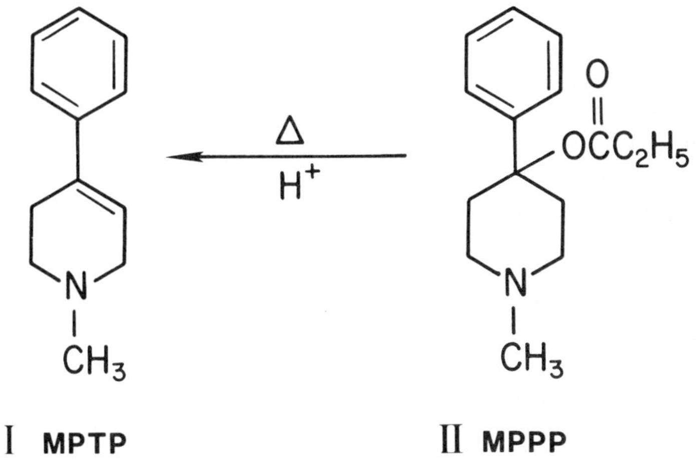

I MPTP   II MPPP

FIGURE 1.   Formation of MPTP as a side product in the synthesis of MPPP.

syndrome similar to that seen in humans and in the destruction of dopamine-containing neurones in the substantia nigra.[3]

These important studies, demonstrating the involvement of MPTP in an irreversible, drug-induced Parkinsonism, provided the impetus for the initiation of studies on the neurotoxin in many laboratories. Numerous research publications have since appeared describing the pharmacological and toxicological effects of MPTP in various animal species.

The initial interest of our laboratories in MPTP originated from considerations of its molecular structure, which give no immediate indications of its potential chemical reactivity and which give no clues as to why its cytotoxic actions should be selective for dopamine-containing nigrostriatal neurons. However, based on our previous investigations on the oxidative metabolism of psychoactive tertiary amines, including nicotine and phencyclidine, it appeared possible that MPTP migh be bioactivated in vivo to unleash its potential for neurotoxicity via the formation of reactive metabolites. As will be described below, our attempts to substantiate this working hypothesis led to the identification of a bioactivation pathway for MPTP involving monoamine oxidase B (MAO B) that appears to be obligatory in the processes leading to expression of its neurotoxic actions.

In this chapter the primary focus is on mechanistic aspects of the neurotoxicology of MPTP. The effects of MPTP on various animal species and its actions on isolated cells and cell organelles of neuronal and nonneuronal origin that appear to be relevant to elucidating its mechanism of action will be discussed. Particular emphasis will be placed on the metabolism of MPTP, its bioactivation mediated by MAO, and the possible role of its metabolites in the molecular events leading to its neurotoxic actions. Finally, consideration will be given to the known and potential neurotoxic effects of MPTP congeners and other structurally related compounds. Research investigations on the neurotoxin prior to July 1985 are described at some length in a recent monograph.[4]

II. PHARMACOLOGICAL EFFECTS OF MPTP IN VIVO

Acute behavioral effects of MPTP have been observed in most animal species studied, including subhuman primates, canines, and rodents, often accompanied by changes in the levels of brain amines (DA, NE, 5HT) and their metabolites. While certain of these biochemical changes may presage the subsequent neurotoxic effects seen with chronic exposure to MPTP, they have not proved to be of predictive value in this regard. When administered to subhuman primates in regimens that result in cumulative doses of between approximately

1 to 10 mg/kg, depending on the particular species, MPTP causes classical signs of Parkinsonism reaching their maximum expression between 10 and 14 days.[3,5,6] In such animals MPTP appears to cause highly selective damage to neurons in the substantia nigra with marked depletion of DA levels,[3,7-9] but other neurons may also be vulnerable including those in the ventral tegmentum and locus ceruleus.[10,11] Chronic exposure of nonprimate species to MPTP leads to nigrostriatal cell loss in the beagle,[12] the cat,[13] and the mouse,[14,15] but these species do not appear to develop a permanent Parkinsonism. For example, the mouse (particularly the C57 Black strain) is the most sensitive of the rodent species to MPTP, but there is slow recovery of the initial dramatic depletion of striatal DA,[10,16] and the observed motor deficits are only temporary. Note also, that while the C57 Black mouse is more responsive to MPTP than other rodents, the cumulative dose required is approximately one order of magnitude more than that required to elicit neurotoxic effects in primates. While it may not be a species immune to the effects of MPTP, the rat is certainly very resistant as judged by criteria of striatal DA depletion, nigrostriatal cell loss, and motor dysfunction,[17-19] In considering which laboratory animal species is most appropriate for characterizing the neurotoxic actions of MPTP, primates appear to be the only species where neuropathological and behavioral effects parallel those observed in humans. Practical and humanistic concerns limit the use of monkeys in MPTP research and, with some reservation, the mouse has become accepted by many investigators as a useful experimental model for in vivo studies. Regard must be given to variations in responsiveness to MPTP in the mouse, due to factors including dosage regimen, route of administration, strain and source of the animals,[20] and age, since older animals appear to be more sensitive to the neurotoxin.[21] The rat, while of limited value for most in vivo studies, may prove to be useful for the study of possible mechanisms involved in protection or resistance to the neurotoxin.

III. METABOLISM AND BIODISPOSITION OF MPTP

Considerations of the chemical structure of MPTP give little indication that the molecule itself has cytotoxic potential, but do raise the possibility of its metabolic activation to form more chemically reactive products, possibly by mechanisms that have been described for other psychoactive cyclic tertiary amines including nicotine and phencyclidine.[22-23] These compounds undergo cytochrome P-450-catalyzed oxidations at carbon atoms alpha to their nitrogen atoms to form reactive electrophilic iminium species which appear to be involved in covalent interactions with tissue macromolecules. By analogy, allylic carbon oxidation of MPTP alpha to the nitrogen atom would be expected to generate the compound $MPDP^+$ (1-methyl-4-phenyl-2,3-dihydropyridine, III; see Figure 2), a potentially reactive and toxic species. Initial attempts to demonstrate this metabolic pathway using rabbit liver microsomes were not successful. However, in vitro metabolic studies with MPTP and mitochondrial preparations[24] led to the recognition that the neurotoxin undergoes rapid oxidation, and that its metabolism was inhibited by inhibitors of MAO B. From NMR and mass spectral data, the structure of a principal mitochondrial metabolite of MPTP was shown to be the species MPP^+ (1-methyl-4-phenylpyridine, IV), the same compound that has been isolated from nigrostriatal structures of monkeys suffering from MPTP-induced Parkinsonism.[9,25] Using brain mitochondrial preparations, this pathway of oxidative metabolism of MPTP was shown to involve alpha carbon oxidation leading initially to the formation of the two-electron oxidation product $MPDP^+$, identified by mass spectral and diode array analytical methods and confirmed by synthesis of the compound and by trapping with cyanide anion as its alpha cyano tetrahydropyridine adduct.[24,26]

The 2,3-dihydropyridine intermediate (III) was shown to undergo disproportionation to form MPTP and MPP^+.[27] This chemical reaction, in addition to generating MPP^+, a major brain metabolite of the neurotoxin, suggested the possibility of involvement of $MPDP^+$ in

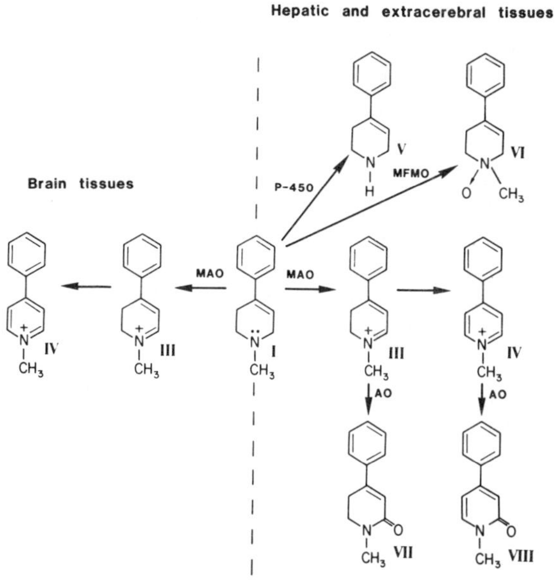

FIGURE 2. Metabolic pathways of MPTP.

redox reactions that could lead to the formation of neurotoxic products. Our proposal that brain MAO B was involved in the bioactivation of MPTP[24] was subsequently confirmed in cultured neurons where MAO inhibitors blocked the toxic effects of the compound[28] and by in vivo studies demonstrating that the prior administration of MAO B inhibitors protected animals against the neurotoxic effects of MPTP.[7,29,30] Is is now generally accepted that the initial two-electron oxidation of MPTP by brain MAO B, resulting in the formation of MPDP$^+$, is a critical step in the biochemical processes leading to the selective cytotoxicity of the neurotoxin.

While microsomal cytochrome P-450 enzymes do not appear to metabolize MPTP to MPDP$^+$, rodent hepatic microsomal preparations catalyze its NADPH-dependent metabolism to form 4-phenyl-1,2,3,6-tetrahydropyridine (V) and 1-methyl-4-phenyl-1,2,3,6-tetrahydro-pyridine-N-oxide (VI). Formation of the N- demethylated metabolite V is dependent on cytochrome P-450[31] and the N-oxide VI on flavin monooxygenase,[32] and such oxidations may represent routes for detoxification of MPTP. Lactam and pyridone metabolites (e.g., VII and VIII) have also been detected in incubations of mouse liver with MPTP.[33] Their formation is possibly the result of MAO-catalyzed alpha carbon oxidation that also leads to the formation of MPDP$^+$ and MPP$^+$ in rodent liver mitochondrial preparations,[31] followed by oxidation of these metabolites by soluble aldehyde oxidases. A scheme of the pathways for oxidative metabolism of MPTP by enzymes present in brain and in peripheral tissues, particularly the liver, is shown in Figure 2. It is not known if the metabolites V and VI, or other products from alpha carbon oxidation of MPTP, such as lactams, are formed in brain tissues. This is of interest because regional differences in the metabolic fate of MPTP could be a factor determining its selective cytotoxicity.

Concerning the in vivo biodisposition of MPTP, there is no evidence that the variable sensitivities of animal species to the neurotoxin are due to quantitative differences in the rate of its peripheral metabolism or to differences in the ability of MPTP to cross the blood-brain barrier.[25,34] These studies, using radiolabeled MPTP, showed that the compound enters the brain of all species very rapidly, as should be the case, given its high lipophilicity. Species differences were noted, however, in the time course of retention of radioactivity in the brain (presumably due to metabolites including MPP$^+$), with prolonged retention a characteristic feature of primates compared to rodents. In the brain of the rhesus monkey, radioactivity was selectively localized in the caudate, putamen, and nucleus accumbens and also the locus ceruleus, a brain area rich in NE-containing cell bodies.[25] In the squirrel monkey, MPP^+ has been reported to be selectively accumulated in the substantia nigra,[35] the pars compacta of which contains DA cell bodies, rather than in dopaminergic cell terminal areas of the brain. The reasons for selective localization and retention of the metabolites of MPTP in specific regions of the primate brain are not fully established. Possible explanations include (1) regional variations in the rates of MPTP-oxidizing activity catalyzed by MAO and perhaps other enzymes yet to be identified, (2) binding of the metabolites of MPTP to macromolecular components located specifically in distinct cell populations, and (3) the active accumulation of MPTP, or its metabolites, by specific cells or cell organelles.

Direct proof for the involvement of MAO forms in the metabolic activation of MPTP has been obtained from experiments with purified A and B forms of the enzyme.[36-38] The determination of true initial oxidation rates revealed that the turnover number of MAO B with MPTP as substrate was approximately 200, compared with 530 for benzylamine, the most rapidly oxidized substrate for the enzyme in steady-state assays. This was a surprisingly rapid oxidation rate, given that tertiary amines were not hitherto considered to be effective substrates for MAO. The K_m value for MPTP in this reaction was 0.30 mM, lower than that for benzylamine (0.38 mM). With purified MAO A, turnover numbers of MPTP and kynuramine, a preferred substrate for this form of the enzyme, were 14 and 200, respectively. The two-electron oxidation product formed during the MAO-catalyzed metabolism of MPTP, $MPDP^+$, was also found to be a substrate for MAO B, with a turnover number of 6, forming MPP^+. MPTP, as well as its two- and four-electron oxidation products were shown to be competitive inhibitors of both forms of MAO.[37] The K_i values of 3 μM for MPP^+ and 6 μM for $MPDP^+$ in the case of MAO A suggest the possibility that the intracellular accumulation of these metabolites of MPTP could exert inhibitory effects on this form of the enzyme in vivo. Both MPTP and $MPDP^+$ caused a mechanism-based irreversible inactivation of MAO A and MAO B[37,38] and, therefore, act as "suicide" substrates for these enzymes. A similar conclusion has been reached from studies of the effects of MPTP on rodent brain preparations containing MAO B.[39]

While mechanism-based inactivation of MAO may have little relevance to the development of the neurotoxicity of MPTP, its occurrence does indicate that potentially reactive intermediates are formed during its oxidation. The precise chemical nature of such intermediates remains speculative and their molecular identification may be difficult if they are unstable compounds.

These biochemical studies demonstrating the rapid oxidation of MPTP by MAO B, presumably generating toxic products, are compatible with in vivo animal experiments showing that prior administration of inhibitors of the B form of the enzyme had protective effects against the development of the neurotoxicity of MPTP. However, it subsequently became apparent that while the four-electron oxidation product of MPTP, MPP^+, accumulates in nigrostriatal neurons, such cells contain little or no MAO B activity, this form of the enzyme being localized mainly in glial cells and serotonin-containing neurons.[40] The observed localization of MAO B in nondopaminergic cells caused a number of problems in considerations of the selective neurotoxicity of MPTP towards dopaminergic neurons. It became necessary to explain how a bioactivation event taking place in one cell type could lead to toxic effects in another type of cell. A plausible explanation would also be needed for the apparent resistance of those cells in which the bioactivation processes took place. A possible answer to the first problem was afforded by studies demonstrating the active accumulation of radiolabeled MPP^+ by synaptosomes prepared from striatal tissues.[41,42] In such preparations, MPP^+ accumulation exhibited a K_m and V_{max} similar to those for dopamine, was competitive with dopamine, and was inhibited by dopamine uptake blockers. It appeared, therefore, that the uptake of MPP$^+$ via the dopamine uptake system could account for its selective accumulation in dopaminergic neurons. To establish whether or not this accumulation process had relevance to the neurotoxicity of MPTP, evidence was sought for protective effects of dopamine uptake blockers in vivo. Such compounds do protect against the dopamine-depeleting effects of MPTP on the mouse striatum,[21,43,44] but there appear to have been no reports documenting protective effects against the development of permanent Parkinsonism in primates. Why such an MPP$^+$ uptake process should be specific for nigrostriatal dopaminergic neurons, as opposed to other DA neurons in the CNS, is not easily understood, but could be rationalized by assuming a higher density of MAO B-containing cells adjacent to striatal DA nerve endings. Active accumulation of MPP$^+$ is not restricted to DA cells of the nigrostriatal system, since it also occurs in NE-containing cells, including those of the cerebral cortex.[41] It may be relevant that both the substantia nigra and locus ceruleus in higher animals (but not rodents) contain neuromelanin which binds MPP$^+$ with high affinity[45] and which may also facilitate the oxidation of MPDP$^+$ to MPP$^+$.[46] Regarding the second problem, no satisfactory explanation of the apparent resistance of MAO B-containing brain cells to MPTP has been volunteered, and we have little idea of how the permanently charged MPP$^+$ species exits from such cells to gain access to the dopamine uptake systems of DA cells. Do cells that contain MAO B have mechanisms for the active extrusion of potentially reactive metabolites of MPTP, or do they perhaps lack the "target" macromolecules or biochemical functions, specific to sensitive cells, which are required for expression of cytotoxicity?

IV. POSSIBLE MECHANISMS OF MPTP CYTOTOXICITY

While it is reasonably well accepted that in order to express its neurotoxic actions, MPTP must initially undergo bioactivation, the molecular events that follow which lead to nigrostriatal cell lesions are less well understood. Most of the research attention concerning the possible mechanisms of neurotoxicity of MPTP has been directed towards the characterization of biochemical properties of its metabolite MPP$^+$. Reasons for this include the fact that MPP$^+$ is a major brain metabolite of the neurotoxin and that it appears to accumulate in target cells, particularly in the brains of the more sensitive primate species. As a quarternary compound which does not readily cross the blood-brain barrier, it is not easy to assess the possible selective neurotoxicity of MPP$^+$ in vivo. However, the metabolite causes dopamine depletion and certain behavioral effects similar to Parkinsonism following intracerebral injection,[14,47] and is also cytotoxic to cells of neuronal and nonneuronal origin in culture.[48-50] A number of biochemical hypotheses have been suggested involving MPP$^+$ as the neurotoxic species, including mechanisms based on its actions on mitochondrial functions and on its possible involvement in the production of "oxidative stress".

In experiments with rat liver and brain mitochondrial preparations, MPP$^+$, at a concentration of 0.5 mM, was observed to inhibit the oxidation of NADH-linked substrates, but had no effects on succinate oxidation.[51] Based on these observations, it was proposed that the compound by inhibiting mitochondrial respiration would cause ATP depletion and result in cell death. These effects of MPP$^+$ on NADH-linked oxidation in intact mitochondria have been confirmed and extended to investigations on mitochondrial membrane preparations.[52] After brief sonication of mitochondria to invert the inner membrane, respiration was no longer inhibited by 0.5 mM MPP$^+$. A similar loss of sensitivity to the inhibitory effects of MPP$^+$ was observed in mitochondrial ETP preparations (respiratory chain components minus the coupling factors) and in Complex I, its initial segment. Such preparations, used commonly to study inhibitors of NADH-linked oxidation, could be inhibited by higher concentrations of MPP$^+$,[53] and these effects were reversible on dilution, appearing to require the continued presence of MPP$^+$ for inhibitory action. Since the concentrations of MPP$^+$

in striatal tissues of MPTP-treated animals are lower by several orders of magnitude than those used in these in vitro experiments, the possible relevance of the observed inhibitory effects of the compound might be questionable. However, intact mitochondria have been shown to concentrate MPP^+ at micromolar external concentrations via an energy-dependent uptake system.[54] This novel mitochondrial uptake system requires the presence of oxidizable substrates and is dependent on the membrane electrical potential. MPP^+ also accumulates in isolated brain mitochondria, and its uptake can be distinguished from its binding to synaptosomal components by the lack of effects of dopamine or the dopamine uptake blocker mazindole.[55] This site of inhibitory action of MPP^+ on the respiratory chain components of the inner mitochondrial membrane appears to be between the high potential Fe-S cluster of NADH dehydrogenase and coenzyme Q, which is also similar to the locus of action of the respiratory poison rotenone. Interestingly, the stereotaxic injection of rotenone into the median forebrain bundle of rats is reported to cause an 80% depletion of striatal DA after 21 days.[56] The active accumulation of MPP^+ appears to be a characteristic property of mitochondria prepared from brain and peripheral tissues, and its possible relevance to the selective neurotoxicity of MPTP presumably depends on other features of the biodisposition of the metabolite, particularly its accumulation in DA cells and/or its sequestration in such cells via binding to neuromelanin. Such processes could provide an intracellular concentration of MPP^+ in nigrostriatal cells favorable to its mitochondrial accumulation, with subsequent inhibition of NADH dehydrogenase and decreased aerobic ATP synthesis.

MPP^+ bears a striking structural resemblance to the herbicide paraquat (methylviologen) and, in fact, was itself marketed for agricultural use (Cyperquat®) until withdrawn because of its toxicity. Thus, it is hardly surprising that interest in the possible mechanisms of action of MPTP has been directed towards the biochemical reactions involved in the toxic effects of paraquat, which are thought to involve "redox cycling" and the generation of oxygen radical.[57] Paraquat, a bis-methylpyridinium, readily undergoes a single-electron reduction (redox potential: -446 mV) to form a radical which, in the presence of oxygen, is immediately reoxidized, generating toxic oxygen species including the superoxide and hydroxyl radicals. Biological systems catalyze the one-electron reduction of paraquat, the NADPH-cytochrome P-450 reductase of lung microsomes being particularly effective in this regard, and the reaction is considered to be an initial event in the chain of biochemical effects leading to lipid peroxidation and pulmonary cytotoxicity.[57] The possibility of occurrence of similar biochemical events in the case of neurotoxic effects of MPTP is suggested by studies reporting protective actions of antioxidants against the striatal DA-depleting and cytotoxic effects of the compound.[58-60] DA-depleting effects of MPTP in mouse brain also appear to be enhanced by pretreatment of animals with the superoxide dismutase inhibitor diethyldithiocarbamate (DDC, Antabuse®) which is presumed to enhance the vulnerability of cells to oxidative stress.[61] None of these studies directly implicate MPP^+ in redox reactions, but systemic administration of this compound to rodents is reported to cause lung toxicity by a mechanism similar to that proposed for paraquat.[34] However, from the results of recent comparative studies of the biochemical effects of paraquat and MPP^+ on isolated hepatocytes, it has been concluded that the two compounds do not exert cytotoxic actions by identical mechanisms,[49,50] the MPTP metabolite failing to cause lipid peroxidation. In order to participate in redox cycling, the MPP^+ molecule should be capable of one-electron reduction to form a radical species. Since the half-wave reduction potential for MPP^+ is -1180 mV,[62] compared to -440 mV for paraquat, the likelihood of its one-electron reduction by biological systems is significantly less than the herbicide. In vitro spectral studies of MPP^+ exposed to various chemical and enzymic reduction conditions performed by Caldera in our laboratory[63] failed to provide evidence for radical formation, though each consistently caused the formation of a characteristic radical from paraquat. Such results do not exclude the possible formation of a carbon-centered radical from the one-electron reduction of MPP^+, since such a species could be unstable under the experimental conditions used, but they fail to add any theoretical support to hypotheses of a mechanism for neurotoxicity of MPTP that involves the redox recycling of its metabolite MPP^+.

Other hypothetical mechanisms have been proposed to explain the neurotoxic actions of MPTP, including an action of the neurotoxin to promote autooxidation of DA, possibly involving trace metals known to be present in basal ganglia structures.[64,65] However, studies designed to test this suggestion, involving manipulations of brain DA levels in vivo, have failed to demonstrate any effects on the neurotoxicity of MPTP.[66] An early hypothesis which suggested the possible involvement of the reactive, electrophilic intermediate $MPDP^+$ in a neurotoxic mechanism[26,42] becomes less tenable if its generation from the two-electron oxidation of MPTP by MAO occurs only in nondopaminergic cells and if the active accumulation of its further oxidation product MPP^+ by dopaminergic cells proves to be a crucial event in the steps leading to neurotoxicity. $MPDP^+$ is certainly a potentially reactive species, since it can undergo nucleophilic attack by cyanide to form its cyano adduct. Its disproportionation at physiological pH[27] and its half-wave reduction potential of -605 mV[62] suggest that $MPDP^+$ is more likely to be involved in redox reactions in biological systems than MPP^+. In addition, the mechanism-based inactivation of MAO by $MPDP^{+}$[38] points to the participation of this intermediate in one-electron transfer reactions leading to the formation of radical species, since such reactions appear to occur during the inactivation of this enzyme by other cyclic amines.[67] Finally, it may prove to be more than simple coincidence that the rate of oxidation of $MPDP^+$ is greatly accelerated by synthetic dopamine-neuromelanin or by neuromelanin extracted from human brain tissues.[46]

V. MPTP STRUCTURE-ACTIVITY RELATIONSHIPS

The precise structural determinants of MPTP neurotoxicity have yet to be characterized. A number of analogues of the molecule have been synthesized and tested for MPTP-like properties including their activities in depleting brain striatal DA levels following administration in vivo[68-70] and their potential for oxidations catalyzed by MAO forms.[71] The addition of methyl groups at one or more positions of the tetrahydropyridine ring (see Figure 3) resulted in compounds that had no effects on striatal DA, though they reached brain levels after intraperitoneal injection in the mouse similar to those with MPTP.[69] It was not reported whether such compounds were substrates for MAO B, but similar molecules synthesized in our laboratories[74] proved to be poor substrates for this form of the enzyme. The substitution of alkyl groups other than methyl on the nitrogen atom abolished brain DA-depleting activity in mice,[68] and such congeners have been reported to be inactive as substrates for MAO-catalyzed oxidations in brain mitochondrial preparations[68] or for human liver MAO B.[72] Since oxidations occur at carbon atoms alpha to the nitrogen atom, it is probably not surprising that substituent effects of this type are seen with MAO and such analogues. Methyl substitutions in the phenyl ring at the 3' and 4' carbon atoms result in compounds that are inactive in terms of striatal DA depletion in mice, but the 2'-methyl-MPTP analogue is more active than MPTP itself.[70] Two other analogues have been shown to be neurotoxic in the mouse, 3'-methoxy-MPTP and 1-methyl-4-cyclohexyl-1,2,3,6-tetrahydropyridine.[73] Each of the three active analogues appears to be a substrate for MAO B present in brain mitochondrial preparations, with the rank order of rates of their oxidation paralleling their effectiveness as apparent neurotoxins. However, capacity to act as a substrate for MAO B does not automatically result in neurotoxic properties, since the nonactive congeners 3'-methyl-MPTP, 2'-methoxy-MPTP, and 1-methyl-4-benzyl-1,2,3,6-tetrahydropyridine are all oxidized rapidly by mouse brain mitochondrial preparations.[73] It has not yet been established whether MAO B-catalyzed oxidation of those congeners that are apparently neurotoxic leads to the formation of the analogous dihydropyridine and pyridinium metabolites. It is also possible

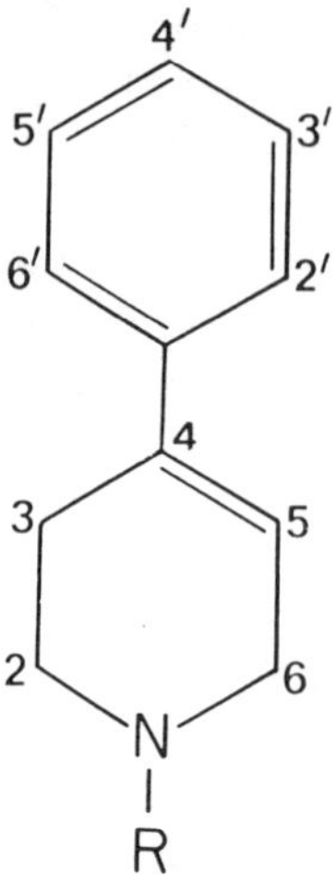

FIGURE 3.   The molecular template for MPTP structure-activity relationships.

that structural congeners of MPTP could be more effective substrates for the A form of the enzyme.

The striking neurotoxicity of MPTP has prompted consideration of the possibility that other structurally related compounds in the environment or endogenous to the brain could account for idiopathic Parkinson's disease. A large number of molecules containing the *N*-alkylated tetrahydropyridine substructure are mentioned in the chemical literature. Most of these have not undergone direct testing for their neurotoxic potential, but the probability that the generalized nigrostriatal toxicity seems remote. A large number of pyridinium-containing compounds exist containing substructures resembling MPP$^+$, and while many of these are quite toxic, their quaternized nature precludes ready access to the CNS. Several pharmacological agents, including haloperidol, reserpine, and the antihistamine pheninda-mine, which have CNS actions that can include effects on extrapyramidal functions, also have chemical structures that bear similarities to that of MPTP. The parkinsonian-like effects of these compounds appears to be more readily reversible than those of MPTP, but could be related to the generation of reactive intermediates through their metabolism by MAO or other enzymes involved in the oxidation of amines. It may also be pertinant to consider the possible involvement of bioactivation processes in the CNS effects of other psychotropic amines that are important in the drug abuse field. Phencyclidine, like MPTP, undergoes alpha carbon oxidation to generate potentially reactive intermediates[23] which could be involved in the expression of untoward CNS effects of the drug.

VI. CONCLUSION

The "MPTP story" is by no means completed, but is has already had far-reaching implications at both a scientific and societal level. Research into the mechanisms of its selective neurotoxicity has revealed that enzyme-mediated bioactivation processes involving exogenous chemicals can occur in the CNS, and that such reactions can be detrimental to brain functions. In the case of the protoxin MPTP, its metabolic activation involves the mediation of monoamine oxidases, enzymes that hitherto had been regarded as having a primary functional role in the metabolic regulation of endogenous CNS neurotransmitter substances. Appreciation of a bioactivation role of brain enzymes may prove to have significance to our understanding of CNS drug actions that extends far beyond the specific involvement of MPTP in nigrostriatal toxicity. MPTP has revitalized research into the etiology of Parkinson's disease and the possibility that environmental chemicals can act as causative agents. In this regard it is of interest to note that approval has now been given in the U.S. for clinical trials of the selective MAO B inhibitor, deprenyl, a drug that has been used for the treatment of Parkinsonism in Europe for a number of years. In the context of the abuse of psychoactive drugs, the MPTP narrative, in revealing the exquisite selectivity with which an apparently innocuous molecule can be converted into a devastating neurotoxin, represents far more than "a cautionary tale". It has furnished a dramatic validation of the expressed concerns of many investigators in the drug abuse field of the potential hazards of illicit designer drug chemistry.

ACKNOWLEDGMENTS

Research support for this work was provided in part by NIDA research grant DA 03405, NINCD research grant NS 23066, NIH program project HL 16251, NSF grant DM 846967, and the Veterans Administration.

REFERENCES

1. **Davis, G. C., Williams, A. C., Markey, S. P., Ebert, M. H., Caine, E. D., Reichert, C. M., and Kopin, I. J.,** Chronic parkinsonism secondary to intravenous injection of meperidine analogues, *Psychiatry Res.,* 1, 249, 1979.
2. **Langston, J. W., Ballard, P. A., Tetrud, J. W., and Irwin, I.,** Chronic parkinsonism in humans due to a product of meperidine-analogue synthesis, *Science,* 219, 979, 1983.
3. **Burns, R. S., Chiueh, C. C., Markey, S. P., Ebert, M. H., Jacobowitz, D. M., and Kopin, I. J.,** A primate model of parkinsonism: selective destruction of dopaminergic neurons in the pars compacta of the substantia nigra by N-methyl-4-phenyl-1,2,3,6-tetrahydropyridine, *Proc. Natl. Acad. Sci., U.S.A.,* 80, 4546, 1984.
4. **Markey, S. P., Castagnoli, N., Jr., Trevor, A. J., and Kopin, I. J.,** *MTPP: A Neurotoxin Producing a Parkinsonian Syndrome.* Academic Press, New York, 1986.
5. **Chiueh, C. C., Markey, S. P., Burns, R. S., Johannessen, J. N., Jacobowitz, D. M., and Kopin, I. J.,** Selective neurotoxic effects of N-methyl-4-phenyl-1,2,3,6-tetrahydropyridine (MPTP) in subhuman primates and man: a new animal model of Parkinson's disease, *Psychopharm. Bull.,* 20, 548, 1984.
6. **Langston, J. W., Irwin, I., Langston, E. B., and Forno, L. S.,** 1-methyl-4-phenylpyridinium ion (MPP$^+$): identification of a metabolite of MPTP, a toxin selective to the substantia nigra, *Neurosci. Lett.,* 48, 87, 1984.
7. **Cohen, G., Pasik, P., Cohen, B., Leist, A., Mytilineou, C., and Yahr, M. D.,** Pargyline and deprenyl prevent the neurotoxiciy of 1-methyl-4-phenyl-1,2,3,6-tetrahydropyridine in monkeys, *Eur. J. Pharmacol.,* 106, 209, 1984.
8. **Jenner, P., Nadia, M. T., Rupniak, S. R., and Marsden, C. D.,** 1-methyl-4-phenyl-1,2,3,6-tetrahydropyridine induced parkinsonism in the common marmoset, *Neurosci. Lett.,* 50, 85, 1984.
9. **Langston, J. W., Forno, L. S., Rebert, C. S., and Irwin, I.,** 1-methyl-4-phenyl-1,2,3,6-tetrahydropyridine causes selective damage to the zona compacta of the substantia nigra in the squirrel monkey, *Brain Res.,* 292, 390, 1984.
10. **Melamed, E. Rosenthal, J., Clobus, M, Cohen, O., Frucht, Y., and Uzzan, A..** Mesolimbic dopaminergic neurons are not spared by MPTP neurotoxicity in mice, *Eur. J. Pharmacol.,* 114, 970, 1985.
11. **Mitchell, I. J., Cross, A. J., Sambrook, M. A., and Crossman, A. R.,** Sites of the neurotoxic action of 1-methyl-4-phenyl-1,2,3,6-tetrahydropyridine in the macaque monkey include the ventral tegmentum area and the locus ceruleus, *Neurosci. Lett.,* 61, 195, 1985.
12. **Parisi, J. E. and Burns, R. S.,** MPTP-induced parkinsonism in man and experimental animals, *J. Neuropathol. Exp. Neurol.,* 44, 325, 1985.
13. **Schneider, J. S., Yuwiler, A., and Markham, C. H.,** Production of a parkinson-like syndrome in the cat with N-methyl-4-phenyl-1,2,3,6-tetrahydropyridine (MPTP): behavior, histology and biochemistry, *Exp. Neurol.,* 91, 293, 1986.

14. **Heikkila, R. E., Hess, A., and Duvoisin, R. C.,** Dopaminergic neurotoxicity of 1-methyl-4-phenyl-1,2,3,6-tetrahydropyridine in mice, *Science,* 224, 1451, 1984.

15. **Gupta, M., Felten, D. L., and Gash, D. M.,** MPTP alters central catecholamine neurons in addition to the nigrostriatal system, *Brain Res. Bull.,* 13, 737, 1984.

16. **Hallman, H., Lange, J., Olson, L., Stromberg, I., and Jonsson, G.,** Neurochemical and histochemical characterization of neurotoxic effects of 1-methyl-4-phenyl-1,2,3,6-tetrahydropyridine on brain catecholamine neurons in the mouse, *J. Neurochem.,* 44, 117, 1985.

17. **Boyce, S., Kelly, E., Reavill, C., Jenner, P., and Marsden, C. D.,** Repeated administration of N-methyl-4-phenyl-1,2,3,6-tetrahydropyridine to rats is not toxic to striatal dopamine, *Biochem. Pharmacol.,* 33, 1747, 1984.

18. **Jarvis, M. F. and Wagner, G. C.,** Neurochemical and functional consequences following 1-methyl-4-phenyl-1,2,3,6-tetrahydropyridine (MPTP) and methamphetamine, *Life Sci.,* 36, 249, 1985.

19. **Chiueh, C. C., Markey, S. P., Burns, R. S., Johannessen, J., Pert, A., and Kopin, I. J.,** Neurochemical and behavioral effects of systemic and intranigral administration of N-methyl-4-phenyl-1,2,3,6-tetrahydropyridine in the rat, *Eur. J. Pharmacol.,* 100, 189, 1984.

20. **Heikkila, R. E.,** Differential neurotoxicity of 1-methyl-4-phenyl-1,2,3,6-tetrahydropyridine (MPTP) in Swiss-Webster mice from different sources, *Eur. J. Pharmacol.,* 117, 131, 1985.

21. **Ricaurte, G. A., Langston, J. W., Irwin, I., Delanney, L. E., and Forno, L. S.,** The neurotoxic effect of MPTP on the dopaminergic cells of the substantia nigra in mice is age-related, *Soc. Neurosci. Abstr.,* 11, 635, 1985.

22. **Ward, D. P., Trevor, A. J., Kalir, A., Adams, J. D., Baillie, T. A., and Castagnoli, N., Jr.,** Metabolism of phencyclidine: the role of iminium ion formation in covalent binding to rabbit microsomal protein, *Drug Metab. Dispos.,* 10, 690, 1982.

23. **Hoag, M. K. P., Trevor, A. J., Asscher, Y., Weissman, J., and Castagnoli, N., Jr.,** Metabolism-dependent inactivation of liver microsomal enzymes by phencyclidine, *Drug Metab. Dispos.,* 12, 371, 1984.

24. **Chiba, K., Trevor, A. J., and Castagnoli, N., Jr.,** Metabolism of the neurotoxic tertiary amine MPTP by brain monoamine oxidase, *Biochem. Biophys. Res. Commun.,* 120, 574, 1983.

25. **Markey, S. P., Johannessen, J. N., Chiueh, C. C., Burns, R. S., and Herkenham, M. A.,** Intraneuronal generation of a pyridinium metabolite may cause drug-induced parkinsonism, *Nature (London),* 31, 464, 1984.

26. **Castagnoli, N., Jr., Chiba, K., and Trevor, A. J.,** Potential bioactivation pathways for the neurotoxic 1-methyl-4-phenyl-1,2,3,6-tetrahydropyridine, *Life Sci.,* 36, 225, 1985.

27. **Peterson, L. A., Caldera, P. S., Trevor, A. J., Chiba, K., and Castagnoli, N., Jr.,** Studies on the 1-methyl-4-phenyl-2,3-dihydropyridinium species, 2,3-MPDP$^+$, the monoamine oxidase catalyzed oxidation product of the nigrostriatal toxin 1-methyl-4-phenyl-1,2,3,6-tetrahydropyridine (MPTP), *J. Med. Chem.,* 28, 1432, 1985.

28. **Mytilineou, C. and Cohen, G.,** 1-methyl-4-phenyl-1,2,3,6-tetrahydropyridine destroys dopamine neurons in explants of rat embryo mesencephalon, *Science,* 225, 529, 1984.

29. **Heikkila, R. E., Manzino, L., Cabbat, F. S., and Duvoisin, R. C.,** Protection against the dopaminergic toxicity of 1-methyl-4-phenyl-1,2,3,6-tetrahydropyridine by monoamine oxidase inhibitors, *Nature (London),* 311, 467, 1984.

30. **Langston, J. W., Irwin, I., Langston, E. B., and Forno, L. S.,** Pargyline prevents MPTP-induced parkinsonism in primates, *Science,* 225, 1480, 1984.

31. **Weissman, J., Trevor, A. J., Chiba, K., Peterson, L. A., Caldera, P., and Castagnoli, N., Jr.,** Metabolism of the nigrostriatal toxin 1-methyl-4-phenyl-1,2,3,6-tetrahydropyridine by liver homogenate fractions, *J. Med. Chem.,* 28, 997, 1985.

32. **Cashman, J. R. and Zeigler, D. M.,** Contribution of N-oxygenation to the metabolism of MPTP (1-methyl-4-phenyl-1,2,3,6-tetrahydropyridine) by various liver preparations, *Mol. Pharmacol.* 29, 163, 1986.

33. **Baker, J. K., Borne, R. F., Davis, M. M., and Waters, I. W.,** Metabolism of 1-methyl-4-phenyl-1,2,3,6-tetrahydropyridine (MPTP) in mouse liver preparations, *Biochem. Biophys. Res. Commun.,* 125, 484, 1984.

34. **Johannessen, J. N., Chiueh, C. C., Burns, R. S., and Markey, S. P.,** Differences in the metabolism of MPTP in the rodent and primate parallel differences in sensitivity to its neurotoxic effects, *Life Sci.,* 36, 219, 1985.

35. **Irwin, I. and Langston, J. W.,** Selective accumulation of MPP in the substantia nigra: a key to neurotoxicity?, *Life Sci.,* 36, 207, 1985.

36. **Salach, J. I., Singer, T. P., Castagnoli, N., Jr., and Trevor, A. J.,** Oxidation of the neurotoxic amine 1-methyl-4-phenyl-1,2,3,6-tetrahydropyridine (MPTP) by monoamine oxidases A and B and suicide inactivation of the enzymes of MPTP, *Biochem. Biophys. Res. Commun.,* 125, 831, 1984.

37. **Singer, T. P., Salach, J. I., and Crabtree, D.,** Reversible inhibition and mechanism-based irreversible inactivation of monoamine oxidases by 1-methyl-4-phenyl-1,2,3,6-tetrahydropyridine (MPTP), *Biochem. Biophys. Res. Commun.,* 127, 341, 1985.

38. **Singer, T. P., Salach, J. I., Castagnoli, N., Jr., and Trevor, A. J.,** Interactions of the neurotoxic amine 1-methyl-4-phenyl-1,2,3,6-tetrahydropyridine with monoamine oxidases, *Biochem. J.,* 235, 785, 1986.

39. **Fuller, R. A. and Hemrick-Luecke, S. K.,** Inhibition of types A and B monoamine oxidase by 1-methyl-4-phenyl-1,2,3,6-tetrahydropyridine, *J. Pharmacol. Exp. Ther.,* 232, 696, 1985.

40. **Westlund, K. N., Denney, R. M., Kochenperger, L. M., Rose, R. M., and Abell, C. W.,** Distinct monoamine oxidase A and B populations in primate brain, *Science,* 230, 181, 1985.

41. **Javitch, J. A., D'Amato, R. J., Strittmatter, S. M., and Snyder, S. H.,** N-methyl-4-phenyl-1,2,3,6-tetrahydropyridine: uptake of the metabolite N-methyl-4-phenylpyridine by dopamine neurons explains selective toxicity, *Proc. Natl. Acad. Sci., U.S.A.,* 82, 2173, 1985.

42. **Chiba, K., Trevor, A. J., and Castagnoli, N., Jr.,** Active uptake of MPP^+, a metabolite of MPTP, by brain synaptosomes, *Biochem. Biophys. Res. Commun.,* 128, 1228, 1985.

43. **Melamed, E., Rosenthal, J., Cohen, O., Globus, M., and Uzzan, A.,** Dopamine but not epinephrine or serotonin uptake inhibitors protect mice against neurotoxicity of MPTP, *Eur. J. Pharmacol.,* 116, 179, 1985.

44. **Sundstrom, E. and Jonnson, G.,** Pharmacological interference with the neurotoxic actions of 1-methyl-4-phenyl-1,2,3,6-tetrahydropyridine (MPTP) on central catecholaminergic neurons in the mouse, *Eur. J. Pharmacol.,* 110, 293, 1985.

45. **D'Amato, R. J., Lipman, Z. P., and Snyder, S. H.,** Selectivity of the parkinsonian neurotoxin MPTP: toxic metabolite MPP^+ binds to neuromelanin, *Science,* 231, 987, 1986.

46. **Wu, E. Y., Chiba, K., Trevor, A. J., and Castagnoli, N., Jr.,** Interactions of the 1-methyl-4-phenyl-2,3-dihydropyridinium species with synthetic dopamine-melanin, *Life Sci.,* 39, 1695, 1986.

47. **Bradbury, A. J., Costall, B., Domeney, A. M., Jenner, P., Kelly, M. E., Marsden, C. D., and Naylor, R. J.,** 1-methyl-4-phenylpyridine is neurotoxic to the nigrostriatal dopamine pathway, *Nature (London),* 319, 56, 1986.

48. **Mytilineou, C., Cohen, G., and Heikkila, R. E.,** 1-methyl-4-phenylpyridine (MPP^+) is toxic to mesencephalic dopamine neurons in culture, *Neurosci. Lett.,* 57, 19, 1985.

49. **Di Monte, D., Sandy, M. S., Ekstrom, G., and Smith, M. T.,** Comparitive studies on the mechanisms of paraquat and 1-methyl-4-phenylpyridine toxicity, *Biochem. Biophys. Res. Commun.,* 137, 303, 1986.

50. **Di Monte D., Jewell, S. A., Ekstrom, G., Sandy, M. S., and Smith, M. T.,** 1-methyl-4-phenyl-tetrahydropyridine (MPTP) and 1-methyl-4-phenylpyridine (MPP^+) cause rapid ATP depletion in isolated hepatocytes, *Biochem. Biophys. Res. Commun.,* 137, 310, 1986.

51. **Nicklas, W. J., Vyas, I., and Heikkila, R. E.,** Inhibition of NADH-linked oxidation in brain mitochondira by 1-methyl-4-phenylpyridine, a metabolite of the neurotoxin 1-methyl-4-phenyl-1,2,3,6-tetrahydropyridine, *Life Sci.,* 36, 2503, 1985.

52. **Ramsay, R. R., Salach, J. I., and Singer, T. P.,** Uptake of the neurotoxin 1-methyl-4-phenylpyridine (MPP^+) and its relation to the inhibition of mitochondrial NADH-linked substrates by MPP^+, *Biochem. Biophys. Res. Commun.,* 134, 743, 1986.

53. **Ramsay, R. R., Salach, J. I., Dadgar, J., and Singer, T. P.,** Inhibition of mitochondrial NADH dehydrogenase by pyridine derivatives and its possible relation to experimental and idiopathic parkinsoniam, *Biochem. Biophys. Res. Commun.,* 135, 269, 1986.

54. **Ramsay, R. R. and Singer, T. P.,** Energy-dependent uptake of N-methyl-4-phenylpyridinium, the neurotoxic metabolite of 1-methyl-4-phenyl-1,2,3,6-tetrahydropyridine, by mitochondria, *J. Biol. Chem.,* 261, 7585, 1986.

55. **Ramsay, R. R., Dadgar, J., Trevor, A. J., and Singer, T. P.,** Energy-driven uptake of N-methyl-4-phenylpyridine by brain mitochondria mediates the neurotoxicity of MPTP, *Life Sci.,* 39, 581, 1986.

56. **Heikkila, R. E., Nicklas, W. J., and Duvoisin, R. C.,** Dopaminergic toxicity after stereotaxic administration of the 1-methyl-4-pyridinium ion (MPP^+) to rats, *Neurosci. Lett.,* 59, 135, 1985.

57. **Bus, J. S., and Gibson, J. E.,** Paraquat: model for oxidant-initiated toxicity, *Environ. Health Perspect.,* 55, 37, 1984.

58. **Perry, T. L., Yong, V. W., and Clavier, R. M.,** Partial protection from the dopaminergic neurotoxin N-methyl-4-phenyl-1,2,3,6-tetrahydropyridine by four different antioxidants in the mouse, *Neurosci. Lett.,* 60, 109, 1985.

59. **Sershen, H., Reith, M. E. A., Hashim, A., and Lajtha, A.,** Protection against 1-methyl-4-phenyl-1,2,3,6-tetrahydropyridine neurotoxicity by the antioxidant ascorbic acid, *Neuropharmacology,* 24, 1257, 1985.

60. **Wagner, G. C., Jarvis, M. F., and Carelli, R. M.,** Ascorbic acid reduces the dopamine depletion induced by MPTP, *Neuropharmacology,* 24, 1261, 1985.

61. **Corsini, G. U., Pintus, S., Chiueh, C. C., Weiss, J. F., and Kopin, I. J.,** 1-methyl-4-phenyl-1,2,3,5-tetrahydropyridine neurotoxicity in mice is enhanced by pretreatment with diethyldithiocarbamate, *Eur. J. Pharmacol.,* 119, 127, 1985.

62. **Sayre, L. M., Arora, P. K., Feke, S. C., and Urbach, F. L.,** Mechanism of induction of Parkinson's disease by 1-methyl-4-phenyl-1,2,3,6-tetrahydropyridine (MPTP). Chemical and electrochemical characterization of a geminal-dimethyl-blocked analogue of a postulated toxic metabolite, *J. Am. Chem. Soc.,* 108, 2464, 1986.

63. **Trevor, A. J., Castagnoli, N., Jr., Caldera, P., Ramsay, R. R., and Singer, T. P.,** Bioactivation of MPTP: reactive metabolites and possible biochemical sequelae, *Life Sci.,* 40, 713, 1987.

64. **Poirier, J. and Barbeau, A.,** A catalyst function of MPTP in superoxide formation, *Biochem. Biophys. Res. Commun.,* 131, 1284, 1985.

65. **Poirier, J., Donaldson, J., and Barbeau, A.,** The specific vulnerability of the substantia nigra to MPTP is related to the presence of transition metals, *Biochem. Biophys. Res. Commun.,* 128, 25, 1985.

66. **Schmidt, C. J., Bruckwick, E., and Lovenberg, W.,** Lack of evidence supporting a role for dopamine in 1-methyl-4-phenyl-1,2,3,6-tetrahydropyridine neurotoxocity, *Eur. J. Pharmacol.,* 113, 149, 1985.

67. **Silverman, R. B. and Zieske, P. A.,** 1-phenylcyclobutylamine, the first in a new class of monoamine oxidase inactivators. Further evidence for a radical intermediate, *Biochemistry,* 25, 341, 1986.

68. **Heikkila, R. E., Manzino, L., Cabbat, F. S., and Duvoisin, R. C.,** Effects of 1-methyl-4-phenyl-1,2,3,6-tetrahydropyridine (MPTP) and several of its analogues on the dopamine nigrostriatal pathway in mice, *Neurosci. Lett.,* 58, 133, 1985.

69. **Fries, D. S., de Vries, J., Hazelhoff, B., and Horn, A. S.,** Synthesis and toxicity toward nigrostriatal dopamine neurons of 1-methyl-4-phenyl-1,2,3,6-tetrahydropyridine (MPTP) analogues, *J. Med. Chem.,* 29, 424, 1986.

70. **Youngster, S. K., Duvoisin, R. C., Hess, A., Sonsalla, P. K., Kindt, M. V., and Heikkila, R. E.,** 1-methyl-4-(2'-methyl-phenyl)-1,2,3,6-tetrahydropyridine is a more potent dopaminergic neurotoxin than MPTP in mice, *Eur. J. Pharmacol.,* 122, 283, 1986.

71. **Brossi, A., Gessner, W. P., Fritz, R. R., Bembenek, M. E., and Abell, C. W.,** Interaction of monoamine oxidase B with analogues of 1-methyl-4-phenyl-1,2,3,6-tetrahydropyridine derived from prodine-type analgesics, *J. Med. Chem.,* 29, 445, 1986.

72. **Gessner, W. P., Brossi, A., Fritz, R. R., Patel, N. T., and Abell, C. W.,** Monoamine oxidase B inhibitory effects of MPTP analogs, in *MPTP: A Neurotoxin Producing a Parkinsonian Syndrome,* Markey, S. P., Castagnoli, N., Jr., Trevor, A. J., and Kopin, I. J., Eds., Academic Press, New York, 1986, 557.

73. **Youngster, S. K., Sonsalla, P. K., and Heikkila, R. E.,** Evaluation of the biological activity of several analogues of the dopaminergic neurotoxin MPTP, *J. Neurochem.,* 48, 929, 1987.

74. **Johnson, A.,** Personal communication.

Chapter 16

METHYL-PHENYL-TETRAHYDROPYRIDINE NEUROTOXICITY: FROM CLANDESTINE DRUG SYNTHESIS TO A MODEL FOR PARKINSON'S DISEASE

Jordi Cami

TABLE OF CONTENTS

I. CLANDESTINE SYNTHESIS OF NEW DRUGS

In the past 5 years, the toxicological problems derived from drug consumption have multiplied due to the introduction of the so-called synthetic drugs, consisting of new heroin, cocaine, amphetamine, and hallucinogenic compounds. This phenomenon is presently limited to certain geographic zones of the Western world, particularly the state of California in the U.S., but how far it will spread is unknown. According to declarations by California professionals, 20% of the heroin presently consumed in this area is of synthetic origin.[1] Although these substances are not easily produced, their clandestine manufacture is mainly motivated by the fact that when first introduced, their possession and/or manufacture is not illegal. This is because the legal identification of a drug is defined precisely by its chemical formula, and these new variants differ appreciably in structure from the drugs officially classified as illegal.[2]

A common characteristic of these new "homemade" products is that they are generally much more potent, the risk of overdose being much greater with synthetic heroin. The cost of synthetic products is usually similar to that of the classic preparations. Many heroin addicts know they are stronger and some think that these substances are less adulterated and, thus, less dangerous. In any case, addicts find it difficult to differentiate these substances with respect to traditional products by their effects.

The first opiate molecule modified in clandestine laboratories was fentanyl, a widely used anesthetic in surgery. Some researchers recognize the existence of several variants on the market. In 1980, one of them, alpha-methyl-fentanyl, was detected for the first time as a drug of illegal commerce in San Francisco.[1] This product turned out to be 100 times more potent than the original drug and caused numerous overdose deaths, obliging the Drug Enforcement Agency (DEA) to classify it as a controlled substance. Another variant, trimethylfentanyl, has recently appeared on the streets of California and is 3000 times more active than heroin. Specialists agree in indicating that these new products are difficult to detect in routine urine tests since they are consumed in minute quantities and are easy to distribute illegally.

II. DESCRIPTION OF THE CLINICAL CASES OF MPTP NEUROTOXICITY

In 1979, Davis and colleagues[3] described the sudden appearance 3 years earlier of an irreversible Parkinson syndrome in a 19-year-old male who had regularly injected for several months a petidine analogue he elaborated himself. After 2 years of treatment with levodopa and bromocriptine, the patient committed suicide. Anatomopathologic study of his brain revealed the presence of a severe degeneration of the neurons of the substantia nigra with abundant extraneuronal melanin pigment and marked astrocyte response. The changes were evident throughout the zona compacta of the substantia nigra, but were more severe in the caudad portion. A single eosinophilic inclusion, perhaps a Lewy body, was found. In contrast with idiopathic Parkinson disorder, the locus coeruleus and vagal dorsal motor nucleus were intact. In the clinical description of the case, it was reported that the symptomatology responded well to the usual anti-Parkinson treatment, but the process was irreversible. Although at this time the association was not established, this was the first clinical report of selective neurotoxicity by methyl-phenyl-tetrahydropyridine (MPTP).[4]

In 1983, in another area of California, Langston et al.[5] described an outbreak of four new cases identical to the one described by Davis a few years before.[3] The only common antecedent among these addicts was "synthetic heroin" consumption. This led the authors to demonstrate by diverse chemical analyses that heroin samples consumed by the patients contained elevated MPTP concentrations. As far as could be determined, it was a product created in 1982 by a California chemist who was addicted to parenteral drugs and synthesized

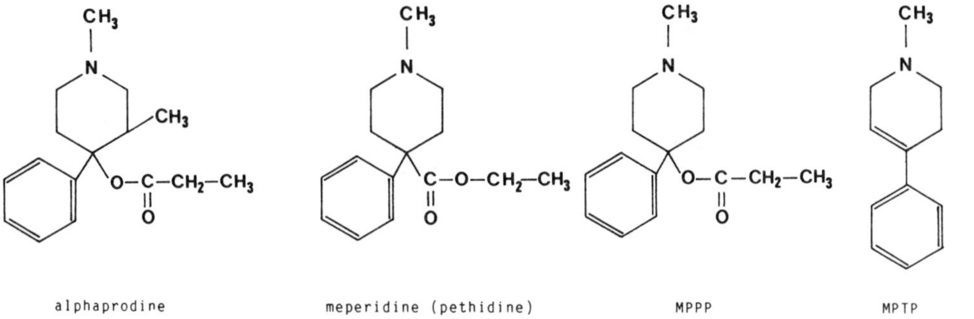

FIGURE 1

a variant of petidine, an opiate widely used in clinical practice to treat pain. The new molecule was 1-methyl-4-phenyl-4-propionoxipiperidine (MPPP), a structural analogue of petidine similar to another opiate analgesic, alphaprodine (Figure 1). MPPP has effects similar to those of heroin, although it differs from heroin in its more intense disorientation effects. A by-product of the process of MPPP synthesis was an intermediate product, 1-methyl-4-phenyl-1,2,5,6-tetrahydropyridine (MPTP), that contaminated samples. As would soon be seen, MPTP was a potent neurotoxin that would be responsible for production of irreversible lesions. MPTP is a commercially available reactant, as a chemical intermediate, but its biological effects had never been systematically studied in animals or humans.

Langston's[5] patients presented virtually all the motor alterations typical of Parkinson's disease, including the triad of bradykinesia, tremor, and muscular rigidity. The symptoms responded well to levodopa therapy, but were considered irreversible because after 2 to 3 years, the patients not only could not discontinue medication, but evidenced worsening of signs.[4] After this outbreak, the potentially affected addict community was specially informed with the object of avoiding new cases and to establish a follow-up program of the exposed population. At the time it was thought that about 100 heroin addicts might have taken similar doses of the same product without developing clinical disorders. As will be commented later, this observation favors the existence of an individual susceptibility for the development of clinical manifestations, contributing another element to the discussion of the etiology of Parkinson's disease.[6] At one moment, it was estimated that about 300 heroin addicts were exposed to MPTP, 20 of whom developed an acute Parkinson syndrome, 7 of them severe.[7]

III. CAN AN EXOGENOUS TOXIN CAUSE PARKINSON'S DISEASE?

The outbreak described in California led to the description of similar cases in the occupational sphere.[8-11] A singular case was that of a 37-year-old chemist who developed chronic Parkinsonism while working at a pharmaceutical company where certain benzomorphine analogues were synthesized using a process that required repeated preparation of MPTP.[8] This and other cases[9,11] confirm that chronic Parkinsonism can develop as a consequence of accidental inhalation or skin contact during MPTP manipulation as well as by intravenous administration. Barbeau et al.[12] realized a study in a pharmaceutical laboratory where MPTP was occasionally prepared in industrial quantities, exhaustively examining 12 employees, and demonstrated that there is a narrow relationship between the intensity and duration of exposure to MPTP and the presentation of extrapyramidal signs. Not all employees exposed were equally susceptible, but after this study the company suspended MPTP manufacture and initiated a specific follow-up program. After the detection and observation of these chemical tragedies, it is not illogical to suspect that many people exposed to MPTP in an occupational capacity could have developed late chronic Parkinsonism directly related to involuntary ingestion of the neurotoxin.

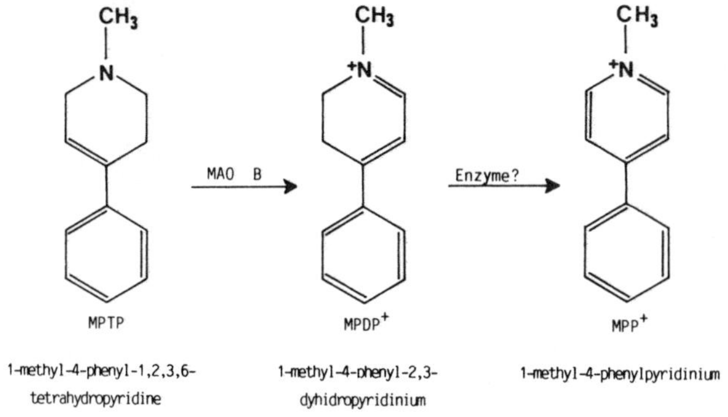

FIGURE 2

IV. SELECTIVE MPTP TOXICITY

After the description of Langston[5] of the clinical cases attributed to MPTP, it was quickly thought that this product could open new horizons in the study of the etiology of Parkinson's disease. The neurotoxin was studied as a tool for producing an animal model of the disease. Within a short time it was demonstrated that other primates were as sensitive to the neurotoxin as humans, but it was surprising that the neurotoxicity criteria for MPTP (structural, neurochemical, and behavioral) were not strictly satisfied in rodents.[10,13,14]

As for the neurochemical alterations, it has been shown that MPTP can cause central dopaminergic depletion in different experimental animals.[4] In the CSF of lower primates and humans exposed to MPTP, a reduction in the principal metabolite of dopamine, homovanyllic acid, has been demonstrated.[10] However, this depletion does not necessarily mean that all the species studied showed lesions of the nervous cells. MPTP also produces other neurochemical changes, like inhibition of serotonin uptake, but they are generally less intense than the effects produced on dopamine release.[4]

Histologically, research confirms that the neurotoxin selectively destroys neurons of the zona compacta of the substantia nigra in both humans and lower primates. MPTP is apparently highly selective of the dopaminergic neurons of this zone since it has not been shown to affect other areas normally injured in idiopathic Parkinson's disease, or other cathecholaminergic neurons.[15] Histologic studies of MPTP neurotoxicity in nonprimate species are less demonstrative with respect to cellular loss (as in the rat, for example, and further down the phylogenetic scale). For example, in the mouse. MPTP elicits a different histologic pattern reflecting a specific lesion of the nerve endings.[16] This observation is interesting since it represents a model of partial neuronal lesion, perhaps retarded in the absence of cell loss. This concept could be relevant in the case of addictive drugs and environmental toxins to which humans are being exposed in even greater amounts.[4]

V. MECHANISM OF ACTION OF MPTP

MPTP is transformed in vitro[17] and in vivo[18,19] into the ion 1-methyl-4-phenyl-piperidinium (MPP$^+$) (Figure 2). After systemic administration of toxic doses of MPTP in monkeys, this transformation takes place in practically all the organs and regions of the brain except the eye.[18] Conversion of MPTP into a charged chemical species could explain the sequester of the metabolite by certain areas of the CNS[18,20] and would account for its absence in CSF.[19] The enzyme responsible for this biotransformation seems to be monoamine oxidase, since pargyline blocks the conversion of MPTP to MPP$^+$.[17,19,21-24] The fact that selegiline but not chlorgiline (IMAO selective), blocks the conversion of MPTP to MPP$^+$ suggests that the enzyme responsible for this biotransformation would be type B monoamine oxidase.[25]

Numerous studies confirm that the mentioned biotransformation is essential for MPTP neurotoxicity. In effect, if the 3-4 double bond is lacking in the nitrogenated ring of MPTP, conversion of MPP[+] is blocked, resulting in another compound, 1-methyl-4-phenyl-py-peridine, which does not have the neurotoxic effects described.[18] Moreover, treatment with MAO inhibitors prior to MPTP administration blocks both dopamine depletion in rodents.[19,26] and parkinsonian symptoms and neuronal loss in primates.[21] In primates, pargyline induces a central elevation of MPTP concentration, but the animals do not present any symptomatology, which suggests that MPTP per se is not neurotoxic.[21]

One of the main hypotheses states that a highly reactive intermediate metabolite is formed during biotransformation of MPTP into MPP[+]. Figure 2 shows this supposed compound, identified by Chiba et al.[27] as the ion 1-methyl-4-phenyl-2,3-dihydropyridinium (MPDP[+]). It seems that type B MAO is only involved in the transformation of MPTP into MPDP[+]; the enzyme responsible for conversion of MPDP[+] to MPP[+] still remains unknown. A complementary hypothesis is that during the process of conversion of MPTP into MPP[+], highly toxic intermediate products of the peroxide type are generated.[18,19] Both hypotheses are interesting, but none explains the selectivity of the compound, since the conversion of MPTP into MPP[+] (presumably by way of MPDP[+]) takes place in all the organic tissues where it has been studied.[18] The exact mechanism involved in the selective toxicity has yet to be clarified, and it is not known to what degree dopamine itself may be a key factor. Markey et al.[19] have demonstrated that MPTP is fixed extraneuronally. However, MPP[+] is selectively fixed by the substantia nigra of primates.[28-30] In contrast, type B MAO is located fundamentally in the serotonergic neurons, which are not affected by MPTP. It could be that these neurons or astrocytes containing type B MAO could selectively capture MPDP[+] and MPP[+] and release them directly into the substantia nigra or striate.[31]

VI. IMPLICATIONS FOR THE ETIOLOGY OF PARKINSON'S DISEASE

Calne and Langston suggest that many cases of Parkinson's disease could be due to environmental factors, possibly a toxin, in addition to the natural, slow and sustained neuronal loss due to age.[6]

In an excellent review of the etiology of Parkinson's disease, after considering genetic predisposition and simple aging as causal factors, Calne and Langston underline the importance of environmental factors. Among them, the infectious etiology is discussed (although none of the histologic patterns are characteristic of infection by conventional or slow virus), although the role of neurotoxins is considered the most consistent physiopathologic hypothesis at present. The environmental aggression would precede presentation of symptoms. This would mean the appearance of a slow degenerative process and would concur with the observation made in idiopathic Parkinsonism: until striatal dopamine is not reduced by 70 to 80%, extrapyramidal symptoms do not appear.

Neurotoxin aggression would be accompanied by lesions caused by free radicals accumulated by different mechanisms. This change in the aging process could occur in early or mid-term stages of life without symptoms appearing. The wide disparity observed in the speed of progression of Parkinson's disease in different patients would be the result of individual variations in the available compensatory mechanisms in the injured brain.[4,6,32,33] Along this line of study, Langston[4] is following up the drug addicts who were exposed to MPTP, but did not develop symptoms: some have begun to present late extrapyramidal disorders. If these preliminary observations are confirmed, they would validate a new and important concept relative to neurodegenerative processes in general: from a simple aggression to the CNS could develop a slow and progressive process that would manifest years later.[4]

VII. THE IMPORTANCE OF FREE RADICALS IN MPTP TOXICITY

One of the other hypotheses that have been considered in the etiology of Parkinson's disease is that the nigrostriatal lesions may result from an accumulation of free radicals and peroxides originated by dopamine oxidation. The lesions obtained in experimental animals using 6-OH-dopamine and those observed in chronic inhalers of manganese (whose parkinsonian symptoms are alleviated with levodopa) both consist in cytolysis resulting directly from the accumulation of highly toxic free radicals of the superoxide type.[34-38] Cerebral oxidation metabolism, much of which results from catecholamine synthesis, leads to generation of free radicals or superoxides that are taken up by the superoxide dysmutase before they cause damage. Catalase and glutathione peroxidase also inactivate free radicals, and it has been demonstrated that their concentrations in the substantia nigra of Parkinson patients are inferior to those found in undiseased subjects.[36,38,39]

One of the few epidemiological correlations observed in series of Parkinson patients is the low percentage of smokers in comparison with the unaffected population.[40,43] It has been suggested that Parkinson's disease would be less frequent in smokers because they maintain sufficient carbon monoxide concentrations in the organism to facilitate rapid elimination of superoxides and other free radicals. As such, the presence of free radicals would generally constitute the final state of the mechanism of action of the exogenous toxins. Compensatory mechanisms, like increased catecholamine synthesis and especially dopamine oxidations, would also contribute to advancing the lesions by producing accumulation of free radicals and peroxides. Some of the findings of Blair et al.[44] suggest a combined system of free radicals and exogenous toxins. These authors have demonstrated that MPTP inhibits dihydropteridine reductase, an enzyme that regenerates tetrahydrobiopterine coenzyme, which is necessary for dopamine formation. A mechanism of compensation would lead to increased intraneuronal levels of tetrahydrobiopterine, a substance that reacts with oxygen and produces superoxide and hydrogen peroxide.

VIII. HYPOTHESIS OF THE ORIGIN AND FORMATION OF THE NEUROTOXIN

According to Williams,[33] a toxin can be ubiquous, can be responsible for a greater geographical or occupational incidence, and can be a relatively new product. MPTP is a simple molecule constituted by a benzene ring and a piperidinic ring, structures found separately in many compounds in plants, animals, and humans. For example, certain tryptamine metabolites are very similar to MPTP. In this respect, an improbable mechanism has been described that would lead to production of a MPTP-like compound in nature as a result of an anomalous tryptamine metabolism pathway[45] Other authors suggest an alternative mechanism by which an MPTP-like molecule would be originated parting from tryptophan and using well-known metabolic pathways.[46] Finally, as shown in Figure 3, other authors sustain the hypothesis of the presence of endogenous toxins due to the structural similarities of MPTP with *n*-methylated derivatives of the 1,2,3,4-tetrahydro-beta-carbolines and certain characteristics of their pharmacological effects.[47] The beta-carbolines have been identified in many animal and plant species in nature. Some indolic alkaloids like reserpine and yohimbine contain partial beta-carboline structures. Beta-carbolines have also been identified in urine and human platelets, and their formation in the human brain has been proposed.[48]

IX. IMPLICATIONS IN THE PREVENTION AND TREATMENT OF PARKINSON'S DISEASE

Parting from what is known of the neurotoxic mechanism of MPTP, diverse alternatives have been proposed for the prevention and treatment of Parkinson's disease. Due to the

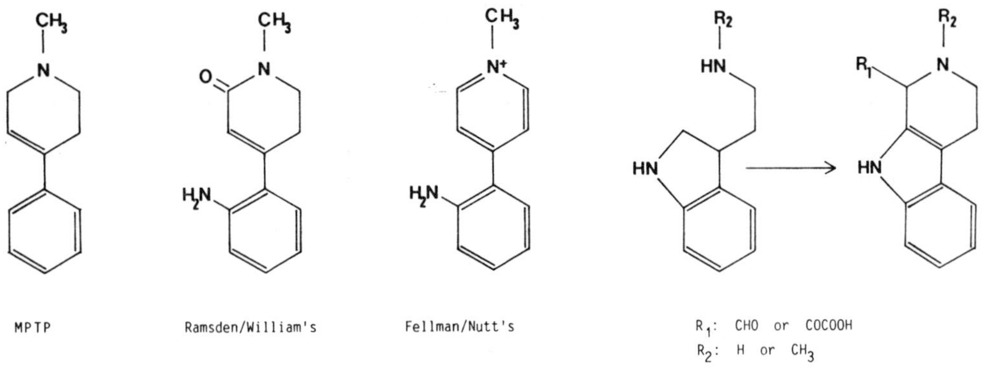

| MPTP | Ramsden/William's | Fellman/Nutt's | R_1: CHO or COCOOH |
| | | | R_2: H or CH_3 |

FIGURE 3

intraneuronal metabolic requirement of MPTP to exercise its neurotoxicity, various authors have been proposed the utilization of inhibitors of dopamine uptake, substances like benzotropine and mazindol that also inhibit neuronal MPP^+ uptake.[29,49]

Nonetheless, the two most consistent proposals derive from observation of the participation of type B MAO in MPTP metabolism and from the hypothesis of the accumulation of free radicals and peroxides originated from dopamine oxidation. This motivated an important controlled clinical trial in which for 3 years were studied the efficacy of vitamin E as an antioxidant, of selegiline as type B IMAO specific, and of the combination of both.[50]

Clinical cases of neurotoxicity due to MPTP have also led to another reconsideration. For example, it was observed that all the drug addicts affected by MPTP responded well to levodopa, but rapidly presented the typical complications of its chronic use (dosis-related fluctuations, dyskinesias at peak levels, psychiatric complications). All these disorders could thus be related to the severity of the disease and not to the duration of levodopa therapy.[32,33] This would contradict the opinion that levodopa use should be postponed as long as possible because it injures the brain. On the contrary, levodopa treatment should be initiated soon because otherwise the patient is deprived of the most satisfactory period of therapeutic response.[4,51]

One of the most important aspects of investigation presently is the identification of possible toxicological risks in the history of patients with Parkinson's disease. To do so, it would be helpful to have a standardized system for detecting and cataloging preparkinsonian cases. In the opinion of Langston, cerebral positron-emission tomography could be a good system, since it has been observed that the population of subjects exposed to MPTP presents low dopamine activity.[52]

It has been demonstrated that Parkinson patients as a group have a higher incidence of "slow" oxidative metabolizers in comparison with a control population.[53] This phenotypical study, realized by analysis of 4-hydroxylation of debrisoquine, concludes that this population is also at greater risk for deficient metabolization of some potentially neurotoxic compounds. As such, "slow" oxidators would have more of a tendency to suffer the disease. Another recent commentary discusses the toxicity of a pyridine derivative commonly used as a herbicide, paraquat, and its similarity to MPTP.[54] Paraquat is one of the herbicides most used at present. Barbeau observed that in nine hydrographic zones of Quebec there is a narrow correlation between use of this herbicide and the incidence of Parkinson's disease.

Based on the possibility that there are environmental factors that cause neurodegeneration, it is important to continue research to determine their role and, if possible, to prevent the disease and act early on its genesis and development. In any case, the unfortunate consequences of MPTP will at least contribute to serious advances in the therapy of Parkinson's disease. MPTP is an unprecedented experimental model for advancing study in the field of nerve tissue transplantation.

REFERENCES

1. **Blaskeslee, S.,** California addicts use legal, synthetic narcotics, *New York Times,* March 24, 1985.
2. **Multilingual Dictionary of Narcotic Drugs and Psychotropic Substances Under International Control,** United Nations, New York, 1983.
3. **Davis, G. C., Williams, A. C., Markey, S. P., Ebert, M. H., Caine, E. D., Reichert, C. M., and Kopin, I. J.,** Chronic parkinsonism secondary to intravenous injection of meperidine analogues, *Psychiatr. Res.,* 1, 249, 1979.
4. **Langston, J. W.,** MPTP and Parkinson's disease, *Trends Neurol. Sci.,* February, 79, 1985.
5. **Langston, J. W., Ballard, P., Tetrud, J. W., and Irwin, I.,** Chronic parkinsonism in humans due to a product of meperidine-analog synthesis, *Science,* 219, 979, 1983.
6. **Calne, D. B. and Langston, J. W.,** Aetiology of parkinson's disease, *Lancet,* ii, 1457, 1983.
7. **Bianchine, J. R. and McGhee, B.,** MPTP and Parkinsonism, *Ration. Drug Ther.,* 19, 5, 1985.
8. **Langston, J. W. and Ballard, P. A.,** Parkinson's disease in a chemist working with 1-methyl-4-phenyl-1,2,5,6-tetrahydropyridine, *N. Engl. J. Med.,* 309, 310, 1983.
9. **Wright, J. J., Wall, R. A., Perry, T. L., and Patty, D. W.,** Chronic parkinsonism secondary to intranasal administration or a product of meperydine-analogue synthesis, *N. Engl. J. Med.,* 310, 325, 1984.
10. **Burns, R. S., Markey, S. P., Phillips, J. M., and Chiueh, C. C.,** The neurotoxicity of 1-methyl-4-phenyl-1,2,3,6-tetrahydropyridine in monkey and man, *Can. J. Neurol. Sci.,* 11 (Suppl.), 166, 1984.
11. **Burns, R. S., Le Witt, P. A., Ebert, M. H., Pakkenberg, H., and Kopin, I. J.,** The clinical syndrome of striatal dopamine deficiency; parkinsonism induced by 1-methyl-4-phenyl- 1,2,3,6-tetrahydropyridine (MPTP), *N. Engl. J. Med.,* 312, 1418, 1985.
12. **Barbeau, A., Roy, M., and Langston, J. W.,** Neurological consequences of industrial exposure to 1-methyl-4-phenyl-1,2,3,6-tetrahydropyridine, *Lancet,* i, 747, 1985.
13. **Burns, R.S., Chiueh, C. C., Markey, S. P., Ebert, M. H., Jacowitz, D. M., and Kopin, I. J.,** A primate model of parkinsonism: selective destruction of dopaminergic neurons in the pars compacta of the substantia nigra by *N*-methyl-4-phenyl-1,2,3,6-tetrahydropyridine, *Proc. Natl. Acad. Sci. U.S.A.,* 80, 4546, 1983.
14. **Langston, J. W., Forno, L. S., Rebert, C. S., and Irwin, I.,** Selective nigral toxicity after systemic administration of 1-methyl-4-phenyl-1,2,5,6-tetrahydropyridine (MPTP), *Brain Res.,* 292, 390, 1984.
15. **Jacobowitz, D. M., Burns, R. S., Chieuh, C. C., and Kopin, I. J.,** *N*-methyl-4-phenyl-1,2,3,6-tetrahydropyridine (MPTP) causes destruction of the nigrostriatal but not the mesolimbic dopamine system in the monkey, *Psychopharmacol. Bull.,* 20, 416, 1984.
16. **Hess, A., Yamasaki, D., Bretschneider, A., Meadows, I., Adamo, P., Heikkila, R. E., and Duvoisin, R. C.,** *Soc. Neurosci. Abstr.,* 10, 705, 1984.
17. **Chiba, K., Trevor A., and Castagnoli, N., Jr.,** Metabolism of the neurotoxic tertiary amine, MPTP, by brain monoamine oxidase, *Biochem. Biophys, Res. Commun.,* 120, 574, 1984.
18. **Langston, J. W., Irwin, I., Langston, E. B., and Forno, L. S.,** 1-Methyl-4-phenylpyridinium ion (MPPT): identification of a metabolite of MPTP, a toxin selective to the substantia nigra, *Neurosci. Lett.,* 48, 87, 1984.
19. **Markey, S. P., Johannessen, J. N., Chiueh, C. C., Burns, R. S., and Herkenham, M. A.,** Intraneural generation of a pyridinium metabolite may cause drug-induced parkinsonism, *Nature (London),* 311, 464, 1984.
20. **Bodor, N., Farag, H. H., and Brewster, M. E.,** Site-specific, sustained release of drugs to the brain, *Science,* 214, 1370, 1981.
21. **Langston, J. W., Irwin, I., and Langston, E. B.,** Pargyline prevents MPTP-induced parkinsonism in primates, *Science,* 225, 1480, 1984.
22. **Salach, J. I., Singer, T. P., Castagnoli, N., Jr., and Trevor, A.,** Oxidation of the neurotoxic amine 1-methyl-4-phenyl-1,2,3,6-tetrahydropyridine (MPTP) by monamine oxidases A and B and suicide inactivation of the enzymes by MPTP, *Biochem. Biophys. Res. Commun.,* 120, 574, 1984.
23. **Cohen, G., Pasik, P., Cohen, B., Leist, A., Mytilineou, C., and Yahr, M. D.,** Deprenyl and pargyline prevent the destruction of dopaminergic substantia nigra neurons by 1-methyl-4-phenyl-1,2,3,6-tetrahydropyridine (MPTP) in monkeys, *Fed. Proc. Fed. Am. Soc. Exp. Biol.,* 44, 1825, 1985.
24. **Fuller, R. W., and Hemrick-Luecke, S. K.,** Inhibition of types A and B monoamine oxidase by 1-methyl-4-phenyl-1,2,3,6-tetrahydropyridine, *J. Pharmacol. Exp. Ther.,* 232, 696, 1985.
25. **Steranka, L. R., Polite, L. N., Perry, K. W., and Fuller, R. W.,** Dopamine depletion in rat brain by MPTP (1-methyl-4-phenyl-1,2,3,6-tetrahydropyridine, *Res. Commun. Subst. Abuse,* 4, 315, 1983.
26. **Heikkila, R. E., Manzino, L., Cabbat, F. S., and Duvoisin, R. C.,** Protection against the dopaminergic neurotoxicity of 1-methyl-4-phenyl-1,2,3,6-tetrahydropyridine by monoamine oxidase inhibitors, *Nature (London),* 311, 467, 1984.

27. **Chiba, K., Peterson, L. A., Castagnoli, K. P., Trevor, A. J., and Castagnoli, N.,** Studies on the molecular mechanism of bioactivation of the selective nigrostriatal toxin 1-methyl-4-phenyl-1,2,3,6-tetrahydropyridine (MPTP), *Drug Metab. Dispos.,* 342, 1985.

28. **Heikkila, R. E., Youngster, S. K., Manzino, L., Cabbat, F. S., and Duvoisin, R. C.,** Effects of 1-methyl-4-phenyl-1,2,5,6-tetrahydropyridine and related compounds on the uptake of [3H]3,4-dihydroxyphenylethylamine and [3H]5-hydroxytryptamine in neostriatal synaptosomal preparations, *J. Neurochem.,* 44, 310, 1985.

29. **Javitch, J. A. and Snyder, S. H.,** Uptake of MPP$^+$ by dopamine neurons explains selectivity of parkinsonism inducing neurotoxin, MPTP, *Eur. J. Pharmacol.,* 106, 455, 1985.

30. **Uhl, G. R., Javitch, J. A., and Snyder, S. H.,** Normal MPTP binding in parkinsonian substantia nigra evidence for extraneuronal toxin conversion in human brain, *Lancet,* i, 956, 1985.

31. **Westlund, K. N., Denney, R. M., Kochersperger, L. M., Rose, R. M., and Abell, C. W.,** Distinct monoamine oxidase A and B populations in primate brain, *Science,* 230, 181, 1985.

32. **Anon.,** Parkinson's disease, 1984, *Lancet,* i, 829, 1984.

33. **Williams, A.,** MPTP Parkinsonism, *Br. Med. J.,* 289, 1401, 1984.

34. **Heikkila, R. E. and Cohen, G.,** Inhibition of biogenic amine uptake by hydrogen peroxide: a mechanism for toxic effect of 6-hydroxydopamine, *Science,* 172, 1257, 1971.

35. **Understedt, U.,** Postsynaptic supersensitivity after 6-hydroxydopamine induced degeneration of the nigrostriatal dopamine system, *Acta Physiol. Scand.,* 367 (Suppl.), 69, 1971.

36. **Ambani, L. M., Van Woert, M. H., and Murphy, S.,** Brain peroxidase and catalase in Parkinson's disease, *Arch. Neurol.,* 32, 114, 1975.

37. **Donaldson, J., McGregor, D., and La Bella, F.,** Manganese neurotoxicity: a model for free radical mediated neurodegeneration, *Can. J. Physiol. Pharmacol.,* 60, 1309, 1982.

38. **Bannon, M. J., Goedet, M., and Williams, B.,** The possible relation of glutathione melanin and 1-methyl-4-phenyl-1,2,5,6-tetrahydropyridine (TP) to Parkinson's disease, *Biochem. Pharmacol.,* 33, 2697, 1984.

39. **Perry, T. L., Godin, D. Y., and Hansen, S.,** Parkinson's disease: a disorder due to nigral glutathione deficiency?, *Neurosci. Lett.,* 33, 305, 1982.

40. **Kessler, I. I.,** Parkinson's disease in epidemiologic perspective, *Adv. Neurol.,* 19, 355, 1978.

41. **Baumann, R. J., Jameson, H. D., McKean, H. E., Haack, D. G., and Weisberg, L. M.,** Cigarette smoking and Parkinson's disease. A comparison of cases with matched neighbours, *Neurology,* 30, 839, 1980.

42. **Haack, D. E., Baumann, R. J., McKean, H. E., Jameson, H. D., and Turbeck, J. A.,** Nicotine exposure and Parkinson's disease, *Am. J. Epidemiol.,* 114, 191, 1981.

43. **Ringwald, E.,** What causes Parkinson's disease?, *Lancet,* i, 336, 1984.

44. **Blair, J. A., Parveen, H., Barford, P. A., and Leeming, R. J.,** Aetiology of parkinson's disease, *Lancet,* i, 167, 1984.

45. **Ramsden, D. B. and Williams, A. C.,** Production in nature of compound resembling methylphenyltetrahydropyridine, a possible cause of Parkinson's disease, *Lancet,* i, 215, 1985.

46. **Fellman, J. H. and Nutt, J. N.,** MPTP-like molecules and parkinson's disease, *Lancet,* i, 924, 1985.

47. **Ohkubo, S., Hirano, T., and Oka, K.,** Methyltetrahydro-beta-carbolines and parkinson's disease, *Lancet,* i, 1271, 1985.

48. **Bloom, F., Barchas, J., Sandler, M., and Usdin, E.,** *Beta-Carbolines and Tetrahydroisoquinolines Proc.,:* Prog. in Clinical and Biological Res., Vol. 90, Alan R. Liss, New York, 1982.

49. **Bradbury, A. J., Kelly, M. E., Costall, B., Naylor, R. J., Jenner, P., and Marsden, C. D.,** Benztropine inhibits toxicity of MPTP in mice, *Lancet,* i, 1444, 1985.

50. **Lewin, R.,** Clinical trial for Parkinson's disease?, *Science,* 230, 527, 1985.

51. **Muenter, M. D.,** Should levodopa therapy be started early or late?, *Can. J. Neurol. Sci.,* 11 (Suppl.), 195, 1984.

52. **Calne, D. B., Langston, J. W., Martin, W. R., et al.,** Positron emission tomography after MPTP: observations relating to the cause of Parkinson's disease, *Nature (London),* 317, 246, 1985.

53. **Barbeau, A., Roy, M., Paris, S., Cloutier, T., Plasse, L., and Poirier, J.,** Ecogenetics of Parkinson's disease: 4-hydroxilation of debrisoquine, *Lancet,* ii, 1213, 1985.

54. **Anon.,** Paraquat spraying of marijuana, *Lancet,* ii, 770, 1985.

Chapter 17

USES AND ABUSES OF ANABOLIC STEROIDS BY ATHLETES

Sayed M. H. Al-Habet, Kinfe K. Redda, and Henry J. Lee

TABLE OF CONTENTS

I. INTRODUCTION

The two principal biological activities of the male sex hormones (androgens) are clearly distinguishable yet inseparable. These are androgenic (male sex characteristic promoting) and anabolic (muscle building). The latter activity has been a particularly attractive property to athletes. However, the use of anabolic steroids by athletes with the hope of enhancing muscle development is still a very controversial issue since the early work of Kochakian and Murlin in 1935.[1] They demonstrated a decrease in the catabolism (breakdown) of protein with a positive nitrogen balance in castrated dogs following the administration of androgen. A few years later, it was shown that injection of testosterone into female or castrated male dogs increased muscular development.[2] During World War II, anabolic steroids were used to enhance the aggressive behavior of troops as well as to build up the weight of those who survived severe starvation.[3]

In the early 1950s, anabolic steroids were introduced to athletes in the U.S.S.R., and a few years later, some athletes in the U.S. started experimenting with these hormones.[3,4] Since that time, the use of anabolic steroids has become increasingly popular among athletes, particularly among weight lifters. Today the anabolic steroids are abused by athletes involved in many types of sports.

II. CHEMISTRY OF ANDROGENS AND ANABOLIC STEROIDS

All anabolic steroids can simply be classified into two major chemical groups: 17-alpha-alkylated and 17-esterified estrogenic steroids.[5] The esters are mainly given intramuscularly, which will be slowly released from the depot following parenteral administration, hence, producing a longer duration of action than the orally administered alkylated derivatives (see Section III.D).[6]

A. Structural Modifications of Testosterone

Structural modifications of testosterone are necessary to produce steroids that are suitable for oral or parenteral administration. There is extensive hepatic first-pass effect (first metabolism of the drug by the liver after absorption) on testosterone following its oral administration.[6,7] Structural modifications of testosterone were introduced to improve both the bioavailability and the duration of action. Table 1 shows the structures of some of the commonly available anabolic steroids.

1. Esterification

The slow release formulations of anabolic steroids were obtained by esterification of the 17-beta-hydroxyl group with relatively simple carboxylic acids.[6] The esterified steroids which have increased lipid solubilities have longer duration of action following intramuscular administration.

2. Alkylation

Alkylation at the 17-alpha position with methyl or ethyl groups protects hepatic metabolic oxidation of 17-beta-hydroxyl function following oral administration. For example, methyltestosterone and fluoxymesterone (Table 1) are more effective than testosterone when given orally.[6] However, absorption through oral mucosa following sublingual (under the tongue) administration of testosterone will avoid the first inactivation of the hormone by the liver. The alkylated derivatives are not as safe as testosterone itself due to higher risk of hepatic toxicity (see Section V.B).[5,6]

B. Structure-Activity Relationships

The total structural requirements for selective androgenic or anabolic activities are not

Table 1

SOME ANDROGENIC AND ANABOLIC STEROIDS USED IN THERAPY AND ABUSED BY ATHLETES

Generic and trade names	Structure	Formulation	Dose
Oral preparations			
17-alpha-methyl derivatives			
Methyltestosterone[a]		Tablets buc-cal	10—40 mg daily
Metandren® (Ciba)			
Oreton® (Schering)			
Fluoxymesterone[a]		Tablets	2—10 mg daily
Halotestin® (Upjohn)			
Android-F® (Brown)			
Oxandrolone[a]		Tablets	5—10 mg daily
Anavar® (Searle)			
Oxymethanolone[a]		Tablets	1—5 mg/kg daily
Andarol-50 (Syntex)			
Stanozolol[a]		Tablets	6 mg daily
Winstrol® (Winthrop)			
17-alpha-ethyl derivatives			
Ethylestrenol		Elixir and tablets	4—8 mg daily
Maxibolin® (Organon)			
Orabolin (Organon)			
Parenteral preparations			
Testosterone[a]		Suspension	10—50 mg 3 times weekly
Testoject-50			
Esters of testosterone			
Propionate, $R = OCCH_2CH_3$ (Oreton)		Solution	10—25 mg, 2—3 times weekly
Cypionate, $R = OCCH_2CH_2$ (Upjohn)		Solution	50—400 mg, 2—4 times weekly
Enanthate[a], $R = OC(CH_2)_5CH_3$ (Squibb)		Solution	50—400 mg, 2—3 times weekly
Esters of 19-nortestosterone			
Nandrolone[a], $R = OC(CH_2)_8CH_3$ decanoate		Solution	50—100 mg, 3—4 times weekly
Deca-Durabolin® (Organon)			
Nandrolone[a], $R = OCH–(CH_2)_2PH$ phenpropionate		Solution	25—50 mg, weekly
Durabolin® (Organon)			
17-alpha-ethinyl derivatives			
Danazol		Capsules	200—800 mg daily
Danocrine® (Winthrop-Breon)			

[a] Commonly abused by athletes.

yet completely clear. The 17-beta-hydroxyl group, which is important for androgenic activity, has been maintained in most of the structures of the available androgens (Table 1). However, if this is oxidized to a 17-oxo group (as in 4-androstenedione), there is a loss of approximately 80% of androgenic potency.[8] The presence of 17-alpha-hydroxyl group or absence of the oxygen function at C-17 also significantly reduce the androgenicity. In addition, either a 4-en-3-oxo configuration (as in testosterone) or a 3-oxo group with saturated ring A (as in 5-alpha-dihydrotestosterone — DHT) are required for their activities.[8]

Androgenic activity may be enhanced by introducing an oxygen atom as part of a six-membered A-ring (as in oxandrolone, Table 1). Introducing a double bond at C-14 also causes a marked enhancement in androgenicity (e.g., 14-dehydrotestosterone and 19-nor-testosterone analogues); 7-alpha-methyl or 14-dehydro modification, as in 19-nortestoster-one, makes a more effective compound than testosterone, particularly when both modifications are present in the structure. The correlation between receptor binding and the androgenicity of the compounds is not always consistent, for example, 19-nortestosterone has greater affinity to the receptor than DHT, but its androgenicity is weaker than DHT.[9]

There are species differences in the receptor binding affinities to androgens. Removal of 19-methyl group of testosterone was found to increase the relative binding affinity for the receptor in rat prostate and in rabbit (but not rat) muscle four- and threefold, respectively.[9] The anabolic-androgenic ratio varies in the different studies, from 0.4 to 1.9 for DHT, 1.5 to 15 for 19-testosterone, 1.8 to 10.6 for oxymetholone, and 1.4 to 10.6 for stanzolol.[9]

Androgens can be divided into four groups based on the binding affinities to the receptor:[9] those that bind well to both muscle and prostate receptors, but have lower affinities to sex hormone binding globulin (SHBG) or testosterone estradiol binding globulin (TEBG); those with higher affinity to SHBG than the receptor; those that bind equally to SHBG and the receptors; and those with very low binding affinities to both SHBG and the receptor.

III. PHYSIOLOGY AND PHARMACOLOGY OF ANDROGENS

A. Regulation of Synthesis and Secretion

The endocrine system consists of a diverse group of ductless glands that synthesize, store, and secrete chemicals called hormones (from Greek word meaning "to urge on" or "to set in motion"). Many of the endocrine glands in the body are regulated by the pituitary and the hypothalamus glands.

Steroid hormones secreted by the gonads and adrenal glands include androgen, estrogen, progestins, glucocorticoids, and mineralocorticoids. All of the steroid hormones are synthesized from cholesterol (Figure 1), and the overall rate of synthesis in each case is regulated by one or more of the pituitary tropic hormones such as luteinizing hormone (LH), follicle-stimulating hormone (FSH), adrenocorticotropin (ACTH), or prolactin.

Plasma gonadotropin levels are controlled by hypothalamus releasing hormones, genetic, and environmental factors.[10] Since the steroid hormones have a common precursor, choles-terol, and depend upon a fairly limited series of structural modifications for their biological properties, it is not surprising that a degree of overlap occurs in the actions of the structurally similar steroid molecules. In general, the gonadal steroids are predominantly involved in regulation of growth and function in reproductive tissues, whereas the adrenal steroids serve mainly as metabolic regulators of intermediary metabolism and electrolyte balance. Testos-terone is the principal male androgenic steroid secreted by the testes. However, the ovary and adrenal cortex in women also synthesize a small amount of testosterone. The production of testosterone in the female is regulated by LH and FSH (Figure 2). However, the production of testosterone in the male is regulated by LH (also called ICSH — interstitial cells-stim-ulating hormone).

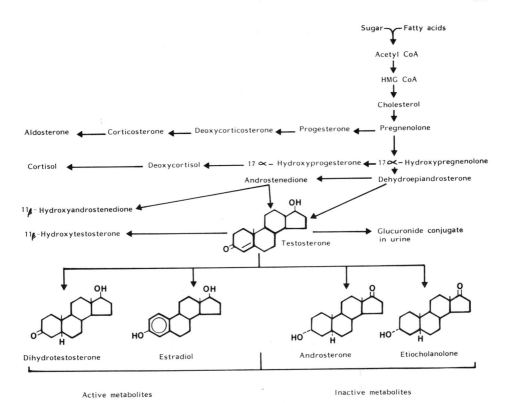

FIGURE 1. Biosynthesis and metabolism of testosterone.

B. Androgenic and Anabolic Effects

The androgens comprise a group of 19 carbon steroids. Testosterone, the major androgen in human is secreted mainly by the Leydig cells of the interstitial tissues of the testes. Androgens exert diversified biological effects which are age dependent. In the embryonic life period, androgens are involved in the development of the reproductive and urogenital tract of the male phenotype.[6] The action of androgens during the neonatal period is not well defined, but they are involved in behavioral and functional actions within the central nervous system. At puberty, the effects of androgens are manifested most markedly.[8] They are responsible for the normal functioning and structural development of the prostate gland and the seminal vesicles, particularly with spermatogenesis and the maturation of sperm. Furthermore, they are involved in the regulation of body weight and the development of skeletal muscles. At this stage, male sex characteristics will start to appear. Androgens stimulate the development of the testes, scrotum, penis, seminal vesicles, prostate, vas deferens, and epididymis.[8]

Overproduction of androgens in adults is responsible for the aggressive sexual behavior in males.[11] The anabolic effects of androgens can be noted especially during the puberty period. The increase in muscle proteins is reflected by the increase in urinary creatinine and the positive nitrogen balance. Androgens affect the length of the vocal cords causing deepening of the voice.[8] One of the unwanted effects of androgens during this period is the stimulation of the sebaceous glands, resulting in oily skin and, hence, acne may develop in some individuals. The body hair starts to grow at a later stage of puberty and includes axillary, trunk, limbs, and finally the beard. At this time, the major spurt in growth is almost completed and the epiphyses of the large bones start to close.[6]

Administration of a physiological dose of androgen to hypogonadal males has a significant positive effect on muscle mass and body weight. It was assumed (but never proven) that

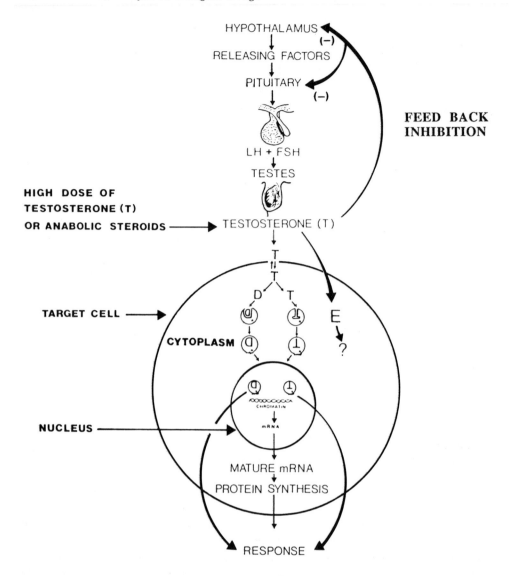

FIGURE 2.   Mechanism of action of endogenous and exogenous androgens (testosterone). (E) denotes estrogens, (D) dihydrotestosterone, (LH) luteinizing hormone, and (FSH) follicle-stimulating hormone.

the administration of a large pharmacological dose might stimulate the growth of the muscle mass above the normal development.[6] Administration of such a large dose will result in dual effects, the androgenic and anabolic effects. Since no anabolic steroid is free from androgenic effects, the hope for such a compound may not be possible because the androgenic and anabolic effects do not result from different actions of the same hormone, but represent the same actions in different tissues.[12] The actions of these steroids are less specific because the androgen responsive muscles contain the same androgen receptor system as the other androgen target tissues.[9,13] Thus, it is not surprising to see that all anabolic agents have androgenic activity, and in appropriate doses they can be used in replacement therapy of androgens.[14,15] It is known that body proteins are broken down more rapidly than they are formed following injury. This results in a negative nitrogen balance. Anabolic steroids can restore this inbalance in well-nourished patients, but the effects last for a short period of time.[16]

C. Mechanism of Action of Androgens

In the body, testosterone is converted to more active metabolites such as dihydrotestosterone (DHT) and estradiol (Figure 1). These conversions appear to occur mainly in the target tissues.[17,18] About 98% of testosterone in the circulation binds to the specific plasma proteins, TEBG or SHBG and albumin.[6] Only 1 to 2% of the hormone remains unbound (free). The free hormone enters the target cell by a simple (passive) diffusion. Inside the cell, it converts to DHT by the action of 5-alpha-reductase enzyme, and both forms probably bind to the same receptor in the cytosol.[17-20] The metabolite DHT has a higher affinity to the receptor than testosterone.[17] The hormone receptor complex binds to a specific acceptor site on the nucleus which generates a new mRNA (Figure 2). Thus, new specific proteins will be synthesized by the ribosomes. It appears that DHT is probably responsible for the sexual maturation at puberty (i.e., virilization in males).[13] However, testosterone receptor complex mediates functions such as gonadotropin regulation, spermatogenesis, and sexual differentiation.[17] The role of estrogen at this stage appears to augment or block the androgen action and, thus, the mechanism of action of estrogen at this level is not yet completely clear. The administration of high doses of anabolic steroids to athletes causes a significant decrease in serum LH, FSH, and ACTH.[21] This is due to the hypothalamic negative feedback effects as a result of administering large doses of exogenous steroids (Figure 2). The synthesis of proteins causes a positive nitrogen balance, increases lean body mass, and enhances muscle growth in castrated animals and castrated or hypogonadal human males.[22,23] These effects do not occur in normal laboratory animals, but in normal adult men it was shown that the effects are about half of those seen in hypogonadal men.[24,25] The mechanisms by which anabolic steroids increase nitrogen retention is not completely clear. However, it was suggested that the effect of anabolic steroids is probably mediated by the action of insulin which increases the cellular uptake of glucose and amino acids.[26]

D. Pharmacokinetics of Androgens

Testosterone is rapidly absorbed following oral administration, and its poor bioavailability due to rapid first-pass effect has been circumvented by structural modifications as discussed earlier.[24] Only about 50% of the testosterone dose reaches the circulation following oral administration as a result of first-pass effect.[27] Thus, in order to achieve clinically effective plasma levels for full replacement therapy, an oral dose as high as 400 mg/day may be needed.[27] Methyltestosterone, a synthetic androgen, is less extensively metabolized by the liver and has a longer half-life, which makes it suitable for oral administration. Buccal administration of methyltestosterone avoids the first-pass TEBG, effects by direct absorption into the systemic venous return. This route may double the potency of the orally administered hormone. Testosterone esters are less polar than free testosterone and are slowly absorbed from the lipid phase when injected intramuscularly in oily vehicles. Thus, testosterone cypionate and enanthate can be given at intervals of 2 to 4 weeks.[6] Suspension of testosterone or its esters in aqueous media may cause local irritation. There is a considerable variation of the half-life of testosterone, as reported in the literature, ranging from 10 to 100 min.[27] This is due to various factors including intersubject variation, formulation differences, analytical, and technical variations.

The pharmacokinetics of nandrolone decanoate were studied following intramuscular injection into healthy human volunteers.[28] The mean half-life of nandrolone decanoate release from the muscle depot into general circulation following intramuscular injection was found to be 6 days. This was comparable to that found in rats which was 4 to 5 days.[29] However, the half-life of serum hydrolysis and elimination of nandrolone decanoate was less than 1 hr.[28] In this study, it was concluded that nandrolone exhibit a linear pharmacokinetic behavior (dose independent). This latter observation was similar to other types of steroids, including prednisolone[30] and methylprednisolone.[31,32]

As mentioned earlier, 98% of testosterone binds to SHBG, and to albumin in a concentration-dependent manner. Generally the concentration of the binding proteins in plasma determines the distribution of testosterone between free (unbound) and bound forms. The free testosterone concentration will determine its elimination half-life. About one third of the variation in the free levels of androgens (e.g., testosterone) are controlled by genetic factors.[10] The abuse of anabolic steroids by athletes who tend to administer repeated high doses of different preparations (particularly the long-acting forms) leads to the accumulation of the hormones in the body. Accumulation occurs when the administered dose is greater than the eliminated amount. This occurs when the drug level reaches a steady state due to the saturation of elimination processes. The times required to achieve the steady-state levels depend upon the half-lives of the hormones.

In the presence of liver diseases, there will be some decrease in both the rate of metabolism of the anabolic steroids and the synthesis of the plasma proteins responsible for their binding.[33] Since anabolic steroids are known to cause liver damage, repetitive use of large doses of these steroids by athletes will increase their plasma free concentration, leading to oversaturation of the receptor binding sites and resulting in more serious side effects. Drug interactions may also increase the incidence of side effects. Recently, it was reported that alcohol interferes with the metabolism of certain androgens which result in increased levels of conjugated estradiol.[34,35] This tends to cause feminization in males.

The main catabolic steps of testosterone are oxidation of the 17-hydroxyl group and reduction of 3-keto groups.[36] Four main enzymes are involved in the metabolism of testosterone. These are 17-beta-hydroxysteroid dehydrogenase, 5-alpha-reductase, 3-alpha-, and 3-beta-hydroxysteroid oxidoreductases.[37] The affinity of these enzymes vary with different androgens; for example, testosterone has a higher affinity to 5-alpha-reductase and 17-beta-hydroxysteroid dehydrogenase than nandrolone.[6] It can be noted from Figure 1 that testosterone produced four main metabolites which are DHT, estradiol (E), androsterone (A), and etiocholanolone (ET). Testosterone and its metabolites are excreted mainly in urine as glucuronic and sulfuric acid conjugates.[27,38] About 90% of the administered isotope-labeled testosterone appears in urine and 6% in feces.[6,7] The plasma levels of androsterone glucuronide (A-G) and estradiol (3-alpha-diol) glucuronide (E-G) are good markers of androgen metabolism since the latter is considered as the end metabolite of androgen metabolism.[38] The predominant C-19 steroid glucuronide derivatives in the plasma of adult males is A-G.[39] The plasma level of A-G is age dependent; it is negligible in children under the age of 7 years, highest during adult life (20 to 35 years), and reduced after the age of 55 years.[39] A similar pattern was also shown for the E-G metabolites. A positive correlation was reported between the plasma levels of testosterone and its metabolite estradiol in athletes.[21] The production of testosterone and its metabolites DHT and E were significantly higher in obese and hirsute women than normal women, more in women with hirsutism as compared to obese.[40] However, the metabolic clearance rate (MCR) of testosterone and its metabolites in obese women were higher than both the normal and the hirsute women. Recently, it was found that peripheral aromatization of testosterone to produce estrogen correlates positively with obesity (adiposity).[41] Aging and obesity were found to account for approximately 15% of the factors that influence the variations of plasma levels of androgens.[10]

IV. ABUSE OF ANABOLIC STEROIDS BY ATHLETES

A. Controversy in the Use of Anabolic Steroids by Athletes

Today, it is almost an impossible task to monitor the number of athletes using anabolic steroids. It is suggested that anabolic steroids are used by more than 80% of athletes worldwide in various types of sports.[3,42-44] Some athletes became interested in using steroids following the Olympic Games in Tokyo in 1964.[45] Anabolic steroids were believed to be a regular part of training in both men and women athletes in the U.S.S.R. and eastern Europe.[46] However, at present, the extent of anabolic steroid use in these countries is not easy to assess. In a surveyed study in the U.S., 90% of body builders were found to use anabolic steroids.[47] Most of the athletes assumed that anabolic steroids increase their performance, strength, muscle mass, and aggressiveness. Body builders in particular are obsessed with anabolic steroids with the belief that these hormones increase the muscular development and reduce the subcutaneous fat so that the musculature is more clearly defined. This group of athletes prefers the injectable forms of the steroids which are normally given intramuscularly.

Most athletes, particularly body builders and weight lifters, believe that anabolic steroids improve their performance.[24,48-50] However, most medical and scientific communities assert that anabolic steroids in athletes do not improve athletic performance and only cause body hormonal imbalances. In the literature, there are few reports that support the use of anabolic steroids by athletes based on limited observations of improved performance. Most of the available data in the literature appear to be biased for lack of adequate study protocols such as a double-blind control design. A number of reports demonstrated no significant effects of anabolic steroids on either aerobic performance or maximal oxygen uptake in athletes.[49,51-80] These results were almost consistent. Some investigators reported, however, that there is a significant increase in muscular strength, by athletes using anabolic steroids.[44,54,57-67] Most of these studies were done on weight lifters who were already using anabolic steroids and continued their training during the study period. Thus, the observed increase in their strength could be a result of the training alone and not due to the effect of the steroids. Other studies showed that subjects who were not involved in athletic training prior to steroid treatment do not seem to increase their strength significantly.[48] In addition, some reports suggested that severe muscle stress and high protein diet must accompany anabolic steroids in order to produce a significant effect.[44,56,72] The wide variability and the inconsistency in the literature appear to be due to the differences in the study protocols. It is interesting to note that most of the controlled double-blind design studies reported significant improvements in athletic strength after using anabolic steroids.

Anabolic steroids appear to have some psychological effects such as motivation, a state of euphoria, and reduced fatigue.[4,42,44] However, those psychological effects were also demonstrated in some experienced weight lifters following trial of placebo.[73] Interestingly, in other studies some athletes were able to differentiate between placebo and anabolic steroids in double-blind studies.[49,44] Other studies which compared physical education students and experienced weight lifters demonstrated significant steroid effects on strength of the latter groups compared to the former.[52,61]

At present, the analysis of the scientific research could not be conclusive for a number of reasons:

- The studied populations are often not properly randomized or matched.
- The potential side effects of these hormones do not encourage individuals to participate or continue the study for a long period.
- Some of the athletes selected in the study were already using or have been using steroids.
- Anabolic steroids cause irritability and aggressiveness in some athletes which result in the drop out of some of the participants.
- It is difficult at the present time to know the duration of the pharmacological action of these steroids and the effect of placebo in some studies which could be due to the delayed effects of steroids taken previously.
- The number of athletes participating in most studies is relatively small.
- Athletes often take a higher dose of steroids than is recommended. Megadoses or stack-high doses of three or four steroids are often taken by athletes simultaneously.

The usual replacement dose of testosterone should match the amount secreted by male testes which is about 4 to 10 mg/24 hr.[74] The plasma level of testosterone is variable but about 10 nmol/ℓ (350 ng/100 mℓ).[7] Various doses of steroids were being used by weight lifters which in the literature vary from 10 to 300 mg/24 hr or even higher.

B. Response of Athletes to Anabolic Steroids

In addition to the anabolic effects, these steroids have an anticatabolic effect. Anabolic steroids can reverse the catabolic effects of glucocorticosteroids (e.g., cortisol) which are increasingly released by stress during the training periods.[77-80] The release of cortisol during stress causes breakdown of protein, and in the presence of anabolic steroids this effect may be blocked.[80,81] Some of the observed improvements in muscle development and performance may be due to exercise alone and not necessarily due to the effects of the large doses of anabolic steroids taken by athletes. It is known that exercise alone causes a number of the following physiological changes.[81-83] These changes include

- Increase in androgen receptor levels in muscle tissue.
- Increase in endogenous androgen levels in blood.
- Changes in glucocorticoid receptor levels in muscle tissues.
- Elevation in serum growth hormone which acts as a synergistic agent with endogenous androgen.
- Increases in cortisol and adrenocorticotropic hormone (ACTH) levels and decreases in testosterone concentration in the body.

Using anabolic steroids may result in a positive nitrogen balance in well-nourished subjects, but not in those that have protein deficiency.[6,76] However, in posttraumatic patients the effect of anabolic steroids on nitrogen balance is inconsistent, being positive in patients following brain injuries[84] and various types of surgery,[84,85] and negative (50%) following total hip replacements.[86] No significant effects are observed in other types of surgery and catabolic illnesses.[88] The negative effect on nitrogen balance suggests that anabolic steroids may act directly on muscle to reduce the protein catabolism.[86] The observed increases in total body weight and size are partially due to the retention of salt and water and not to the increase of muscle mass.[44,48,61,72] Consequently, the blood volume of athletes taking anabolic steroids tends to increase.[24] The administration of a small subcutaneous dose (1 mg/kg body weight per day for a few days) of testosterone to female rats increased the growth rate.[89] However, a tenfold increase in the dose failed to produce further increase in growth. In this study, the increase in growth rate was found to occur in whole body weight and not specifically in muscle. In two types of athletes (body builders and weight lifters), there was an increase in their lean body mass (LBM) following a large dose of different preparations of anabolic steroids over a period of 4 to 5 months.[90]

The increase in motivation and reduction in fatigue claimed by athletes using anabolic steroids could be a consequence of many other factors including the increase in the number of red blood cells, hence, resulting in corresponding increase of hemoglobin concentration.[91-95] The hormones were shown to enhance erythropiesis due to the stimulation of the erythropoietin production.[24,94] This will increase the amount of oxygen available to the muscle cells and, hence, reduce fatigue.

C. Control of Abuse of Anabolic Steroids

At present, very few sports organizations around the world routinely carry out the complex and expensive testing of anabolic steroids. In 1977, the American College of Sports Medicine issued a statement about the abuse of anabolic steroids in sports which reads as follows, "There is no conclusive scientific evidence that extremely large doses of anabolic-androgenic steroids either aid or hinder athletic performance.''[96] The first urine testing was carried out in 1974 at the British Commonwealth Games in Auckland, New Zealand.[97] There were 9 positive results out of 55 urine samples. Testing was continued at the Pan-American Games in 1975. The cost of drug testing at the Olympic Games in Montreal in 1976 was well over $2 million.[97] At this game, athletes, mostly winners, were randomly selected for testing. In the 1980 Moscow Olympics, there was no positive result of the presence of the anabolic steroids in 831 tested athletes.[63] This could be true, but athletes and their associates are getting well educated about the limitation of the testing protocols and know that oral preparation might not be detected after withdrawal 2 weeks prior to the test.[42] Since testosterone is normally present in the body fluids, athletes often use it with the hope of avoiding its detection. Scientists are, however, aware of the illegal use of testosterone since it can be detected from the ratios of the concentrations of testosterone to those of pituitary gonadotropins (i.e., LH and FSH). Still some athletes attempt to avoid detection by injecting themselves with human gonadotropins to stimulate the secretion of testosterone and also balance the testosterone-gonadotropin ratios.[75,98] However, there is another way of detecting abuse of testosterone. The ratio of testosterone and its metabolites epitestosterone in urine is normally one to one, and a significant increase in this ratio is an evidence of increased testosterone use.[46] Often athletes are using the growth hormone hoping to obtain an anabolic effect.[99] To control the abuse of anabolic steroids more effectively, the following methods are recommended:

- Random testing of athletes not only during competition but during training periods.
- Educating athletes, their coaches, and associates about the risk of using anabolic steroids.
- Make an effective control of the distribution of anabolic steroids by medical and pharmaceutical personnel. The law against steroid abuse must be strictly enforced.
- Carrying out more research to fully understand the mechanism of action and the various aspects of possible use, misuse, and abuse of anabolic steroids.

V. CLINICAL EVALUATIONS

A. Therapeutic Uses

Since their introduction, anabolic steroids were used in a number of clinical conditions, and occasionally the rationale for their therapeutic use was not always clear. The possible clinical applications of androgen-anabolic steroids are discussed below.

1. Replacement Therapy in Hypogonadal Males

In appropriate doses, all anabolic steroids are androgenic and can be employed in a replacement therapy in males with deficient function of the testes.[6] In fact this is the most appropriate clinical application of androgens. It should be noted that androgen therapy in these conditions does not restore spermatogenesis to normal levels.[24] It was suggested that the volume of ejaculate (derived largely from the prostate and seminal vesicles) and other sex characteristics return to normal.[24,100] When there is severe testicular dysfunction leading to a delay in puberty, prolonged therapy is required. For these conditions, long-acting esters of testosterone are useful, e.g., the cypionate or enanthate preparations. In some situations, growth hormone can be used concurrently with testosterone to enhance the action of the latter.

2. Disorders of the Skeleton
a. Stunted Growth

Growth hormone is the drug of choice in the treatment of stunted growth. However, the high cost of production of this hormone has limited its long-term therapy. Therefore, anabolic steroids can be substituted for the growth hormone in the treatment of this condition. Anabolic steroids should be administered prior to the epiphyseal closure to promote linear growth.[6] This increase in growth following treatment with anabolic steroids is the result of increase in the release of growth hormone.[101,102] The age of the individual is very critical when starting therapy with anabolic steroids. It was shown that anabolic steroids may be useful in the treatment of growth retardation in uremic children who are on regular hemodialysis.[26] The mean growth velocity was significantly increased following the administration of the anabolic steroid, oxandrolone, over a period of 0.4 to 1.3 years.[26]

b. Osteoporosis

Anabolic steroids produce a rapid improvement of bone tissue in patients with osteoporosis. The causes of osteoporosis include gonadal hormone deficiency, malabsorption disorders, hyperthyroidism, and excess of corticosteroids. Osteoporosis is characterized by the loss of bone mass (osteopenia) which may result in the increase of the incidence of fractures of the spine, hip and the wrist. Anabolic steroids were shown to have a place in the treatment and/ or prevention of osteoporosis in some patients.[103] Due to their anabolic effects, these hormones can also be used postoperatively and in certain types of fractures, e.g., hip replacement.[84,86]

3. Mammary Carcinoma

The combination of testosterone with conventional chemotherapy has a palliative effect in some women with carcinoma of the breast. The detailed mechanism is unknown, but the androgen may act as an antiestrogen.[5]

4. Anemias

Anabolic steroids have been found effective in various malignant hematological disorders like lymphoma and leukemia.[95] They enhance the erythropoiesis by increasing the production of erythropoietin.[5,24,104,105] They may also have a direct effect on the bone marrow and, hence, increase the responsiveness of hematopoietic tissues. Anabolic steroids may have some benefits in other hematological disorders that are associated with bone marrow depression such as profound anemia and myelofibrosis.

5. Hereditary Angioneurotic Edema (HAE)

This is an autosomal dominant condition which is characterized by an increase in the permeability of the vessels causing swelling of the face, extremities, genitalia, bowel wall, and upper respiratory tract. This is probably caused by deficiency or malfunction of the inhibitor of the first component of the complement system.[24,27] It appears that from all of the available anabolic steroids, only 17-alpha-alkylated derivatives, e.g., danazol, is the most effective derivative.[106] The danazol action is likely due to its side effects.

6. Deficiency States and Catabolic Conditions

Anabolic steroids as adjuvants in therapy are used not only for their anabolic effects, but also for their additional actions such as increase in appetite, psychic stimulation, and improving the patient's immune defense mechanism.[24,107] Anabolic steroids are used to accelerate the tissue repair mechanism in various injuries such as major surgery, burns, and trauma.

7. Thrombosis and Fibrinolysis

Anabolic steroids may be used as adjuvants in the treatment of vascular disorders. They increase the fibrinolytic activity and decrease the level of fibrinogen, cholesterol, and platelet adhesiveness.[108]

8. Miscellaneous

Hyperlipidemia — This is an expected effect since androgens decrease total plasma levels of cholesterol and decrease low-density lipoproteins (LDL) in certain patients with hyperlipidemia.[5,24]

Protective agents — In some animal experiments, male anabolic steroids may be used to protect the bone marrow from deleterious effects of irradation and cytotoxic drugs.[5]

Autoimmune diseases — Anabolic steroids may be used in the treatment of certain autoimmune diseases such as systemic lupus erythematosus (SLE), myasthenia gravis, and lupus glomerulonephritis.[109,110] The mechanism of their actions are not yet known.

B. Side Effects

The side effects of anabolic steroids are varied and depend on many factors such as age, sex, and the type of hormone being administered. Different hormones are metabolized by different pathways and consequently produce different side effects. Table 2 lists some of the possible side effects of anabolic steroids.

1. Side Effects in Children

It is well known that anabolic steroids are contraindicated in children as they cause premature closure of the epiphyses of the long bones.[6,24] Children may also experience virilization and feminine breast development (gynecomastia) in both sexes. Male children have a higher incidence of feminizing side effects than adult males, which could be related to a higher metabolic rate in children, hence, androgens will be converted to estrogen at a faster rate.[6] These steroids are also teratogenic and, hence, they are contraindicated in pregnant women since they tend to cause abnormal growth of the embryo.

2. Side Effects in Women

All androgens carry the risk of inducing virilization in women. Other side effects include acne, hirsutism (growth of facial hair), male-pattern baldness, hoarsening or deepening of the voice, shrinking breast size, enlargement of the clitoris, uterine atrophy, menstrual irregularities, amenorrhea, and oligomenorrhea.[6,27,48] Most of these changes are not reversible.

3. Side Effects in Men

Feminization in men is a very common side effect following administration of anabolic steroids. As mentioned earlier, this is due to the production of the estrogenic metabolites of anabolic steroids (Figure 1). Men experience enlargement in the breasts (gynecomastia), which can be a very disturbing appearance. The development of gynecomastia in men is a good indication of liver damage caused by the anabolic steroids, since androgens are mainly metabolized by the liver. Thus, in a damaged liver, estrogen will not be inactivated. During initial androgen-replacement therapy in hypogonadal males, sustained erections may be seen which may lead to some sexual aggression. However, this effect does not last long and subsides with continued therapy.[6] Prolonged use of anabolic steroids at a large dose can cause a frightening effect on the reproductive system such as testicular atrophy and decrease in sperm count and possibly infertility. In one study, following administration of 15 mg of metadienone, an anabolic steroid, daily for 2 months to athletes, there was a reduction of the sperm density and motility to an extent of 73 and 30%, respectively.[97,111] In addition, the percentage of sperm with amorphous heads increased by 100%. Some athletes become azoospermic. The effect of anabolic steroids on spermatogenesis is associated with the decrease in plasma testosterone level, which may occur by the following mechanisms.[48]

Central mechanism — Anabolic steroids depress the release of gonadotrophins (both LH and FSH) and, hence, decrease testosterone production. It is believed that anabolic

Table 2
SUMMARY OF THE POSSIBLE SIDE EFFECTS OF ANABOLIC STEROIDS

Side Effects	Children	Adult males	Adult females
I. Endocrine urogenatal			
A. Amenorrhea	— [a]	—	+ + [b]
B. Oligomenorrhea	—	—	+ [c]
C. Menstrual irregularities	—	—	+ +
D. Inhibition of gonadotropin secretion (LH and FSH)	± [d]	+	+
E. Virilization	±	+	+ +
1. Deepening of the voice	±	+	+ +
2. Clitorial enlargement	—	—	+ +
F. Teratogenic (virilization of external genitalia of the female fetus)	—	—	+ +
G. Shrinking of breast size	±	±	+
H. Feminization (gynecomastia)	+ +	+	—
I. Alteration of libido	—	+ +	+
J. Erection	—	+	—
K. Impotence	—	+	—
L. Uterine atrophy	—	—	+
M. Testicular atrophy	—	+	—
N. Inhibition of spermatogenesis	—	+	—
O. Infertility	—	+ +	±
P. Masculinization	±	+	+ +
II. Cardiovascular			
A. Fluid and electrolyte disturbances	±	+	+
B. Edema (peripheral and pulmonary)	±	±	±
C. Hypertension	±	±	±
D. A V block	±	±	±
E. Bradycardia	±	±	±
III. Gastrointestinal and liver			
A. Hepatic toxicity (jaundice, peliosis, tumor, necrosis)	±	+	+
B. Liver function tests (increase serum bromosulphalein, bilirubin, SGOT, SGPT, and alkaline phosphatase)	±	+	+
C. Nausea, vomiting, and constipation	±	±	±
IV. Central nervous system			
A. Headache, anxiety, depression, and dizziness	—	+	+
B. Generalized paresthesia	+	+	+
V. Metabolic			
A. Increase in plasma low-density lipoprotein (LDL)	±	+	+
B. Decrease plasma high-density lipoprotein (HDL)	±	+	+
C. Increase in creatine and creatinine excretion	±	±	±
D. Increase in plasma level of creatinine phosphokinase (CPK)	±	±	±
E. Decrease in glucose tolerance	±	±	±
VI. Hematological			
A. Suppression of clotting factors (II, V, VII, and X)	—	+	+
B. Bleeding during anticoagulant therapy	—	±	±
C. Polycythemia	—	±	±
VII. Skin and appendages			
A. Hirsutism	—	±	+ +
B. Baldness	—	+	+
C. Skin hypersensitivity	—	+	+
D. Acne	—	+	+ +
VIII. Skeletal			
A. Premature closure of epiphyses	+	±	±
IX. Miscellaneous			
A. Muscle cramps	—	±	±
B. Muscle abnormalities	—	+	±
C. Inflammation and pain at the site of intramuscular injection	±	±	±

Table 2 (continued)
SUMMARY OF THE POSSIBLE SIDE EFFECTS OF ANABOLIC STEROIDS

Side Effects	Children	Adult males	Adult females
D. Anaphylactoid reactions	±	+	±
E. Bladder irritability	±	+	±
F. Stomatitis (buccal preparation)	±	+	+
G. Insomnia	±	+	+
H. Diarrhea	±	+	+

[a] — Unknown or no effect.
[b] + + More pronounced effect.
[c] + Known effect.
[d] ± Undetermined positive effect.

steroids reduce testosterone production through the negative feedback system which is mediated by the pituitary and the hypothalamus (Figure 2). This supresses the release of gonadotropin by the pituitary which, in turn, decreases testosterone formation by the testes.

Local mechanisms — Anabolic steroids may increase the free fraction of the endogenous testosterone in plasma by two possible mechanisms: (1) displace testosterone from its binding sites in plasma protein (SHBG or TEBG) by competitive binding mechanism, or (2) decrease in the synthesis of binding proteins (SHBG or TEBG) by the liver. Whatever the mechanism might be, the ultimate effect is the increase in the free fraction of plasma testosterone.[48,111]

4. Hepatic Toxicity of Anabolic Steroids

Prolonged administration of anabolic steroids causes a number of hepatic complications including jaundice, cholestatic hepatitis, peliosis hepatitis, and hepatic carcinoma.[48,72] Liver tumors associated with the use of anabolic steroids are much more vascular than other tumors and may be silent until life-threatening intra-abdomen hemorrhage develops.[27]

Most of these liver complications are associated with the use of oral preparations of 17-alpha alkylated anabolic steroids.[24,72] Alterations in normal liver functions have been found in about 80% of those using C17-alkylated testosterone derivatives.[97] The abnormalities of liver functions induced by anabolic steroids include retention of bromosulphalein (BSP), elevation of plasma levels of glutamic pyruvic transaminases (SGPT), glutamic oxaloacetic transaminase (SGOT), bilirubin, lactic dehydrogenase (LDH), and alkaline phosphatase. The latter two enzymes are used in the determination of specific liver function tests.[48] These biochemical changes contribute to the obstruction of the bile canals (cholestases) and jaundice. If jaundice occurs, it generally develops after 2 to 5 months of therapy.[6] The severity of the side effects depends on the dose and the duration of action.

The development of peliosis hepatitis (blood filled sacs in the liver) can be life threatening when these sacs rupture causing severe hemorrhage and liver failure. Other life-threatening complications that may result from the use of anabolic steroids are hepatic carcinoma and hepatoma. However, these develop following prolonged use of anabolic steroids.[24,48,82]

5. Cardiovascular Side Effects of Anabolic Steroids

Athletes normally have higher levels of high-density lipoproteins (HDL) than the general population. However, when these athletes start taking anabolic steroids, the HDL level decreases with higher risk of atherosclerosis and coronary heart diseases.[112,114] Fluid and electrolyte retention which is associated with the use of anabolic steroids can lead to edema and hypertension. This action appears to be consistent with the observed increase in body weight of some athletes.

C. Contraindications and Precautions[24,27,28]

1. Unnecessary use of anabolic steroids in healthy individuals.
2. Carcinoma of the prostate and carcinoma of the breast.
3. Nephritis.
4. Pregnancy; because of the possibility of masculinization of the fetus.
5. Patients with hypercalcemia.
6. Patients with serious cardiac, hepatic, or renal diseases.
7. Patients making professional use of their voice.
8. Patients with hypersensitivity to anabolic steroids.
9. Nursing mothers because of the possibility of anabolic steroids and/or their metabolites being excreted in milk.
10. Children with growth retardation taking prescribed anabolic steroids.

D. Drug Interactions

Few clinical data on drug interactions are available in the literature. Data on drug interactions of the different preparations of anabolic steroids taken by athletes are not often reported in the literature. The following are some of the known and expected interactions of anabolic steroids with other drugs. Anabolic steroids may[27,34,48]

1. Enhance the effects of anticoagulant agents. Hence, the anticoagulant dose must be adjusted when they are administered concurrently with anabolic steroids. This effect is mainly associated with the C-17-substituted derivatives of testosterone, which tend to inhibit the clotting factors.
2. Interfere with the action of insulin, resulting in a decrease of blood glucose levels.
3. Inhibit the metabolism of oral hypoglycemic agents. Thus, diabetic patients must be closely monitored.
4. Concurrent administration of anabolic and adrenal steroids or ACTH may lead to edema.
5. Increase plasma level of the nonsteroidal anti-inflammatory drug, oxyphenbutazone.
6. Alcohol may interfere with the metabolism of anabolic steroids resulting in increased production of estrogen.

VI. CONCLUDING REMARKS

The financial, personal, and national prestige in competitive sports entices athletes to win at almost any cost. In the past, athletes have depended on high-protein intake in search of muscle strength. With the advent of anabolic steroids, following World War II, thousands of athletes around the world have taken these hormones with the hope of improving muscle strength. Although, the validity of this belief appears illusionary, the use of these anabolic steroids still continues. There is a big gap between the athletes and the medical and scientific communities concerning the use of anabolic steroids. This gap may remain open for the following reasons:

1. Athletes are not well informed about the deleterious side effects of the use of these steroids.
2. Unfortunately, there are differences of opinion within the medical and scientific communities about the effects and/or side effects of anabolic steroids in athletes.
3. The laws in most countries are not very strict and uniform in controlling the abuse of anabolic steroids.

From the literature review, the following conclusions may be drawn:

1. Anabolic steroids have no place in sports and they are therapeutic agents used for the treatment of male hypogonadism, hereditary angioneurotic edema, and selected patients with anemia.
2. The effects of anabolic steroids on the strength of athletes were inconsistent and inconclusive.
3. The discrepancies seen within the literature on the use of anabolic steroids in athletes were due to lack of adequately controlled studies and the differences of study protocols.
4. There is a good degree of agreement within the literature in reporting that there is no improvement in the aerobic performance of athletes following the use of anabolic steroids.
5. The observed beneficial effects of large doses of anabolic steroids in athletes may not be due to a direct pharmacological action of the steroids on muscles, but due to the following:

    a. Psychological effects, since some athletes have responded to placebo administration.
    b. Steroids may cause some central effects such as euphoria and aggressiveness which may increase the athlete's performance.
    c. Anabolic steroids cause fluid and electrolyte retention which tend to increase body weight.

6. Anabolic steroids cause serious side effects following their prolonged use. The most common side effects, which occur in about 30% of male athletes, are alterations in libido, increased aggressiveness, muscle cramps, and gynecomastia. The more serious side effects are liver toxicity, (including peliosis, jaundice, and carcinoma), masculization in female athletes, feminization in male athletes, cardiovascular abnormalities, infertility, and teratogenic effects in women. The liver toxicity is mainly associated with the use of C-17-alpha-alkylated oral derivatives of testosterone. Anabolic steroids should be very carefully administered when given to children.

In conclusion, it must be stated that the risks of using anabolic steroids by athletes by far outweighs their putative benefits.

REFERENCES

1. **Kochakian, C. D. and Murlin, J. R.,** The effect of male hormone on the protein and energy metabolism of castrated dogs, *J. Nutr.,* 10, 437, 1935.
2. **Papanicolaou, G. N. and Falk, E. N.,** General muscular hypertrophy induced by androgenic hormones, *Science,* 87, 238, 1938.
3. **Wade, N.,** Anabolic steroids: doctors denounce them, but athletes aren't listening, *Science,* 176, 1399, 1972.
4. **Meliton, M. B.,** Anabolic steroids in athletes, *Am. Fam. Physician,* 30(1), 113, 1984.
5. **Kopera, H.,** The history of anabolic steroids and a review of clinical experience with anabolic steroids, *Acta Endocrinol. Suppl.,* 271, 11, 1985.
6. **Murad, F. and Haynes, R. C.,** Androgens, in *The Pharmacological Basis of Therapeutics,* 7th ed., Gilman, A. G., Goodman, L. S., Rall, T. W., and Murad, F., Eds., Macmillan, New York, 1985.
7. **Rogers, H. J., Spector, R. G., and Trounce, J. R.,** *A Textbook of Clinical Pharmacology,* Hodder and Stoughton, London, 1981.
8. **Gower, D. B.,** *Steroid Hormones,* Croom Helm, London, 1979.

9. **Saartok, T., Dahlberg, E., and Gustafsson, J. A.,** Relative binding affinity of anabolic-androgenic steroids: comparison of the binding to the androgen receptors in a skeletal muscle and in prostate, as well as to sex hormone-binding globulin, *Endocrinology,* 114(6), 2100, 1984.

10. **Meikle, W. A., Bishop, D. T., Stringham, J. D., and West, D. W.,** Quantitating genetic and nongenetic factors that determine plasma sex steroid variation in normal male twins, *Metabolism,* 35, 1090, 1987.

11. **Wilson, J. D.,** Gonodal hormones and sexual behavior, in *Clinical Neuroendocrinology,* Vol. 2, Martini, L. and Besser, G. M., Eds., Academic Press, New York, 1982, 1.

12. **Desauller, P. A. and Krahenbhl, C.,** Evaluation and mode of action of anabolic steroids: differentiation of action of various anabolic steroids, in *Protein Metabolism,* Springer-Verlag, Berlin, 1962, 185.

13. **Wilson, J. D.,** Sexual differentiation, *Annu. Rev. Physiol.,* 40, 279, 1978.

14. **Van Wayjen, R. G. A. and Buyze, G.,** Clinical pharmacological evaluation of certain anabolic steroids, *Acta Endocrinol. Suppl.,* 63, 18, 1962.

15. **Nowakowski, H.,** Metabolic studies with anabolic steroids, *Acta Endocrinol., Suppl.,* 63, 37, 1962.

16. **Lunde, D. T. and Hamburg, D. A.,** Techniques for assessing the effects of sex steroids in affect, arousal and aggression in human, *Recent Prog. Horm. Res.,* 28, 627, 1972.

17. **Griffin, J. E., Leshin, M., and Wilson, J. D.,** Androgen resistant syndromes, *Am. J. Physiol.,* 243, E81, 1982.

18. **Griffin, J. E. and Wilson, J. D.,** The syndrome of androgen resistance, *N. Engl. J. Med.,* 302, 198, 1980.

19. **Smith, R. G., Nag, A., Syms, A. L., Norris, J. S., II,** Steroid receptor, gene structure and molecular biology, *J. Steroid Biochem.,* 214, 51, 1986.

20. **Mistry, P., Griffiths, K., and Maynard, P.,** Endogenous C_{19}-steroids and estradiol levels in human primary breast tumour tissues and their estrogen receptors, *J. Steroid Biochem.,* 24, 1117, 1986.

21. **Alen, M., Reinila, M., and Vihko, R.,** Response of serum hormones to androgen administration in power athletes, *Med. Sci. Sports Exercise,* 17, 354, 1985.

22. **Tepperman, J.,** *Metabolic and Endocrine Physiology,* Yearbook Medical Publisher, Chicago, 1973, 70.

23. **Kruskemper, H. L.,** *Anabolic Steroids,* Academic Press, New York, 1968.

24. **Wilson, J. D. and Griffin, J. E.,** The use and misuse of androgens, *Metabolism,* 29, 1278, 1980.

25. **Kochakian, C. D. and Endahl, B. R.,** Changes in body weight of normal and castrated rats by different doses of testosterone propionate, *Proc. Soc. Exp. Biol. Med.,* 100, 520, 1959.

26. **Jones, R. W., Bloom, S. R., Carter, J. E., Dalton, R. N., and Chntler, C.,** The effects of anabolic steroids on growth, body composition and metabolism in boys with chronic renal failure on regular hemodialysis, *J. Pediatr.,* 97, 559, 1980.

27. **Physician's Desk References,** 41st ed., Medical Economics, N.J., 1987.

28. **Wijnand, H. P., Bosch, A. M. G., and Donker, C. W.,** Pharmacokinetic parameters of nandrolone (19-nortestosterone) after intramuscular administration of nandrolone decanaote (Deca. — Durbolin) to healthy volunteers, *Acta Endocrinol. Suppl.,* 271, 19, 1985.

29. **Van der, V.,** Implication of basic pharmacology in the therapy with esters of nandrolone, *Acta. Endocrinol. Suppl.,* 271, 38, 1985.

30. **Al-Habet, S. and Rogers, H. J.,** Pharmacokinetics of intravenous and oral prednisolone, *Br. J. Clin. Pharmacol.,* 10, 503, 1980.

31. **Al-Habet, S. M. H.,** Clinical Pharmacokinetic Studies of Prednisolone and Methylprednisolone, Ph.D. thesis, University of London, 1983.

32. **Szelfler, S. J., Ebling, W. F., Georgitis, J. W., and Jusko, W. J.,** Methylprednisolone versus prednisolone pharmacokinetics in relation to dose in adults, *Eur. J. Clin. Pharmacol.,* 30, 323, 1986.

33. **Guechot, J., Vaubourdolle, M., Ballet, F., Giboudeau, J., Darnis, F., and Poupon, R.,** Hepatic uptake of sex steroids in men with alcoholic cirrhosis, *Gastroenterology,* 92, 203, 1987.

34. **Anderson, S. H. G., Cronholm, T., Sjovall, J.,** Effects of ethanol on the levels of unconjugated and conjugated androgens and estrogens in plasma of men, *J. Steroid Biochem.,* 24, 1193, 1986.

35. **Lieber, C. S.,** *Medical Disorders of Alcoholism,* W. B. Saunders, Philadelphia, 1982, 83.

36. **Fotherby, K. and James, F.,** Metabolism of synthetic steroids, *Adv. Steroid Biochem. Pharmacol.,* 3, 67, 1972.

37. **Bergink, E. W., Geelen, J. A. A., and Turpijn, E. W.,** Metabolism and receptor binding of nandrolone and testosterone under in vitro and in vivo condition, *Acta Endocrinol. Suppl,* 271, 31, 1985.

38. **Belanger, A., Brochu, M., Cliche, J.,** Levels of plasma steroid glucuronides in intact and castrated men with prostatic cancer, *J. Clin. Endocrinol. Metab.,* 62, 812, 1986.

39. **Belanger, A., Brochu, M., and Cliche, J.,** Plasma levels of steroid glucuronides in prepubertal, adult and elderly men, *J. Steroid Biochem.,* 24, 1069, 1986.

40. **Samojlik, E., Kirschner, M. A., Silber, D., Schneiderm, G., and Ertes, N. H.,** Elevated production and metabolic clearance rates of androgens in morbidly obese women, *J. Clin. Endocrinol. Metab.,* 59, 949, 1984.

41. **Longcope, C., Baker, R., and Johnson, C. C.,** Androgen and estrogen metabolism: relationship to obesity, *Metabolism,* 35, 235, 1986.
42. **Lucking, M. T.,** Steroid hormones in sports. Special reference: sex hormones and their derivatives, *Int. J. Sports Med.,* 3, 65, 1982.
43. **Lamb, D. R.,** Androgens and exercise, *Med. Sci. Sports,* 7, 1, 1975.
44. **Freed, D. L. G., Banks, A. J., and Longson, F.,** Anabolic steroids in athletics: crossover double-bind trial in weight lifters, *Br. Med. J.,* 2, 471, 1975.
45. **Payne, A. H.,** Anabolic steroids in athletes, *Br. J. Sports Med.,* 9, 83, 1975.
46. **Zurer, P. S.,** Drugs in sports, *Chem. Eng. News,* April, 69.
47. **Wright, J. E.,** Anabolic steroids and athletes, *Exercise Sports Sci. Rev.,* 8, 149, 1980.
48. **Haupt, H. A. and Rovere, G. D.,** Anabolic steroids: a review of the literature, *Am. J. Sports Med.,* 12(16), 169, 1984.
49. **Crist, D. M., Stack Pole, P. J., and Peake, G. T.,** Effects of androgenic-anabolic steroids in neuromuscular power and body composition, *J. Appl. Physiol.,* 54, 366, 1983.
50. **Hervey, G. R.,** Are athletes wrong about anabolic steroid, *Br. J. Sports Med.,* 9, 74, 1975.
51. **Loughton, S. J. and Rubling, R. O.,** Human strength and endurance responses to anabolic steroid and training, *J. Sports Med. Phys. Fitness,* 17, 285, 1977.
52. **Hervey, G. R., Hutchinson, I., and Knibbs, A. V.,** ''Anabolic'' effects of methandienone in men undergoing athletic training, *Lancet,* 2, 699, 1976.
53. **Johnson, L. C., Roundy, B. S., Allsen, P. E.,** Effect of anabolic steroid treatment on endurance, *Med. Sci. Sports,* 7, 287, 1975.
54. **Win-May, M. and Mya-Tu, M.,** The effect of anabolic steroids on physical fitness, *J. Sports Med. Sci. Sports,* 15, 266, 1975.
55. **Stromme, S. B., Meen, H. D., and Aakyaag, A.,** Effects of an androgenic-anabolic steroid on strength development and plasma testosterone levels in normal males, *Med. Sci. Sports,* 6, 203, 1974.
56. **Fahey, I. D. and Brown, C. H.,** The effects of an anabolic steroid on the strength, body composition, and endurance of college males when accompanied by weight program, *Med. Sci. Sports,* 5, 272, 1973.
57. **Bowers, R. W. and Reardon, J. P.,** Effects of methandrostenolone (Dianabol) on strength development and aerobic capacity, *Med. Sci. Sports,* 4, 54, 1972.
58. **Johnson, L. C., Fisher, G., and Silvester, L. J.,** Anabolic steroid: effects on strength, body weight, oxygen uptake and spermatogenesis upon mature males, *Med. Sci. Sports,* 4, 43, 1972.
59. **O'Shea, J. P. and Winker, W.,** Biochemical and physical effects of an anabolic steroid in competitive swimmers and weight lifters, *Nutr. Rep. Int.,* 2, 351, 1970.
60. **O'Shea, J. P.,** Anabolic steroid: effect on competitive swimmers, *Nutr. Rep. Int.,* 1, 337, 1970.
61. **Hervey, G. R., Knibbs, A. V., and Burkinshaw, L.,** Effects of methandienone on the performance and body composition of men undergoing athletic training, *Clin. Sci.,* 60, 457, 1981.
62. **Tahmindjis, A. J.,** The use of anabolic steroids by athletes to increase body weight and strength, *Med. J. Aust.,* 1, 991, 1976.
63. **O'Shea, J. P.,** The effects of anabolic steroids on dynamic strength levels of weightlifters, *Nutr. Rep. Int.,* 4, 363, 1971.
64. **Ariel, G.,** The effect of anabolic steroids (methandrostenolone) upon selected physiological parameters, *Athlet. Train.,* 7, 190, 1972.
65. **Ward, P.,** The effect of anabolic steroid on strength and lean body mass, *Med. Sci. Sports,* 5, 277, 1973.
66. **Ariel, G.,** Residual effect of an anabolic steroid upon isotonic muscular force, *J. Sports Med. Phys. Fitness,* 14, 103, 1974.
67. **Stamford, B. A. and Moffatt, R.,** Anabolic steroid: effectiveness as an ergogenic aid to experienced weight trainers, *J. Sports Med.,* 14, 191, 1974.
68. **Golding, L. A., Freydinger, J. E., and Fishel, S. S.,** Weight size and strength unchanged with steroids, *Phys. Sports Med.,* 2, 39, 1974.
69. **Samuels, L. T., Henschel, A. F., and Keys, A.,** Influence of methyltestosterone on muscular work and creatinine metabolism in normal young men, *J. Clin. Endocrinol. Metab.,* 2, 649, 1942.
70. **Fowler, W. M., Jr., Gardner, G. W., and Egstrom, G. H.,** Effect of an anabolic steroid on physical performance of young men, *J. Appl. Physiol.,* 20, 1038, 1965.
71. **Casner, S. W., Jr., Early, R. G., and Carlson, B. R.,** Anabolic steroid effects on body composition in normal young men, *J. Sports Med. Phys. Fitness,* 11, 98, 1971.
72. **Lamb, D. R.,** Anabolic steroids in athletics. How well do they work and how dangerous are they?, *Am. J. Sports Med.,* 12, 31, 1984.
73. **Ariel, G. and Saville, W.,** Anabolic steroids: the physiological effects of placebos, *Med. Sci. Sports,* 4, 124, 1972.
74. **Vermeulen, A.,** Plasma level and secretion rate of steroids with anabolic activity in LU FC, in *Anabolic Agents in Animal Production,* Rendel, J., Ed., Georg Thieme, Stuttgart, 1976, 171.

75. **Morey, S. W. and Passariello, K.,** *Steroids — A Comprehensive and Factual Report,* S. W. Morey and K. Passariello, Tampa, 1982.
76. **Thomason, D. P., Pearson, D. R., and Costill, D. L.,** Use of anabolic steroids by national level athletes, *Med. Sci. Sports Exercise,* 13, 111, 1981.
77. **Kochkian, C. D.,** Anabolic-androgenic steroids, in *Handbook of Experimental Pharmacy,* New series, Springer-Verlag, Berlin, 1976, 43.
78. **Bullock, G., White, A. M., and Wortington, J.,** The effects of catabolic steroid and anabolic steroids on amino acid incorporation by skeletal muscle ribosomes, *Biochem. J.,* 108, 417, 1968.
79. **MacDougall, J. D., Sale, D. G., Elder, G. C., and Sutton, J. R.,** Muscle ultrastructure characteristics of elite powerlifters and body builders, *Eur. J. Appl. Physiol.,* 48, 117, 1982.
80. **Buchwald, D., Argyres, S., Easterling, R. E., et al.,** Effect of nandrolone decanoate in the anemia of chronic hemodialysis patients, *Nephron,* 18, 232, 1977.
81. **Hickson, R. C., Kurowski, T. T., Capaccio, J. A., and Chatterton, J. R.,** Androgen cytosol binding in exercise induced sparing from muscle atrophy, *Am. J. Physiol.,* 247, E597, 1984.
82. **Lukaszewska, J. H. and Obuchowicz-Fidelus, B.,** Serum and urinary steroids in women athletes, *J. Sports Med.,* 25, 215, 1985.
83. **Bunt, J. C.,** Hormonal alterations due to exercise, *Sports Med.,* 3, 331, 1986.
84. **Mosebach, K. O., Hausmann, D., Caspari, R., Stoeckel, H.,** Deca-Durabolin and parenteral nutrition in post traumatic patients, *Acta Endocrinol. Suppl.,* 271, 60, 1985.
85. **Tweedle, D., Walton, C., and Johnson, I. D. A.,** The effect of an anabolic steroid on postoperative nitrogen balance, *Br. J. Clin. Pract.,* 27, 130, 1972.
86. **Michelsen, C. B., Askanazi, J., Kinney, J. M., Gump, F. E., and Elwyn, D. H.,** Effect of an anabolic steroid on nitrogen balance and amino acid patterns after total hip replacement, *J. Trauma,* 22, 410, 1982.
87. **Young, G. A., Yule, A. G., and Hill, G. I.,** Effects of an anabolic steroid on plasma amino acids, proteins and body composition in patients receiving intravenous hyperalimentation, *J. Parent. Ent. Nutr.,* 7, 221, 1983.
88. **Lewis, L., Dahn, M., and Kirkpatatrick, J. R.,** Anabolic steroids administration during nutritional support, a therapeutic controversey, *J. Parent. Ent. Nutr.,* 5, 64, 1981.
89. **Martinez, J. A., Buttery, P. J., and Pearson, J. T.,** The mode of action of anabolic agents: the effect of testosterone on muscle protein metabolism in the female rat, *Br. J. Nutr.,* 52, 515, 1984.
90. **Forbes, G. B.,** The effect of anabolic steroids on lean body mass: the dose response curve, *Metabolism,* 34(6), 571, 1985.
91. **Cattran, D. C., Fenton, S. S. A., Wilson, D. R., et al.,** A controlled trial of nandrolone decanoate in the treatment of uremic anemia, *Kidney Int.,* 12, 430, 1977.
92. **Von Hartitzch, B., Kerr, D. N. S., Morley, G., et al.,** Androgen in the anemia of chronic renal failure, *Nephron,* 18, 13, 1977.
93. **Hendler, E. D., Goffinet, J. A., Ross, S., et al.,** Controlled study of androgen therapy in anemia of patients in maintenance hemodialysis, *N. Engl. J. Med.,* 291, 1046, 1974.
94. **Evens, R. P. and Amerson, A. B.,** Androgens and erythropoiesis, *J. Clin. Pharmacol.,* 14, 94, 1974.
95. **Gardner, F. H.,** Anabolic steroids in aplastic anemia, *Acta Endocrinol. Suppl.,* 271, 87, 1985.
96. American college of sports in medicine position statement on the use and abuse of anabolic-androgenic steroids in sports, *Med. Sci. Sports,* 9, 11, 1977.
97. **Ryan, A. J.,** Anabolic steroids are fool's gold, *Fed. Proc. Fed. Am. Soc. Exp. Biol.,* 40, 2682, 1981.
98. **Eik-Nes, K. B.,** Human chronic gonadotropin as stimulants for androgen secretion, in *The Endocrine Function of the Human Testis,* Vol. 2, James, V. H. T. and Martini, L., Eds., Academic Press, 1974, 207.
99. **Clark, M., Gelman, D., Gosnell, M., and Hager, M.,** The user's guide to hormones, *Newsweek,* January 12, 50, 1987.
100. **Holma, P. and Aldlercreutz, H.,** Effect of anabolic steroid (metondienone) on plasma LH, FSH, and testosterone and on the response to intravenous administration of LRH, *Acta Endocrinol.,* 83, 856, 1976.
101. **Martin, L. G., Grossman, M. S., Connor, T. B., et al.,** Effect of androgen on growth in boys with short stature, *Acta Endocrinol.,* 91, 201, 1979.
102. **Moore, D. C., Tattoni, D. S., Limbeck, G. A., et al.,** Studies of anabolic steroids: effect of prolonged oxandrolone administration on growth in children and adolescents with umcomplicated short stature, *Pediatrics,* 58, 412, 1979.
103. **Dequeker, J. and Geusen, S. P.,** Anabolic steroids and osteoporosis, *Acta Endocrinol. Suppl.,* 271, 45, 1985.
104. **Alen, M.,** Androgenic steroid effects on liver and red blood cells, *Br. J. Sports Med.,* 19, 15, 1985.
105. **Neff, M. S., Goldberg, J., Slifkin, R. F., Eiser, A. R., Calsmia, V., Kaplan, M., Baez, A., Gupta, S., and Mattoo, N.,** Anemia in chronic renal failure, *Acta Endocrinol. Suppl.,* 271, 80, 1985.
106. Danazol and other androgens for hereditary angiedema, *Med. Lett.,* 23, 83, 1981.

107. **Paul, M. and Turner, R. L.,** Experimental study of the effect of an anabolic steroid on lymphoid cell production and on the natural cytotoxicity of lymphocytes, *Exp. Hematol. (Copenhagen),* 10, 117, 1982.
108. **Cade, J. F., Stubbs, K. P., Stubbs, A. E., and Clegg, E. A.,** Thrombosis, fibrinolysis and ethylestrenol, *Acta Endocrinol. Suppl.,* 271, 53, 1985.
109. **Schuurs, A. H. W. M., Verheul, H. A. M., and Schot, L. P. C.,** Experimental work with anabolics in autoimmunity models, *Acta Endocrinol.,* 7, 97, 1985.
110. **Verheul, H. A. M., Stimson, W. H., Den Hollander, F. C., and Schuurs, A. W. H. M.,** The effects of nandrolone, testosterone and their decanoate esters on murine lupus, *J. Immunol.,* 44, 11, 1981.
111. **Holma, P. K.,** Effect of an anabolic steroid (methandienone) on spermatogenesis, *Contraception,* 15, 151, 1979.
112. **Leeds, E. M., Wilkerson, J. E., Brown, G. D., Kamen, G., and Bredle, D.,** Effects of exercise and anabolic steroids on total and lipoprotein cholesterol concentrations in male and female rats, *Med. Sci. Sports Exercise,* 18, 663, 1986.
113. **Webb, O. L., Laskarzewski, P. M., and Glueck, C.,** Severe depression of high density lipoprotein cholesterol levels in weight lifters and body builders by self-administered exogenous testosterone and anabolic — androgenic steroids, *Metabolism,* 33, 971, 1984.
114. **Haffner, S. M., Kushwaha, R. S., Foster, D. M., Applebaum-Bowden, D., and Hazzard, W.,** Studies on the metabolic mechanism of reduced high density lipoproteins during anabolic steroid therapy, *Metabolism,* 32, 413, 1983.

INDEX